PRENATAL DIAGNOSIS
IN OBSTETRIC PRACTICE

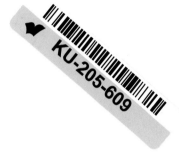

Prenatal Diagnosis in Obstetric Practice

EDITED BY

M. J. WHITTLE

MD, FRCOG, FRCP(Glas.)
Professor of Fetal Medicine,
Department of Obstetrics and Gynaecology,
Birmingham Maternity Hospital,
Edgbaston, Birmingham

AND

J. M. CONNOR

BSc, MB ChB, MD, FRCP
Professor of Medical Genetics,
University of Glasgow,
and Director of the West of Scotland
Regional Genetics Service,
Duncan Guthrie Institute,
Yorkhill, Glasgow

FOREWORD BY

C. R. WHITFIELD

MD, FRCOG, FRCP(Glas.)

SECOND EDITION

b
**Blackwell
Science**

© 1989, 1995 by
Blackwell Science Ltd
Editorial Offices:
Osney Mead, Oxford OX2 0EL
25 John Street, London WC1N 2BL
23 Ainslie Place, Edinburgh EH3 6AJ
238 Main Street, Cambridge
  Massachusetts 02142, USA
54 University Street, Carlton
  Victoria 3053, Australia

Other Editorial Offices:
Arnette Blackwell SA
  1, rue de Lille, 75007 Paris
  France

Blackwell Wissenschafts-Verlag GmbH
  Kurfürstendamm 57
  10707 Berlin, Germany

  Feldgasse 13, A-1238 Wien
  Austria

First published 1989
Second edition 1995

Set by Setrite Typesetters, Hong Kong
Printed and bound in Great Britain
at the University Press, Cambridge

DISTRIBUTORS

Marston Book Services Ltd
PO Box 87
Oxford OX2 0DT
(*Orders*: Tel: 01865 791155
    Fax: 01865 791927
    Telex: 837515)

North America
Blackwell Science, Inc.
238 Main Street
Cambridge, MA 02142
(*Orders*: Tel: 800 215-1000
    617 876-7000
    Fax: 617 492-5263)

Australia
Blackwell Science Pty Ltd
54 University Street
Carlton, Victoria 3053
(*Orders*: Tel: 03 347-0300
    Fax: 03 349-3016)

A catalogue record for this title
is available from the British Library

ISBN 0-632-03838-1

Library of Congress
Cataloging-in-Publication Data

Prenatal diagnosis in obstetric practice
edited by M.J. Whittle, J.M. Connor;
foreword by C.R. Whitfield, — 2nd ed.
    p.   cm.
  Includes bibliographical references
  and index.
  ISBN 0-632-03838-1
  1. Prenatal diagnosis.
  2. Fetus — Abnormalities. 3. Fetus — Diseases.
I. Whittle, Martin J.
II. Connor, J.M. (James Michael), 1951–
  [DNLM: 1. Prenatal Diagnosis.
WQ 209 P9268 1995]
RG628.P735 1995
618.2′2 — dc20
DNLM/DLC
for Library of Congress   94-26804
                                            CIP

Contents

Contents

List of Contributors

D. AITKEN BSc, PhD, *Top Grade Scientist, Duncan Guthrie Institute of Medical Genetics, Yorkhill, Glasgow G3 8SJ*

R. B. BEATTIE MD, MRCOG, *Consultant in Fetal Medicine, University Hospital of Wales, Heath Park, Cardiff CF4 4XW*

A. D. CAMERON MD, MRCOG, *Consultant Obstetrician & Gynaecologist, The Queen Mother's Hospital, Yorkhill NHS Trust, Glasgow G3 8SH*

D. CARRINGTON BSc, MB BS, DTM & H, *Senior Lecturer and Consultant in Clinical Virology, St George's Hospital Medical School, Cranmer Terrace, London SW17 0RE*

J. M. CONNOR BSc, MB ChB, MD, FRCP, *Professor of Medical Genetics, Department of Medical Genetics, Duncan Guthrie Institute of Medical Genetics, Yorkhill, Glasgow G3 8SJ*

J. A. CROSSLEY BSc, PhD, *Principal Clinical Scientist, Duncan Guthrie Institute of Medical Genetics, Yorkhill, Glasgow G3 8SJ*

G. M. DURBIN BA, MB BCh, FRCP, *Consultant Neonatologist, Birmingham Maternity Hospital, Edgbaston, Birmingham B15 2TG*

E. LETSKY MB BS, FRCPath, *Consultant Haematologist, Queen Charlotte's Hospital, Goldhawk Road, London W6 0XG*

J. McHUGO MB BS, MRCP, FRCR, *Consultant Radiologist, X-ray Department, Birmingham Maternity Hospital, Edgbaston, Birmingham B15 2TG*

M. B. McNAY FRCOG, MRCP(Glas.), *Consultant in Obstetric Ultrasound, The Queen Mother's Hospital, Yorkhill NHS Trust, Glasgow G3 8SH*

M. E. I. MORGAN MB ChB, FRCP, *Consultant Neonatologist, Birmingham Maternity Hospital, Edgbaston, Birmingham B15 2TG*

W. J. A. PATRICK MB ChB, FRCS, FRCSE, FRCPath, *Consultant Paediatric and Perinatal Pathologist, Royal Hospital for Sick Children, Yorkhill, Glasgow G3 8SJ*

List of Contributors

J. M. PEARCE MD, FRCS, FRCOG, *Consultant Perinatal Obstetrician, St George's Hospital, Blackshaw Road, London SW17 0QT*

P. A. M. RAINE MA, MB BChir, FRCS(Ed. and Glas.), *Barclay Lecturer in Paediatric Surgery, University of Glasgow, Consultant Paediatric Surgeon, Royal Hospital for Sick Children, Yorkhill, Glasgow G3 8SJ*

L. ROBERTS MB BS, MRCGP, MRCOG, *Senior Registrar in Fetal Medicine, Fetal Medicine Unit, University College London Medical School, 86–89 Chenies Mews, London WC1E 6HX*

M. ROBSON MB BS, MRCOG, *Senior Registrar in Obstetrics and Gynaecology, Royal United Hospital, Coombe Park, Weston, Bath*

C. H. RODECK BSc, MB BS, DSc, FRCPath, FRCOG, *Professor of Obstetrics and Gynaecology, University College London Medical School, 86–89 Chenies Mews, London WC1E 6HX*

J. L. TOLMIE BSc, FRCP(Glas.), *Consultant Clinical Geneticist, Duncan Guthrie Institute of Medical Genetics, Yorkhill, Glasgow G3 8SJ*

M. J. WHITTLE MD, FRCOG, FRCP(Glas.), *Professor of Fetal Medicine, Academic Department of Obstetrics & Gynaecology, Department of Fetal Medicine, Birmingham Maternity Hospital, Edgbaston, Birmingham B15 2TG*

Foreword

In this eagerly awaited second edition, the high standards and integrated and practical approach of the pioneering first volume of six years ago have been fully maintained. These stem from the motivation and active clinical and teaching commitments of the two editors, their experience in directing large regional services and research programmes, and from the expertise and clarity shown by their collaborators. One of the two editors remains at Yorkhill in Glasgow where the original team of authors was based, and where the West of Scotland Medical Genetics Service and a subspeciality referral service for fetal medicine for the same population and beyond continue to operate in close association. There is now a similarly well integrated and comprehensive regional service centred on Birmingham, where the other editor moved as the first Professor of Fetal Medicine in Britain, and from where a new group of contributors has reinforced the Glasgow team, as have several experts who draw mostly on their specialized experience of fetal diagnosis and therapy at hospitals in London where tertiary referral systems are also well established.

The primary aim remains to provide, in a single text, the means whereby obstetricians may keep abreast of continuing refinements, new developments and ever widening opportunities for prenatal counselling, diagnosis and fetal — as well as neonatal — treatment. An increasingly important part of generalist obstetricians' work is to give initial and routine prenatal advice, to provide detailed information and guidance about most of the commoner inherited and other fetal disorders, and to arrange more specialized consultations and investigations when there is a risk of rarer or more complex conditions. Especially with the growing development of special interests and expertise within group practices, some family doctors can and do provide much genetic, prepregnancy and prenatal advice and counselling; they too will find this book a valuable updating source, as will both neonatal and general paediatricians, and also the new community gynaecologists and other doctors specially concerned with women's health. For clinicians and scientists already expert in any of the aspects of this diverse multidisciplinary field, and for those in advanced training for such work, this and expected future editions can serve another important function by helping to promote the mutual understanding and unity of purpose without which no service of real excellence can be achieved.

The editors and their team are to be congratulated on again producing a text that remains unrivalled in meeting so effectively the particular needs of its main intended readership in obstetrics, and of others involved in the science or practice of genetic counselling and prenatal diagnosis.

C.R. WHITFIELD

Preface to the Second Edition

In this new edition we have attempted to maintain the essentially practical style of the first edition. Certainly many changes have occurred in the intervening years with regard to prenatal diagnosis and we have taken the opportunity to invite some new contributors to reflect this. Many of the chapters have been revised or rewritten. The appendices have been amalgamated to form a single database which should be easier to use and now contains 622 entries compared with just under 400 in the first edition.

We are immensely grateful to our contributors, all of whom are busy practitioners in their own right. We hope that both they and the readers feel that all the effort has been worthwhile.

M.J.W., J.M.C.

Preface to the First Edition

The last 20 years have witnessed the growth of prenatal diagnosis from a controversial experimental procedure into a routine component of obstetric management. Nevertheless, although the basic methods of prenatal diagnosis such as ultrasound and amniocentesis are known to most practising obstetricians, the utility of more invasive methods, the information they provide and the various management options available remain unfamiliar territory. Indeed, the whole area of prenatal diagnosis, counselling and treatment is changing so rapidly that it is increasingly difficult to keep abreast of new developments. Currently nearly 400 different genetic and non-genetic conditions can be diagnosed *in utero* and, with the recent development of chorionic villus sampling and DNA diagnosis, this figure will continue to rise.

The contributors to this volume are all directly engaged in the provision of genetic and specialist prenatal diagnostic services for a population of nearly three million. Their backgrounds reflect the diversity of problems encountered in daily practice and emphasize the desirability of a team approach for optimal care of mother and fetus. Chapters are orientated to common prenatal diagnostic problems and cover differential diagnosis, prognosis, management options and potential pitfalls of interpretation. Finally, four appendices are provided which aspire to be comprehensive with regard to conditions which have been diagnosed in the fetus. In the appendices and each chapter selected key recent references are provided. Whilst primarily directed towards the practising obstetrician, this information might also be of value to those involved in other aspects of genetic counselling and prenatal diagnosis.

M.J.W., J.M.C.

Chapter 1
Genetic Assessment and Counselling

J. M. CONNOR

Improvements in control of many environmental agents have resulted in an increased relative importance of genetic diseases. These diseases are now the commonest causes of childhood handicap and mortality and they often carry high recurrence risks for parents and other family members. Hence their recognition is vital but this task is complicated by the large number of distinct conditions which have now been described (Table 1.1).

For the obstetrician, the chromosomal disorders, single gene disorders and congenital malformations due to multifactorial inheritance are most relevant (as most other multifactorial disorders and somatic cell genetic disorders occur after childhood). Table 1.2 indicates the factors evident either before or during a pregnancy which serve to indicate an increased risk for one of these conditions.

IDENTIFICATION OF THE AT-RISK PREGNANCY

Factors identifiable prior to a pregnancy

Elevated maternal age

The commonest identifiable risk factor prior to a pregnancy is elevated maternal age and in the UK about 7% of mothers will be 35 years or older at their estimated date of confinement. Elevated maternal age is related to the incidence of several chromosomal abnormalities (trisomy 21 (see Table 5.2)), 18 and 13, 47,XXX, and 47,XXY).

Table 1.1 Classification of genetic diseases

Type	No. of subtypes	Combined frequency in livebirths (%)
Chromosomal disorders*	>600	0.7
Single gene disorders	>5000	1
Multifactorial disorders	>100	25
Somatic cell genetic disorders	>100	30

* Including disorders of mitochondrial chromosomes.

Table 1.2 Identification of pregnancies at increased risk for fetal abnormality

	Chr	SGD	MCM
Factors identifiable prior to a pregnancy			
Elevated maternal age	+	−	−
Parental consanguinity	−	+	+
Ethnic origin	−	+	(+)
Positive family history	+	+	+
Maternal illness or medication	−	(+)	+
Population carrier screening	−	+	−
Factors identifiable during a pregnancy			
Abnormal ultrasound appearance	(+)	(+)	(+)
Maternal serum screening	+	−	(+)
Maternal exposure to teratogens	−	−	+

Chr, chromosomal disorders; SGD, single gene disorders; MCM, major congenital malformations.
+, associated; (+), may be associated; −, not associated.

Parental consanguinity

Parents often do not realize the importance of consanguinity and will not volunteer that they are blood relatives unless directly questioned. Consanguinity results in an increased frequency of autosomal recessive disorders and multifactorial congenital malformations. If the family history is otherwise negative, the couple can be advised that the risk of a major congenital malformation is 4% (as compared with the general population risk of 2%) and that the added risk for autosomal recessive conditions is about 1%. No special screening is indicated before a pregnancy unless indicated by other factors, such as ethnic origin, but during a pregnancy detailed ultrasound scanning for malformations might be considered. Consanguinity *per se* is not an indication for fetal chromosomal, DNA or biochemical analysis.

Ethnic origin

Certain ethnic groups have high carrier frequencies for particular autosomal recessive conditions (Table 1.3). Hence if a couple belong to one of these ethnic groups screening for carrier status should be considered.

Positive family history

The traditional question 'Is there a family history of tuberculosis, diabetes or epilepsy?' is completely inadequate if a serious attempt is to be made to

Table 1.3 Ethnic associations of genetic diseases

Disease	Populations at risk	Carrier test
Alpha-thalassaemia	Chinese, Thais	Red cell indices
Beta-thalassaemia	African blacks, Chinese, Cypriots, Egyptians, Greeks, Turks	Red cell indices, Hb electrophoresis
Cystic fibrosis	North Europeans	DNA analysis
Gaucher disease	Ashkenazi Jews	Serum β-glucosidase
Sickle cell disease	African blacks, Arabs, West Indians	Sickledex test
Tay–Sachs disease	Ashkenazi Jews	Serum β-N-acetylhexose-aminidase A

Hb, haemoglobin.

identify high-risk pregnancies. Conversely, the construction of a detailed pedigree (Fig. 1.1) would be impractical for every patient in a busy antenatal clinic and a compromise would be, in addition to the standard medical and previous obstetric history, to ask about the above points (maternal age, parental consanguinity and ethnic origin), about malformed and/or handicapped children in the immediate or distant family and whether or not any condition seems to run in the family.

Correct interpretation of a positive family history may be straightforward or be a difficult challenge. Difficulties most frequently arise when the diagnosis in the affected individual has not been adequately documented or is unknown, and where genetic conditions are clinically similar or identical (*genetic heterogeneity*). In view of the potential consequences of faulty advice, referral to a clinical geneticist should be considered if any doubts exist or if more distant family members are at increased risk.

Maternal illness or medication

Maternal illnesses such as insulin dependent diabetes mellitus, epilepsy, spina bifida and congenital heart disease carry an increased risk of fetal abnormality and many drugs have been implicated as teratogens (see Table 10.3).

Population carrier screening

At the present time population carrier screening is confined to ethnic groups with particularly high frequencies for certain autosomal recessive disorders (Table 1.3).

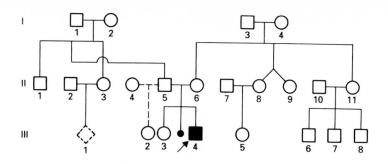

Key:

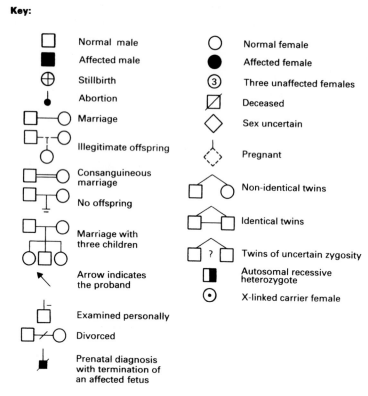

Fig. 1.1 Example of a family pedigree and details of the symbols used in pedigree construction. From Connor and Ferguson-Smith (1993).

Factors identifiable during a pregnancy

There may be no clues to an increased risk of fetal abnormality until it is signalled during the pregnancy by an abnormal ultrasound appearance, an abnormal result on maternal serum screening or exposure to a teratogen (see Chapters 3, 4 and 10 respectively).

Genetic counselling

Identification of an at-risk pregnancy from the preceding approaches will necessitate counselling for the couple. This counselling may occur in the obstetric clinic and/or in a genetic counselling clinic. Adequate time in an appropriate setting is essential and in general 30–45 minutes is required for a new family in order to take the medical history, construct the pedigree, examine key family members, consult appropriate records and counsel the family. Precision of diagnosis is the cornerstone of medical genetics and hence counselling should be deferred until all data from specialized investigations and/or evaluation of medical records or other family members are available. Ideally both parents should be counselled and neither the corner of a hospital ward nor a crowded clinic room is adequate.

Counselling needs to include all aspects of the condition and the depth of explanation should be matched to the educational background of the couple. Generally geneticists consider a risk of more than 1 in 10 as high and of less than 1 in 20 as low but the risks have to be considered in relation to the degree of disability. Couples often feel very guilty or stigmatized and it is important to recognize and allay these and other common misconceptions (Table 1.4).

Table 1.4 Common lay misconceptions about heredity

Absence of other affected individuals means that a disorder is not genetic and vice versa
Any condition present at birth must be inherited
Upsets, mental and physical, of the mother in pregnancy cause malformations
Genetic diseases are always untreatable
If only males or females are affected in the family this indicates sex linkage
A 1 in 4 risk means that the next three children will be unaffected

Table 1.5 Pitfalls in genetic counselling

Incorrect or incomplete diagnosis
Genetic heterogeneity (genetic mimics)
Non-penetrance (clinically normal gene carriers for autosomal dominant traits)
Variable expression (clinical variation of dominant traits)
Unstable mutations (with consequent variable severity in different family members)
Gonadal mosaicism (mutation confined to the gonad — hence high risk to offspring for an autosomal dominant trait or chromosomal disorder despite clinically normal parents)
Inadequate knowledge of the literature
Previously undescribed disease

Counselling must be non-directive; the aim is to provide the couple with a balanced version of the facts which will allow them to reach a decision with regard to their reproductive future. There are several pitfalls for the unwary in this area and the commonest is an inaccurate or incomplete diagnosis (Table 1.5).

Assessment and counselling can often be accomplished in one session and many geneticists follow this with a letter to the couple which summarizes the information given and invites the couple to return if new questions arise.

FURTHER READING

Harper, P.S. (1993) *Practical Genetic Counselling* 4th edn, Butterworth-Heinemann, Oxford, 348 pp.

Connor, J.M. and Ferguson-Smith, M.A. (1993) *Essential Medical Genetics* 4th edn, Blackwell Scientific Publications, Oxford, pp. 113–14.

Chapter 2
Prepregnancy Counselling

M. J. WHITTLE

Prepregnancy counselling probably still remains relatively unfashionable as a component of obstetric care. This seems a pity because unless special arrangements are made it is not usually possible to obtain an 'obstetric' opinion in the absence of a pregnancy. Apart from the antenatal clinic the alternative venue for such counselling might be Gynaecology Outpatients, but this for many reasons is usually very inappropriate.

Prepregnancy advice is not a new concept, although it is unlikely that many units will have a dedicated clinic. Most often mothers or their partners are seen on an *ad hoc* basis out of normal clinic time, circumstances which are not particularly satisfactory.

There can be little doubt, however, that the demand for prepregnancy counselling and care has increased enormously over recent years as a result of the realization that appropriate pregnancy planning can optimize the outcome in difficult cases. Some of the indications for referral to a prepregnancy clinic are shown in Table 2.1.

Table 2.1 Indications for referral to a prepregnancy clinic

Early pregnancy failure
Recurrent first trimester loss
Single second trimester loss
Delivery before 32 weeks

Previous pregnancy complications
Recurrent bleeding in pregnancy
Severe hypertensive complications

Previous fetal abnormalities
Miscarriage/abortion/birth
Family history
High carrier risk

Maternal disease
Diabetes mellitus
Hypertension/renal disease
Auto-immune disorders
Cardiac disease
Maternal drug therapy (epilepsy, anticoagulation etc.)

The increasing capability of prenatal diagnosis, and the increasing availability of genetic services in general, has resulted in a greater number of couples requiring advice before embarking on a further pregnancy. This need holds for a wide variety of genetic disorders and indeed the prepregnancy clinic provides an important interface with the genetic services. Couples want to learn not only the chances of a recurrence for a particular disorder, but also the likelihood that such a recurrence could be identifiable by prenatal diagnostic methods. There can be little doubt that the important decisions that the couple need to make with regard to planning a further pregnancy can only be fully taken once they have this information.

Those mothers who have medical disorders and who are planning a pregnancy undoubtedly benefit from prepregnancy counselling. Because of the uncertainties which inevitably surround the outcome of pregnancy in the presence of a medical disorder, many physicians feel uncomfortable about advising women wishing to become pregnant. A negative view is unhelpful and, to a large extent unwarranted and it can be shown that with adequate planning and case selection the risks arising from pregnancy, both for mother and baby, may be quite small. Careful planning is the key and this is particularly so when the mother is diabetic or has a condition requiring therapy which may be teratogenic, such as anticonvulsants or anticoagulants. The consequences of embarking upon a pregnancy under these circumstances must be fully explained to the mother and her partner so that both are aware of the risks. Only then can the couple decide whether or not they wish to undertake a pregnancy.

PLANNING TO ESTABLISH THE CLINIC

The justification for a prepregnancy clinic will, of course, depend on the estimated workload and, for individual obstetricians with relatively low-risk practices, the need may be minimal. However, most busy district general hospitals delivering between 4000 and 5000 babies a year, and certainly most teaching hospitals, could probably justify the establishment of such a clinic.

Firstly, there is a need for one or, preferably, two obstetricians to agree to run the clinic. Again depending upon workload, one session a week should be perfectly adequate, particularly if the clinic itself is well organized. Secondly, finding a suitable venue can be difficult and certainly a space attached to a normal antenatal clinic is inappropriate. The use of a 'quiet' room is ideal and, as in other counselling situations, it is better to discard the formal doctor/desk/patient arrangement. Appointments can usually be set at half an hour each although occasionally, of course, more time will be required particularly if the problem is distressing.

The assistance of an experienced midwife is invaluable. Clearly, it would be unlikely, unless the clinic was very large, that the midwife would

8

do only prepregnancy counselling, but she may also have involvement in other counselling situations and also in the care and assistance of couples undergoing prenatal diagnosis. Our view is that the presence of such a person provides seamless care between the prepregnancy situation and a future pregnancy.

The development of clear protocols for the management of certain situations is essential, and encouraging the use of consistent management strategies makes subsequent auditing more feasible. In fact it is advantageous for the midwife to see the couple first and initiate all the necessary investigations (Table 2.2) which can then be available when the couple come back to see the midwife, obstetrician and whoever else may be necessary such as the geneticist or physician. Such an arrangement provides an extremely efficient method of managing even very difficult clinical problems. About 90% of couples should need to attend the prepregnancy clinic only twice.

The 'early pregnancy clinic' is an offshoot of prepregnancy counselling. Most couples are exceedingly anxious in the early weeks of pregnancy and need a great deal of support, most suitably from the midwife they have already met and know. An experienced midwife can do all the necessary early pregnancy checks, including ultrasound, to establish early fetal viability and to exclude gross abnormality. The couple do not have to wait in antenatal clinics amongst women with successful pregnancies, something which is exceedingly harrowing for them, and, in addition, often arrangements can be made for them to be seen on an *ad hoc* basis if they have particular bouts of anxiety.

Table 2.2 Prepregnancy clinic investigations

Routine investigations	Special investigations
Haemoglobin	Serum iron and ferritin
Full blood count	Blood group
Haematocrit	Virology (cytomegalovirus, herpes simplex, herpes zoster,
Urine culture	parvovirus)
Calcium	Hepatitis B surface Ag
Phosphate	Haemoglobin A1c
Liver function tests	Random blood sugar
Serum folate	Chromosomes
Rubella serology	Cervical smear
	Cervical culture (*Chlamydia trachomatis, Ureaplasma, Trichomona vaginalis, Mycoplasma hominis, Gardnerella vaginalis, Neisseria gonorrhoeae*)
	Hysterosalpingography
	Cervical resistance studies
	Pelvic ultrasound
	Antinuclear factor, anticardiolipins
	Lupus anticoagulant

Ag, antigen.

Types of problem attending the prepregnancy clinic

Experience indicates that the main indications for referral to a prepregnancy clinic include recurrent miscarriage, previous fetal abnormality and chronic maternal disease.

Previous spontaneous miscarriage

The traditional view that these couples do not need to be seen until they have had three miscarriages seems unnecessarily inhuman. Many women become upset after a single miscarriage, but a second one can cause extreme anxiety. It is important that first and second trimester losses are both thoroughly evaluated. Although an identifiable cause will only be found in about 2% of first trimester losses, this rises to 20% when loss occurs in the second trimester. Furthermore, even though the yield of investigations in the group with first trimester losses is low, they still warrant full investigation, since the couple will much more readily accept the situation if they can be reassured that all necessary investigations have been completed. In the absence of identifiable abnormalities most clinics report an 80% success rate in a subsequent pregnancy without resort to any drugs or other therapeutic strategies.

Previous fetal abnormality

These are usually couples with whom initial contact has been made at the time of prenatal diagnosis of an abnormality in an earlier pregnancy. To some extent, therefore, the prepregnancy clinic acts as a follow-up clinic, but it gives, in addition, the opportunity for the couple to discuss recurrence risks and to provide them with some idea about whether or not an earlier diagnosis would be possible during the next pregnancy.

Medical disorders

Medical disorders can form a major component of the prepregnancy workload. Counselling and evaluation in this group can produce some major improvements in outcome because those patients for whom a further pregnancy is advisable can be more clearly identified. Improvements in the mother's condition, for example better diabetic control, will also enhance the chances of a successful pregnancy if undertaken in the prepregnancy period.

Prepregnancy counselling should provide a multidisciplinary approach, the clinic being organized by a dedicated midwife who can see the couples at almost any time during a working week and who can arrange and initiate preliminary investigations. The midwife also performs an important link in terms of care when the mother eventually achieves a further pregnancy, which is a time of great anxiety.

The advantages of having a single venue, at which the couple can meet all the relevant specialists, are immense. Too often couples are passed from one specialist to another, with little dialogue between the specialists themselves, something which causes enormous confusion between professionals and patients alike. Inconsistent advice is probably more damaging than no advice at all and can often cause anger in patients.

FURTHER READING

Chamberlain, G. (1981) The use of a prepregnancy clinic. *Maternal and Child Health*, 6, 314–16.
Cox, M., Whittle, M., Byrne, A., Kingdom, J. and Ryan, G. (1992) Prepregnancy counselling — does it benefit? Experience from a cohort of 1075 cases. *British Journal of Obstetrics and Gynaecology*, 99, 845–49.

Chapter 3
Prenatal Screening — Biochemical

D. A. AITKEN and J. A. CROSSLEY

Prenatal screening for neural tube defects (NTDs) and chromosome abnormalities is now an established part of routine antenatal care in many pregnant populations. The biochemical screening tests for these two categories of abnormality utilize the same blood sample taken at 15−20 weeks' gestation. However, the tests are neither perfectly sensitive nor specific and in practice 10−15% of open spina bifida pregnancies and around one-third of Down syndrome pregnancies will be missed, while a proportion of various other fetal abnormalities or complications of pregnancy will be identified. The objective of such screening therefore, is to identify, through analysis of various pregnancy markers in maternal blood, a group of women who are at increased risk of having a pregnancy affected by a serious fetal abnormality. Being *screen positive* does not indicate with certainty that the pregnancy is affected but that the risk is high enough to justify the use of a specific diagnostic test to confirm or exclude the presence of a fetal abnormality. Being *screen negative* reduces, but does not exclude the possibility of an affected fetus.

For maximum effectiveness, screening should be applied to the whole pregnant population and this has implications for the demand on laboratory and obstetric resources. It should be noted that, as currently practised, combined NTD and Down syndrome screening programmes may initially classify 1 in 10 women (10%) as screen positive therefore requiring follow-up. The majority of these women will in fact be found to be 'diagnosis negative' on further investigation and can therefore be reassured. However, considerable anxiety may be experienced by women who are screen positive and careful and adequate counselling should be an integral part of all screening programmes. This may often take the form of an explanatory leaflet which can be distributed to women at a clinic visit in advance of the time for the screening test. This may be followed by further discussion before the patient opts to have the test, of the types of abnormality being screened for, the performance of the test, and the options following a positive screening result and positive diagnostic result.

NEURAL TUBE DEFECTS

Without the intervention of prenatal diagnosis and selective termination of affected pregnancies, the birth incidence of neural tube defects may reach 2–3 in 1000 live births in certain regions of the UK. This represents a marked decline from incidences of 6–8 in 1000 in the early 1970s and may be due in part to the improved dietary awareness of the population and the protective role of periconceptional vitamin supplementation (Medical Research Council Vitamin Study Group, 1991). In regions with active screening programmes and adequate ultrasound facilities, birth incidences of NTD have fallen to around 0.6 in 1000 (Cuckle and Wald, 1987). In the west of Scotland, over 450 000 pregnancies have been screened since 1976 and there has been an overall 86% reduction in the birth incidence of open NTD.

Prenatal diagnosis by amniotic fluid biochemistry

Two biochemical tests on amniotic fluid (AF) are used to establish a diagnosis of open NTD: (1) quantitative analysis of alphafetoprotein; and (2) qualitative analysis of acetylcholinesterase.

1. Alphafetoprotein (AFP)

This is normally virtually undetectable in the adult except in the presence of certain types of tumour but is detectable in fetal serum and amniotic fluid by 6 weeks' gestation. In amniotic fluid from unaffected pregnancies, AFP levels rise to a peak of around 20 mg/l at 13 weeks and then fall steadily throughout the second and third trimesters. This change with gestation means that an accurate knowledge of gestation is crucial for interpretation of an amniotic fluid AFP result. The normal route for AFP to enter the amniotic fluid is by permeation from the fetal capillaries through unkeratinized skin in the first trimester and later, once fetal micturition commences, via the fetal urine. Failure of closure of the neural tube increases the passage of fetal proteins from the neural tube and surrounding capillaries into the amniotic fluid thus raising their concentrations. Elevated levels of AFP in amniotic fluid from affected pregnancies were first reported in 1972 (Brock and Sutcliffe, 1972) providing a method for the biochemical diagnosis of open NTD. The sensitivity and specificity of amniotic fluid AFP measurements were defined in the Second UK Collaborative study (1979) in over 13 000 mid-trimester amniotic fluid samples including 385 from pregnancies with open NTD. By defining the upper limit of normal amniotic fluid AFP at each gestation in multiples of the appropriate gestational median (MOM) (Table 3.1), 98% of affected pregnancies could be classified as abnormal while only 0.5% of normal pregnancies were falsely positive due to the small overlap of the distribution of amniotic fluid AFP levels in spina bifida and unaffected pregnancies (Fig. 3.1).

13

Table 3.1 Amniotic fluid AFP cut-off values in multiples of the median (MOM) at different gestations. (From Second Report of UK Collaborative Study, 1979)

Gestation (completed weeks)	Cut-off (AFP MOM)
13–15	2.5
16–18	3.0
19–21	3.5
22–24	4.0

A number of other fetal abnormalities such as anterior abdominal wall defects (AAWD), congenital nephrosis and fetal demise are associated with significantly elevated amniotic fluid AFP levels. Closed NTD lesions, however, are not detectable and twin pregnancies have normal levels of amniotic fluid AFP. Fetal blood contaminating the amniotic fluid is an important source of false positive results. The performance of amniotic fluid AFP measurements as a diagnostic method for open NTD at gestations earlier than 14 weeks has not been fully evaluated.

2. Acetylcholinesterase (AChE)

All amniotic fluid samples contain non-specific (pseudo-) cholinesterase which appears as a single band on polyacrylamide gel electrophoresis. Leakage of cerebrospinal fluid through the open lesion in affected pregnancies causes the appearance of a second, neurospecific AChE in amniotic fluid. A qualitative polyacrylamide gel electrophoresis test which identifies

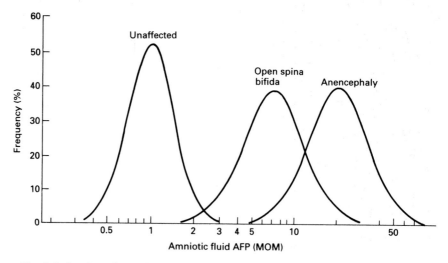

Fig. 3.1 Overlap of AFP values (logarithmic scale) in amniotic fluid from open NTD and unaffected pregnancies.

the presence of the specific AChE as a second band just below the non-specific cholinesterase band (Fig. 3.2) has proved to be an excellent complementary test for open NTD (Collaborative Acetylcholinesterase Study, 1981). Sensitivity is close to 100% and false positive results, even in bloodstained fluids, are rare. During fetal development the closure of the neural tube is not normally complete until around 28 days and residual AChE is still detectable in amniotic fluid from normal pregnancies until 10–12 weeks' gestation. Therefore AChE analysis should not be used as a diagnostic test in first-trimester amniotic fluid.

Affected pregnancies may therefore be diagnosed with a high degree of reliability using mid-trimester amniotic fluid. However, it is clearly impractical to use amniocentesis as a screening method for all pregnancies as this would lead to the loss of many more unaffected fetuses through procedure-related miscarriage than the detection of affected pregnancies. Women who have had a previous pregnancy with NTD have an increased risk of recurrence (approximately 10× population incidence for one previously affected pregnancy, 20× for two previously affected pregnancies) and therefore clearly constitute a high-risk group in whom diagnostic amniocentesis and/or detailed ultrasound scanning may be justified. However, this represents only a small percentage (under 5%) of affected pregnancies. Biochemical screening provides an alternative approach to selection of an at-risk group for diagnostic testing.

Maternal serum screening for neural tube defects

Alphafetoprotein has a molecular weight of 68 000 daltons and is therefore small enough to cross the placenta and enter the maternal circulation.

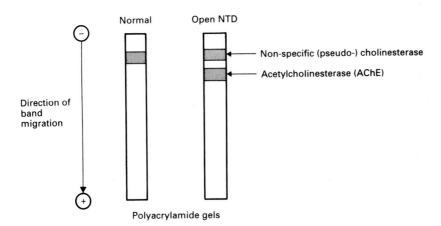

Fig. 3.2 Polyacrylamide gel electrophoretic profile of cholinesterases in amniotic fluid from open NTD and unaffected pregnancies.

Maternal serum AFP (MSAFP) levels rise continuously throughout early pregnancy but at concentrations in the region of 1000-fold lower than in second-trimester amniotic fluid. MSAFP levels reach a peak at around 30 weeks, thereafter falling towards term. The median MSAFP concentration at 16 weeks' gestation is about 30 ng/ml. As with amniotic fluid AFP measurements, accurate gestational dating of pregnancies is necessary for interpretation of MSAFP levels. Table 3.2 lists some of the conditions which are known to be associated with significantly elevated MSAFP levels. The most important category is open NTDs and 90% of all affected pregnancies are associated with MSAFP levels more than twice the normal median level ($\geq$2.0 MOM) at 16−18 weeks' gestation. NTD screening is most sensitive at these gestations (UK Collaborative Study, 1977) as the degree of overlap between the distributions of MSAFP levels in affected and unaffected pregnancies is lowest at this stage (Fig. 3.3). If a cut-off level of 2.0 MOM is used to define the high-risk group, approximately 5% of pregnancies will be classified as being at increased risk necessitating further investigation. Using a cut-off of 2.5 MOM will yield detection rates of around 95% for anencephaly and 75% for open spina bifida at a 3% false positive rate.

Following an elevated MSAFP result, an ultrasound examination should be performed to confirm gestational age, identify any pregnancy complications and to exclude multiple pregnancy and fetal abnormality. Many women may be removed from the high-risk group by upward revision of gestations, or by taking account of lower than average maternal weight to correct the MSAFP level. Twin pregnancies have MSAFP levels approaching double those found in singleton pregnancies although substantially elevated levels (>4.0 MOM) may be indicative of an affected twin. Many abnor-

Table 3.2 Some causes of elevated maternal serum AFP

Anencephaly
Open spina bifida
Anterior abdominal wall defects

Congenital nephrosis
Teratoma
Missed or threatened abortion
Severe fetal compromise
Fetal infection

Chromosomal syndromes (some)
Haemangioma of cord/placenta
Intrauterine diagnostic procedures

Multiple pregnancy
Underestimated gestation
Lower than average maternal weight
Hereditary persistence of AFP

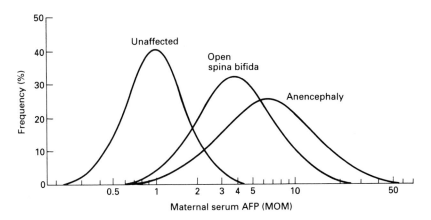

Fig. 3.3 Overlap of AFP values (logarithmic scale) in maternal serum from open NTD and unaffected pregnancies at 16–18 weeks' gestation.

malities are also identified by ultrasound at this stage. For the remainder, it is often useful to repeat the MSAFP test. A second normal MSAFP level backed up by normal ultrasound findings is reassuring but a second elevated result is an indication for further action. If further detailed ultrasound scanning cannot confidently exclude a fetal abnormality, amniocentesis should be considered for AFP and AChE analysis.

Raised MSAFP levels are often associated with fetal abnormalities other than open NTDs (see Table 3.2). For example, over three-quarters of the pregnancies with AAWDs will have raised MSAFP (Morrow *et al.*, 1993) while in Finland, where congenital nephrosis is common in some areas, detection rates by raised MSAFP are comparable to those of anencephaly in the UK. Pregnancies without NTD or other fetal abnormality, but with persistently elevated MSAFP levels, are often associated with poor prognosis such as prematurity, stillbirth or neonatal death (Table 3.3) and such pregnancies should be assigned to a high-risk obstetric category.

CHROMOSOME ABNORMALITIES

Reliable prenatal diagnosis of a fetus with Down syndrome or other chromosome abnormality depends on the analysis of the fetal chromosome constitution using amniotic fluid cell cultures, chorionic villus samples (CVS) or fetal blood samples. Since the early 1970s the association between increasing risk of a pregnancy affected by Down syndrome and advancing maternal age has been used to select pregnancies at high risk for diagnostic amniocentesis. However, maternal age alone is an inefficient method of screening as around 7% of the UK pregnant population would require invasive sampling to detect the 30% of Down syndrome pregnancies which occur in women aged 35 years and over. The predictive value of

Table 3.3 Adverse outcome of pregnancy associated with elevated maternal serum AFP (≥2.5 MOM)

Outcome	Expected rate (%)*	Observed rate (%)†
Abortion		
(2nd trimester)	0.2	7.2
Prematurity	9.6	23.8
Stillbirth	0.7	2.5
First week death	0.53	1.9
Perinatal death	1.23	4.3
Birth weight <2500 g	6.2	18.4

MOM, multiple of the median.
* In the west of Scotland.
† From a study of 793 singleton pregnancies, west of Scotland 1980−1.

maternal age screening is low (1 abnormality detected for every 125 diagnostic tests performed) leading to the possible loss of one normal fetus for each chromosomally abnormal fetus detected. In practice, the uptake of such screening in most populations has been poor, with less than 50% of eligible women having prenatal diagnosis. For example, in the west of Scotland, prior to the introduction of biochemical screening, the average annual uptake of diagnostic testing in women aged 35 years and over was less than 40%, resulting in an average detection rate for Down syndrome of around 12−15% (Aitken and Crossley, 1992).

Screening for Down syndrome by maternal serum markers

In 1984 it was reported that pregnancies with fetal chromosome abnormalities tended to have significantly lower MSAFP values than unaffected pregnancies (Merkatz *et al.*, 1984). Numerous retrospective studies totalling over 800 cases of Down syndrome give a combined reduction in MSAFP levels to 75% of normal. Similar reductions have been noted in a smaller series of trisomy 18 pregnancies. No systematic reduction in MSAFP levels has been found for sex chromosome abnormalities. Although this small shift in median MSAFP level in Down syndrome pregnancies leads to a large overlap of the distributions of MSAFP levels in chromosomally abnormal and unaffected pregnancies compared to spina bifida pregnancies, this property can be exploited to provide an odds ratio (Fig. 3.4) which can be used to modify the age-related risk in individual pregnancies (Cuckle *et al.*, 1987). The risk (likelihood) that a particular MSAFP level (in MOM) is associated with a Down syndrome pregnancy can be calculated from the ratio of the relative heights of the distributions at that AFP level. For example, diagnostic testing in a woman aged 32 years would not be justified if only her age-related risk of Down syndrome (1 : 546 at mid-

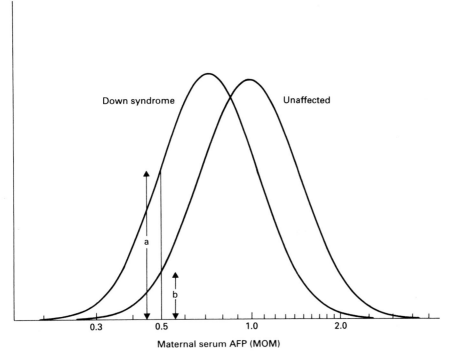

Fig. 3.4 Log Gaussian distributions of maternal serum AFP levels in Down syndrome and unaffected pregnancies. Likelihood of a Down syndrome pregnancy at 0.5 MOM = a/b = 3.10 i.e. risk increased by a factor of 3.1.

trimester) is considered. However, if such a patient had an MSAFP result equivalent to 0.5 MOM this would give a likelihood ratio from the overlapping distributions of 3.10 and a new combined AFP/age risk of 1 : 176 (i.e. 3.10 : 546). This new risk exceeds the age-related risk at 37 years and is high enough to justify the risks of diagnostic amniocentesis.

The use of MSAFP/age screening is more efficient in practice than age-only screening. Setting the intervention risk at 1 : 280 (which is approximately equivalent to the age-related risk at 35 years), screening can be extended to women aged 25 years and over and 1 abnormality will be found for every 100 diagnostic tests carried out. The expected detection rates and corresponding false positive rates vary for different threshold risks and for individual maternal ages. Using locally derived risk tables (Zeitune *et al.*, 1991), over 100 000 pregnancies were screened in the west of Scotland between July 1987 and December 1990 using the MSAFP/age combination. Overall, 43% of autosomal trisomy pregnancies were identified in a screen positive group of 6.2%.

While the use of data from an existing MSAFP screening programme in this way offers a useful improvement in detection of chromosomally abnormal pregnancies at a reduced false positive rate when compared with

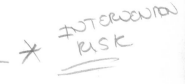

19

age-only screening, around 60% of affected pregnancies, predominately in younger mothers, are not detected. Improved detection can be achieved by using a series of other maternal serum markers in combination with AFP and maternal age. Table 3.4 lists the most extensively investigated markers and the average change in median level associated with Down syndrome and trisomy 18 pregnancies from a series of retrospective studies. The predictive value of a particular marker with respect to Down syndrome depends on three factors: (1) the shift from normal of the median value in chromosomally abnormal pregnancies; (2) the spread of the distribution of values in normal and affected pregnancies; and (3) the degree of correlation between that marker and any other used together. Currently, the most powerful marker known is human chorionic gonadotrophin (hCG), either as the intact molecule (inthCG) or as the free β subunit (FβhCG), which are both increased in Down syndrome pregnancies to over twice the level in unaffected pregnancies (Fig. 3.5). HCG levels are also significantly reduced in trisomy 18 pregnancies. Adding hCG analysis to MSAFP analysis provides a second virtually independent measure of risk of a Down syndrome pregnancy and likelihood ratios derived from the overlapping distributions of hCG levels in Down syndrome and unaffected pregnancies can be combined with the risks derived from the MSAFP result and maternal age. The inclusion of hCG extends screening to the whole pregnant population irrespective of maternal age, although it should be noted that detection rates and false positive rates vary according to maternal age (Table 3.5, Crossley *et al.*, 1991). Overall false positive rates and detection rates are influenced by the age distribution of the screened population, but in most screening programmes around two-thirds of affected pregnancies can be expected to be detected at a false positive rate of 5% (RCOG Report, 1993).

Screening for Down syndrome using this combination of markers has been offered to pregnant women of all ages in the west of Scotland since

Table 3.4 Combined published data on maternal serum marker levels in Down syndrome and trisomy 18 pregnancies in the second trimester

Marker	Down syndrome		Trisomy 18	
	Median MOM	(*n*)	Median MOM*	(*n*)
Alphafetoprotein	0.75	(870)	0.60	(109)
Unconjugated oestriol	0.78	(350)	0.46	(14)
Total or intact hCG	2.12	(440)	0.29	(45)*
Free β hCG	2.30	(148)	0.23	(12)*
Pregnancy specific β-1 glycoprotein	1.28	(168)	1.16	(27)

MOM, multiple of the median from published studies; *n*, total number of cases.
* Includes unpublished data from the west of Scotland.

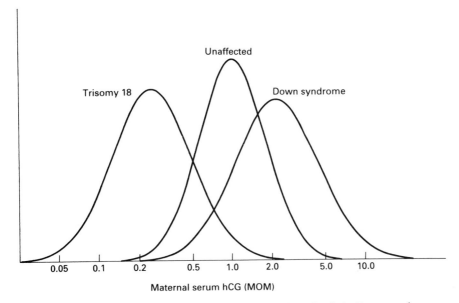

Fig. 3.5 Log Gaussian distributions of maternal serum hCG levels in Down syndrome, trisomy 18 and unaffected pregnancies.

1991. Women are defined as being screen positive if they have a combined risk $\geq 1:220$, a cut-off risk chosen to generate a follow-up rate of about 5%. A summary of the first 30 000 pregnancies screened routinely is presented in Table 3.6 along with a comparison of 'age only' screening and AFP/age screening in the same region. This approach to screening can detect more than twice as many pregnancies with Down syndrome as 'age only' screening for no increase in the number of amniocenteses.

A third marker, unconjugated oestriol (UE3), is also sometimes used in prenatal screening programmes in addition to AFP and hCG (Wald *et al.*, 1988), its value, however, is disputed. Some studies have shown a small

Table 3.5 Age-group specific detection rates for Down syndrome and corresponding false positive rates using AFP/hCG/age

Maternal age (years)	Detection rate (%)	False positive rate (%)	OAPR
<20	35	2.2	1:85
20−24	37	2.6	1:80
25−29	41	3.2	1:75
30−34	58	6.3	1:65
35−37	73	17	1:60
38−40	86	38	1:55
>40	94	70	1:30

OAPR, overall odds of an affected pregnancy for women with screen positive results (i.e. risk $\geq 1:220$).

21

Table 3.6 Summary of performance of screening programmes

	Age (≥35 years)*	Age/AFP	Age/AFP/hCG
No. of pregnancies	35 750	100 481	30 084
No. (%) in high-risk group			
Initial	2321 (6.5%)	6781 (6.8%)†	1904 (6.3%)‡
After gestation reassessed	—	6183 (6.2%)	1523 (5.1%)
Uptake of diagnostic testing	39%	42%	70%
No. of Down syndrome in screened population	39	127	37
Pregnancy prevalence	1.1/1000	1.3/1000§	1.2/1000§
No. (%) in high-risk group (95% confidence interval)	12 (31%) (17–48%)	55 (43%) (35–52%)	26 (70%) (53–84%)
No. (%) of affected pregnancies prenatally diagnosed	5 (13%)	36 (28%)	21 (56%)
Risk of being affected if in high-risk group	1:190	1:112	1:59
Risk of being affected if in low-risk group	1:1240	1:1310	1:2600

* Final year (1986) of screening by maternal age (≥35 years) alone.
† Cut-off risk 1:280.
‡ Cut-off risk 1:220.
§ Excludes some cases diagnosed by first trimester CVS prior to screening.

improvement in detection (Wald *et al.*, 1988) and others no benefit (Crossley *et al.*, 1993), while in clinical practice there seems to be little difference between the performance of the double (AFP/hCG) and triple (AFP/hCG/ UE3) combinations (RCOG Report, 1993). Screening programmes based on the analysis of up to five serum markers have been advocated in some reports (e.g. Ryall *et al.*, 1992). However, there appears to be no significant improvement in the detection rates over and above those achievable by AFP/hCG/age or AFP/hCG/UE3/age and the additional analytical costs and increasing imprecision of the final risk estimate make the use of more than three markers impractical in large scale population screening programmes.

Significant marker variations (notably very low levels of intact hCG and FβhCG) are also found in trisomy 18 pregnancies (see Table 3.4) and these can be used to define a second screen positive group in which detailed ultrasonography and fetal karyotyping are warranted (Palomaki *et al.*, 1992).

A screening protocol for NTD and Down syndrome is shown in Fig. 3.6 and an example of the reporting format for a pregnancy at increased risk of Down syndrome in shown in Fig. 3.7.

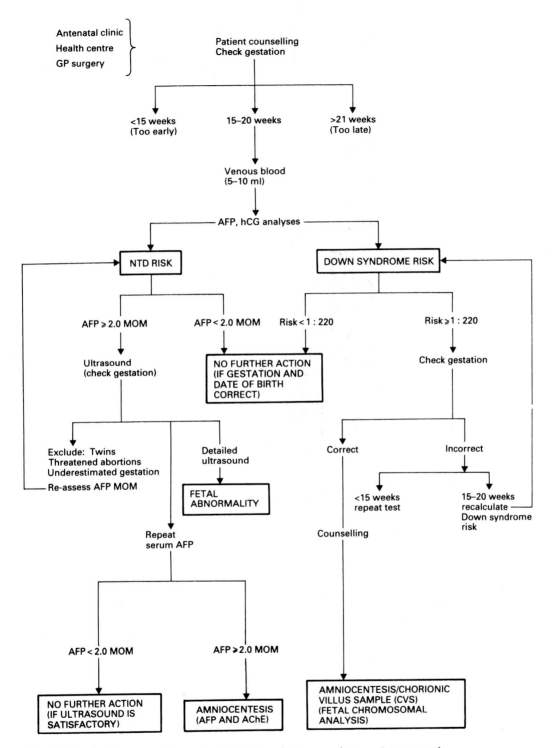

Fig. 3.6 Protocol for prenatal screening for NTD and Down syndrome using maternal serum AFP and hCG.

PRENATAL SCREENING ASSAY REPORT

FROM: DUNCAN GUTHRIE INST. OF MEDICAL GENETICS
YORKHILL, GLASGOW G3 8SJ
Tel: 041-339 8888 ext. 4372

Date Sample Taken	Lab. Ref. No.
16-06-93	314125

Surname:
Forename:
Address:

Weight: 61.0 Kg.   Height: 1.62 m.
Date of Birth: 25-11-61

Hospital:
Address:

Hospital No.
Clinic/Ward:
Consultant:

Previous Serum Report Number   None

L.M.P Certain   17-02-93   Gestation (completed weeks):

	By Dates	Exam[n]	Ultrasound
	17		17

Previous History of Neural Tube Defect   No

Complication of this Pregnancy None

Remarks

Serum AFP result: 36.1   kU/l   Equivalent to 0.97 multiples of median

Serum hCG result: 88   IU/ml   Equivalent to 3.52 multiples of median

Comment AFP value not elevated for stated gestation.

The AFP and hCG results at maternal age 31 give a combined risk of Down's syndrome at mid trimester of 1:100, which exceeds the cut-off risk of 1:220.
(The population mid trimester maternal age risk of Down's syndrome at 31 years is 1:637).

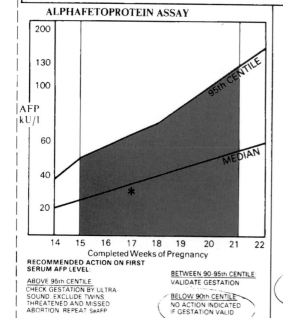

ALPHAFETOPROTEIN ASSAY

DOWN'S RISK (hCG/AFP)

RECOMMENDED ACTION ON FIRST
SERUM AFP LEVEL:

ABOVE 95th CENTILE:
CHECK GESTATION BY ULTRA
SOUND. EXCLUDE TWINS.
THREATENED AND MISSED
ABORTION. REPEAT SeAFP

BETWEEN 90-95th CENTILE:
VALIDATE GESTATION

BELOW 90th CENTILE:
NO ACTION INDICATED
IF GESTATION VALID

DOWN'S RISK ESTIMATE
ONLY VALID IF
GESTATION AND DATE
OF BIRTH CORRECT

Date 24-06-93

Signature

24

INTERPRETATION OF SCREENING RESULTS

Interpretation of the results of the screening tests for NTD and Down syndrome is complicated by a variety of factors.

1. Gestation. If the gestation at the time of sampling is underestimated, AFP and UE3 values converted to MOM will be falsely elevated and hCG MOM falsely reduced. If the AFP level exceeds 2.0 MOM then the pregnancy will be in the high-risk group for NTD. In the case of Down syndrome, underestimated gestation will lead to the derivation of lower likelihood ratios for AFP, UE3 and hCG resulting in calculation of a lower than appropriate risk. Overestimated gestations have the opposite effect. Thus if gestations are revised following a first screening result, a reassessment of the risks for NTD and Down syndrome should be requested from the laboratory.

2. Maternal age. Maternal age is an important component of the combined risk of Down syndrome and is calculated from the difference between the date of birth and date of sampling as recorded on the laboratory request form. Therefore any error in recording this information will affect the accuracy of the calculated risk. There is no known association between the risk of a pregnancy affected by NTD and maternal age.

3. Twin pregnancies. Maternal serum AFP, UE3 and hCG levels are increased in twin pregnancies. While the possibility of fetal structural abnormality should be checked by ultrasound in the case of significantly elevated MSAFP levels (≥4.0 MOM), there are no data on the maternal serum levels of these markers in twin pregnancies concordant or discordant for Down syndrome. Therefore accurate risks for Down syndrome cannot be calculated in twin pregnancies.

4. Threatened abortion. Episodes of bleeding, particularly if recently preceeding the collection of the screening blood sample may cause a rise in MSAFP levels but are less likely to affect the levels of hCG and UE3. This should be taken into account when considering elevated MSAFP results and the possibility of NTD, while in the case of Down syndrome, threatened abortion may cause risks to be underestimated.

5. Maternal weight. Women of lower than average maternal weight tend to have greater than average serum concentrations of AFP, UE3 and hCG.

Fig. 3.7 (*Opposite*) Prenatal screening report showing a low risk of NTD (AFP 0.97 MOM) and high risk of Down syndrome (AFP/hCG/age risk 1 : 100) in a 31-year-old woman at 17 weeks' gestation.

The opposite is found for heavier than average women and the effect is more pronounced as weights move further from the population median (61.5 kg in the west of Scotland). Weight-adjusted MOM can be calculated to compensate, but in practice the effect is small except at significantly lower or higher than average weights.

6. *Race.* Median MSAFP levels are about 15% higher in Black women than in Caucasian women. It is important therefore that normal medians used to convert test results to MOM are appropriate for the population being screened.

7. *Insulin-dependent diabetes mellitus (IDDM).* Reduced levels of MSAFP (0.77 MOM), UE3 (0.92 MOM) and hCG (0.95 MOM) have been reported in pregnancies with IDDM (Wald *et al.*, 1992). Uncorrected serum marker levels may therefore lead to loss of detection of NTD and overestimated risks for Down syndrome. Recent data gathered prospectively in the west of Scotland have shown a smaller effect for AFP (0.93 MOM) in a series of 39 well-controlled diabetics. Two of these (5%) were screen positive for Down syndrome (risk $\geq 1:220$) using uncorrected AFP and hCG results, suggesting that well-controlled IDDM patients are neither significantly over- nor under-represented in the high-risk group.

8. *Smoking.* A 20–25% reduction in maternal serum hCG levels has been found in smokers. A small increase (3%) in AFP levels and a small decrease (3%) in UE3 levels has also been noted and these changes appear to be independent of the level of cigarette consumption. For Down syndrome risk estimation, this leads to a systematic under-representation (by approximately 40%) of smokers in the high-risk group. This can be corrected by adjusting hCG levels for smoking status, which is also predicted to result in a small increase in detection (0.7%) of Down syndrome (Palomaki *et al.*, 1993), although some studies have noted a lower prevalence of Down syndrome among smokers.

CONCLUSION AND FUTURE PROSPECTS

Biochemical screening in the second trimester will, in total, identify about 10% of the screened population as at risk and therefore requiring follow-up diagnostic tests. Under the circumstances, about 90% of pregnancies with open NTD and two thirds of pregnancies with Down syndrome will be identified. The implications of being screen positive for NTD are quite different from those of being screen positive for Down syndrome. Although highly specific and sensitive diagnostic tests exist for the diagnosis of open NTD by amniotic fluid AFP and AChE analysis, in practice these serious structural abnormalities are rarely diagnosed by amniocentesis. The majority of anencephalic pregnancies are detected by ultrasound examination, usually prior to the time for serum screening, while the majority of spina bifida pregnancies are diagnosed by ultrasound scanning following a raised serum AFP result. Most women who are screen positive for NTD but have normal pregnancies can be reassured following a non-invasive ultrasound scan. This option, however, is not available for women who are screen positive for Down syndrome. Fetal karyotyping by amniocentesis, CVS or fetal blood sampling is the only reliable diagnostic measure to confirm or exclude the presence of a fetal chromosome abnormality.

Much effort is required to convey to women the rationale of screening before they decide to be screened. Counselling should include an explanation of the type of abnormalities being screened for, the sensitivity of the tests, the meaning of being screen positive or screen negative and the possible need for follow-up tests. The options following a positive diagnostic result should also be explained and counselling and support should be available for women who choose to terminate or choose to continue an affected pregnancy.

The current timing of prenatal screening for Down syndrome i⁻ by the need to carry out MSAFP screening for NTD at 16- gestation when maximum sensitivity is achieved. However, ther evidence that maternal serum screening for Down syndrome ⁻ in the first trimester which would bring the substantial ⁻ detection and termination of affected pregnancies (A⁻ Brambati *et al.*, 1993). Retrospective studies have ider⁻ which show variation in Down syndrome pregnanc⁻ gestation (Table 3.7) although the pattern of vari⁻ markers between first and second trimester. Fβl⁻

Table 3.7 Combined published data on maternal s⁻ syndrome pregnancies in the first trimester*

Marker		
Alphafetoprotein		
Unconjugated oestriol	0.6∪	
Total hCG	1.17	
Free βhCG	2.20	
Pregnancy associated		
plasma protein A	0.39	(66)
Pregnancy specific		
β-1 glycoprotein	0.77	(35)†

MOM, multiple of the median in Down syndrome pregnancies from published studies; *n*, total number of cases.
* Includes some cases at 14 weeks' gestation.
† Includes unpublished data from the west of Scotland.

27

useful marker and in combination with maternal age, AFP or possibly pregnancy associated plasma protein A (PAPP-A), may yield detection rates approaching those found in the second trimester with AFP/hCG/age. Further studies on larger numbers of affected pregnancies are required to more accurately assess the likely detection and false positive rates before first trimester screening becomes routine. However, detection of open NTD by raised MSAFP levels is not possible in the first trimester and a separate screening protocol using AFP at 16–18 weeks may still be required if the current level of detection in populations with high rates of NTD is to be maintained (Aitken *et al.*, 1993).

REFERENCES

Aitken, D.A. and Crossley, J.A. (1992) Screening for chromosome abnormalities. *Current Obstetrics and Gynaecology*, 2, 65–71.

Aitken, D.A., McCaw, G., Crossley, J.A., Berry, E., Connor, J.M., Spencer, K. and Macri, J.N. (1993) First trimester biochemical screening for fetal chromosome abnormalities and neural tube defects. *Prenatal Diagnosis*, 13, 681–89.

Brambati, B., Macintosh, M.C.M., Teisner, B., Maguiness, S., Shrimanker, K., Lanzani, A., Bonacchi, T., Tului, L., Chard, T. and Grudzinskas, J.G. (1993) Low maternal serum levels of pregnancy associated plasma protein A (PAPP-A) in the first trimester in association with abnormal fetal karyotype. *British Journal of Obstetrics and Gynaecology*, 100, 324–26.

Brock, D.J.H. and Sutcliffe, R. (1972) Alphafetoprotein in the antenatal diagnosis of anencephaly and spina bifida. *Lancet*, ii, 197–99.

Crossley, J.A., Aitken, D.A. and Connor, J.M. (1991) Prenatal screening for chromosome abnormalities using maternal serum chorionic gonadotrophin, alphafetoprotein and age. *Prenatal Diagnosis*, 11, 83–101.

Crossley, J.A., Aitken, D.A. and Connor, J.M. (1993) Second trimester unconjugated oestriol levels in maternal serum from chromosomally abnormal pregnancies using an optimised assay. *Prenatal Diagnosis*, 13, 271–80.

Cuckle, H.S. and Wald, N.J. (1987) The impact of screening for neural tube defects in England and Wales. *Prenatal Diagnosis*, 7, 91–99.

Cuckle, H.S., Wald, N.J. and Thomson, S.G. (1987) Estimating a woman's risk of having a pregnancy associated with Down's syndrome using her age and serum alphafetoprotein level. *British Journal of Obstetrics and Gynaecology*, 94, 387–402.

Medical Research Council Vitamin Study Group (1991) Prevention of Neural Tube Defects: Results of the MRC Vitamin Study. *Lancet*, 238, 131–37.

Merkatz, I.R., Nitowsky, H.M., Macri, J.N. and Johnson, W.E. (1984) An association between low maternal serum alpha-fetoprotein and fetal chromosome abnormalities. *American Journal of Obstetrics and Gynecology*, 148, 886–94.

Morrow, R.J., Whittle, M.J., McNay, M.B., Raine, P.A.M., Gibson, A.A.M. and Crossley, J.A. (1993) Prenatal diagnosis and management of anterior abdominal wall defects in the west of Scotland. *Prenatal Diagnosis*, 13, 111–15.

Palomaki, G.E., Knight, G.J., Haddow, J.E., Canick, J.A., Saller, D.N. and Panizza, D.S. (1992) Prospective intervention trial of a screening protocol to identify fetal trisomy 18 using maternal serum alphafetoprotein, unconjugated oestriol and human chorionic gonadotrophin. *Prenatal Diagnosis*, 12, 925–30.

Palomaki, G.E., Knight, G.J., Haddow, J.E., Canick, J.A., Wald, N.J. and Kennard, A. (1993) Cigarette smoking and levels of maternal serum alphafetoprotein, unconjugated oestriol and hCG: impact on Down syndrome screening. *Obstetrics and Gynaecology*, 81, 657–78.

Report of Collaborative Acetylcholinesterase Study (1981) Amniotic fluid acetylcholinesterase electrophoresis as a secondary test in the diagnosis of anencephaly and open spina bifida in early pregnancy. *Lancet*, **ii**, 321–25.

Report of the RCOG Working Party on Biochemical Markers and the Detection of Down's Syndrome (1993) The Royal College of Obstetricians and Gynaecologists, London.

Ryall, R.G., Staples, A.J., Robertson, E.F. and Pollard, A.C. (1992) Improved performance in a prenatal screening programme for Down's syndrome incorporating serum free hCG subunit analyses. *Prenatal Diagnosis*, **12**, 251–61.

Second Report of the UK Collaborative Study on alphafetoprotein in relation to neural tube defects (1979) Amniotic fluid alphafetoprotein measurement in antenatal diagnosis of anencephaly and open spina bifida in early pregnancy. *Lancet*, **ii**, 625–62.

UK Collaborative Study on Alpha-fetoprotein in Relation to Neural Tube Defects (1977) Maternal serum alpha-fetoprotein measurement in antenatal screening for anencephaly and spina bifida in early pregnancy. *Lancet*, **i**, 1323–32.

Wald, N.J., Cuckle, H.S., Densem, J.W., Nanchahal, K., Royston, P., Chard, T., Haddow, J.E., Knight, G.J., Palomaki, G.E. and Canick, J.A. (1988) Maternal serum screening for Down's syndrome in early pregnancy. *British Medical Journal*, **297**, 883–87.

Wald, N.J., Cuckle, H.S., Densem, J.W. and Stone, R.B. (1992) Maternal serum unconjugated oestriol and human chorionic gonadotrophin levels in pregnancies with insulin-dependent diabetes: implications for screening for Down's syndrome. *British Journal of Obstetrics and Gynaecology*, **99**, 51–53.

Zeitune, M., Aitken, D.A., Crossley, J.A., Yates, J.R.W., Cooke, A. and Ferguson-Smith, M.A. (1991) Estimating the risk of a fetal autosomal trisomy at mid-trimester using maternal serum alphafetoprotein and age: a retrospective study of 142 pregnancies. *Prenatal Diagnosis*, **11**, 847–57.

Chapter 4
Prenatal Screening — Ultrasound

M. J. WHITTLE

The potential for prenatal diagnosis and treatment using ultrasound has increased enormously over recent years and invasive procedures can be directed at those most at risk of carrying an abnormal fetus. Screening methods are particularly important since the majority of abnormalities are unexpected although certain at-risk groups can be identified on the basis of factors such as maternal age or past obstetric history.

Most pregnant women are unaware that potential problems may exist until the possibility is raised at the time of their first visit to the doctor, a circumstance which can lead to much distress. Those mothers at particular risk, such as those with diabetes, on some form of therapy like anticonvulsants or with a positive family history should, ideally, be counselled prior to becoming pregnant so that the various issues can be discussed away from the emotional pressures of pregnancy.

Ultrasound can detect fetal abnormalities, either as the result of a screening procedure or as a specific diagnostic examination.

ROUTINE ANOMALY SCANS

Scans are performed at a variety of gestational ages but the two main times are at booking, which in the UK will be in the first or early second trimester, and around 18 to 20 weeks.

The booking scan can be performed by appropriately trained midwives or doctors and, on average, will take about 5 minutes to complete. The scan has a number of objectives including confirmation of dates, counting number of fetuses, establishing viability and excluding gross abnormalities such as anencephaly.

An ultrasound scan screening for fetal anomalies should usually be performed around 19 to 20 weeks. It takes about 15 to 20 minutes to complete and will often be undertaken by trained radiographers. The examination should include the following anatomical checks:

1 measurement of biparietal diameter, head and abdominal circumference, femur length

2 head, shape, anterior and posterior ventricular and hemispheric ratios, cerebellum diameter, exclusion of intracerebral pathology, face for clefting and neck for cysts and nuchal fold

3 spine longitudinal and transverse section, overlying skin intact
4 heart, four chamber view and outflow tracts, chest contents
5 diaphragm
6 stomach, check on left side
7 anterior abdominal wall and cord insertion. Intra-abdominal masses
or cysts
8 kidneys and bladder
9 genitalia
10 limbs, hands and feet
11 assessment of amniotic fluid
12 placental site and appearance
13 number of cord vessels.

The ability of ultrasound to detect fetal anomalies is dependent on good training, good equipment and a sound technique. The above schedule should ensure that about 70% of anomalies are detected. Most studies have suggested that virtually 100% of neural tube defects should be detectable by a screening ultrasound scan. This contrasts with a possible detection rate for cardiac defects of around 50%, although this may range from 5% to 70%. Other anomalies also have a considerable detection rate range and this may be because certain problems do not develop, or become obvious, until later. This may reflect more our lack of knowledge about the natural history of a condition rather than technical inability. For example, diaphragmatic hernias not seen at 20 weeks may become obvious in later pregnancy and this may be because the passage of gut into the chest is, for some reason, delayed or transient. Similarly, cardiac ventricular hypoplasia may not be apparent at the time of the screening scan because the condition may develop through underperfusion of the relevant ventricle and subsequent failure of the normal 'modelling' processes.

Ultrasound markers of chromosomal abnormalities

It has become apparent that certain fetal anomalies may be found with abnormal karyotypes (Table 4.1). Whilst the exact frequency of these associations remains uncertain because the original descriptions have come from referral centres, there is sufficient evidence to use the markers as an indication for further investigation.

Ultrasound markers of fetal disease

Polyhydramnios

Amniotic fluid is produced from a number of sources but mainly, after 20 weeks, by the fetal kidneys. The amount of fluid in the amniotic cavity is kept in balance by fetal swallowing and probably some exchange across

Table 4.1 Possible rate of karyotypic abnormalities in the presence of ultrasound markers. (Adapted from Nicolaides *et al.*, 1992.)

Marker	Single (%)	Multiple (%)
Ventriculomegaly	4	28
Microcephaly	*	16
Holoprosencephaly	*	29
Choroid plexus cyst	2	46
Facial cleft	*	55
Nuchal oedema	*	40
Cystic hygroma	*	73
Diaphragmatic hernia	*	41
Cardiac defects	*	66
Exomphalos	3	48
Duodenal atresia	16	53
Renal defects	2	24
Abnormal extremities	*	43

* Small numbers.

the fetal membranes. The fetal lungs also contribute some fluid to the amniotic pool.

The abnormal accumulation of fluid is often the result of a defect in swallowing caused by one or more of the following:
- gut atresia (oesophageal, duodenal or jejunal)
- neurological defect (neural tube defect, cerebellar dysfunction)
- neuromuscular defect (congenital myotonia, Pena−Shokeir)
- chondrodysplasias
- fetal hydrops
- diaphragmatic hernia
- cystic adenomatoid malformation of the lung.

Oligohydramnios

Here there is a loss of fluid either as a result of membrane rupture or because amniotic fluid is not being manufactured, causes of which are:
- fetal urinary tract obstruction
- fetal renal failure (bilateral agenesis or cystic dysplasia)
- intrauterine growth retardation.

The value of a routine scan

Although ultrasound has been used for many years, few studies have been done to confirm its usefulness in practice, although few obstetricians doubt its value. Data from a large study in the USA (Ewigman *et al.*, 1993) suggested that, in a low-risk group, no obvious advantages accrued from a routine ultrasound examination. However, the detection rate for anomalies in the scanned group was only 16%, a surprisingly low figure. Conversely, a meta-analysis has shown that ultrasound in the first half of pregnancy allows early diagnosis of multiple pregnancy, the identification of serious fetal abnormality (with subsequent termination) and fewer inductions of labour (Neilson, 1994).

Clear objectives for a scan examination must be defined, and they include assessment of viability, establishing dates, and the exclusion of multiple pregnancy and major structural abnormalities. An additional aspect may be the identification of a nuchal fold as a marker of a trisomic fetus. The evidence that routine ultrasound in pregnancy improves outcome is not extensive but studies confirm its importance in accurate dating, the exclusion of twins and the identification of fetal abnormalities (Saari-Kemppainen *et al.*, 1990; Bucher and Schmidt, 1993).

The preferred schedules for routine ultrasound remain uncertain. Ideally, the first scan should be offered at booking thus establishing the dates, which are inaccurate by more than 2 weeks in about 15% of women with regular menstrual cycles. Gross anomalies can also be diagnosed. The next scan should be timed for 20 weeks as this is probably the optimal stage to exclude anomalies.

Alternative schedules include a scan at booking and biochemical screening alone. Under these circumstances structural abnormalities, such as in the heart or kidneys, will be missed and both these systems can be involved with either fatal anomalies or those anomalies which produce major morbidity.

Although there is often resistance to undertaking both booking and 20 week scans, such a scheme is more efficient because nearly 70% of women first attending have an indication for a scan at this time. It is therefore preferable, from the point of view of organization, to offer everyone a scan. The first scan, by assessing dates, allows the remainder of the screening procedures to be arranged logically and precisely.

Ultrasound provides an important and powerful tool with which to investigate early pregnancy. It is, however, highly operator-dependent and demands high skill levels if optimal results are to be obtained. Although there is little current evidence that ultrasound may have deleterious effects, the fact that it might should always be bourne in mind and the technique should only be used when clinically justified.

REFERENCES

Bucher, H.C. and Schmidt, J.G. (1993) Does routine ultrasound improve outcome in pregnancy? Met-analysis of various outcome measures. *British Medical Journal*, **307**, 13–17.

Ewigman, B.G., Crane, J.P., Frigoletto, F.D. *et al.* (1993) Effect of prenatal ultrasound screening on perinatal outcome. *New England Journal of Medicine*, **329**, 821–27.

Neilson, J.P. (1994) Usefulness of fetal monitoring. *Contemporary Reviews in Obstetrics and Gynaecology*, **6**, 72–78.

Nicolaides, K.H., Snijders, R.J.M., Gosden, C.M., Berry, C. and Campbell, S. (1992) Ultrasonographically detectable markers of fetal chromosome abnormalities. *Lancet*, **340**, 704–707.

Saari-Kemppainen, A., Karjalainen, O., Ylostalo, P., Heinoneu, O.P. (1990) Ultrasound screening and perinatal mortality; controlled trial of systematic one-stage screening in pregnancy. *Lancet*, **336**, 387–91.

Chapter 5
Chromosome Disorders

J. L. TOLMIE

Chromosome disorders affect 6 per 1000 newborn infants and two-thirds of these infants will be disabled, either mentally or physically, as a result. A proportion of the remainder will, in adult life, be at increased risk of either miscarriage or having a disabled child. These chromosomally abnormal liveborn infants comprise only a small proportion of all chromosomally abnormal conceptions. It is estimated that the rate of chromosome abnormality in embryonic and fetal deaths is in the range 32−42% and the proportion of all recognized conceptuses which are chromosomally abnormal is between 5% and 7% (Hook, 1992). In spontaneous abortions and liveborn infants different types of chromosome abnormality predominate, for example trisomy 16 is the commonest autosomal trisomy in abortions whereas trisomy for chromosomes 21, 18 and 13 are the only autosomal trisomies occurring at appreciable frequencies in liveborns; 45,X occurs in about 1% of all conceptions but 98% of those affected do not reach term; triploidy is also frequent in abortions but exceptional in newborns. The high frequency of chromosomally abnormal conceptions is mirrored by results of chromosome analysis in gametes which reveal an approximate abnormality rate of 10% in sperm. The rate in oocytes is more difficult to estimate and one review suggests that 23% are aneuploid (Pellestor, 1991). Since the great majority of chromosome abnormalities are lethal in early gestation, the abnormality rate in stillbirths is considerably lower at about 5%. Amongst embryos from *in vitro* fertilization programmes there are wide estimates of the frequency of chromosome abnormality ranging from 12% to 90%, the recognized high chance of implantation failure may thus be partly attributable to cytogenetic abnormality. An observation with potential practical significance is that the chromosome status of non-transferred embryos from an *in vitro* fertilization (IVF) programme correlated with that of transferred sibling embryos so that there was an increased chance of pregnancy when the non-transferred sibling embryo has normal chromosomes (Zenzes *et al.*, 1992).

PRENATAL CLASSIFICATION

From the standpoint of prenatal diagnosis, fetal chromosome disorders can be divided into two groups: a numerically small group where each case

34

derives from a parent with a chromosomal abnormality; and a larger group where the fetal chromosome abnormality has arisen by new mutation (*de novo*). This chapter concentrates upon identification of at-risk couples and covers genetic counselling issues which arise after diagnosis of specific chromosome disorders.

Identification of at-risk couples

Family history of congenital malformation, Down syndrome or mental disability

This can be an obvious pointer to an increased risk of fetal chromosome abnormality but in practice it is often difficult to verify details of events which may have happened to distant relatives or even close relatives in a previous generation. Less understandable is a lack of information concerning the patient's own past obstetric history. For future genetic counselling it is essential that malformed fetuses are carefully examined with documentation, including photography, of abnormal findings. Permission for a full pathological examination should also be sought. As a general rule, establishing the diagnosis in the index case underpins any subsequent genetic counselling and the appropriateness of prenatal diagnosis in relatives close or distant. Early referral for formal genetic counselling is often indicated if a couple present to the obstetrician with this history.

The commonest problem encountered is 'family history of Down syndrome.' If the affected individual has or had cytogenetically proven trisomy 21 Down syndrome, then all relatives other than the mother of the affected child are *not* at appreciably increased risk on account of the family history. Commonly, however, cytogenetic confirmation of the diagnosis in the affected individual is not available to the obstetrician, in which case the parent with the positive family history should have urgent cytogenetic testing of a peripheral blood sample to exclude the possibility that he or she carries a balanced chromosome 21 translocation. If the affected individual is known to have translocation Down syndrome then unless the translocation was proven to have arisen by a new mutation in the affected person, the at-risk parent should have urgent blood cytogenetic testing and, since other relatives may be at increased risk, the obstetrician should seek advice on genetic counselling implications. The only genetic indication for proceeding directly to prenatal diagnosis given a distant family history of Down syndrome is when a parent of the fetus is known to carry a balanced translocation and has received appropriate genetic counselling; since maternal serum screening tests do not have 100% sensitivity, they should *not* be presented to a known translocation carrier as a substitute for prenatal diagnostic testing by amniocentesis or chorionic villus sampling (CVS).

Parent with a balanced chromosome rearrangement
(translocations and inversions)

Balanced chromosome rearrangements are, by definition, present in clinically normal individuals who have no net gain or loss of genetically active chromosome material. Such rearrangements do, however, predispose to production of chromosomally unbalanced gametes which, if fertilized, result in a pregnancy with duplication or deficiency of specific chromosome segments. Such a pregnancy may spontaneously abort but if it reaches term, the infant is frequently mentally disabled and malformed. If both parents of an individual with a structural chromosome rearrangement are chromosomally normal then the rearrangement is presumed to have arisen by a new mutation (*de novo*); alternatively, a balanced rearrangement may be inherited unchanged through several generations of normal individuals. Cytogenetic testing of the patient's parents will distinguish *de novo* from inherited rearrangements. Non-paternity and gonadal mosaicism (i.e. the rearrangement is not present in the parent's peripheral blood cells but is present in the parent's germ cells and so can be transmitted in balanced or unbalanced forms to further children) are but two phenomena which may disprove confident prediction that a new mutation has occurred. If one parent is found to be a carrier of a balanced rearrangement, then blood cytogenetic testing should be offered to other adult relatives in order to determine if they too are carriers. Responsibility for carrying out an extended family study and giving genetic counselling to carriers is usually assumed by the clinical genetics service.

Chromosome translocations occur if breakage in two non-homologous chromosomes is followed by exchange of chromosome material (Fig. 5.1). If the chromosome breakpoints are within centromeres of acrocentric chromosomes (chromosomes 13, 14, 15, 21 and 22) then Robertsonian (centric fusion) translocations can result, whereas breakpoints within the long or short arms and subsequent exchange, results in reciprocal translocations. Translocation families are usually ascertained through a family history of recurrent miscarriages or of mental disability and/or congenital malformation (Fig. 5.2).

Chromosome inversions exist in two main forms: *Pericentric inversions* have an inverted chromosome segment which includes the centromere. Balanced pericentric inversion carriers have a risk of producing chromosomally abnormal offspring through genetic recombination within the inversion loop which forms at the time of homologous chromosome pairing at meiosis. Small pericentric inversions of chromosome 9, present in about 1% of the population, are an exception to this rule and carriers do not have increased reproductive risks. A second type of inversion, the *paracentric*

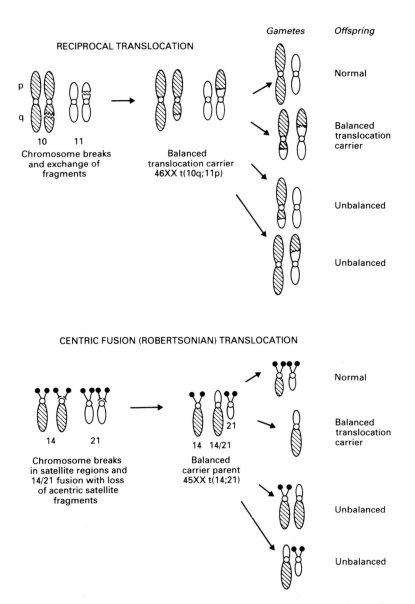

RECIPROCAL TRANSLOCATION

Gametes   Offspring

p

q

10   11

Chromosome breaks
and exchange of
fragments

Balanced
translocation carrier
46XX t(10q;11p)

Normal

Balanced
translocation
carrier

Unbalanced

Unbalanced

CENTRIC FUSION (ROBERTSONIAN) TRANSLOCATION

14   21

Chromosome breaks
in satellite regions and
14/21 fusion with loss
of acentric satellite
fragments

14   14/21

Balanced
carrier parent
45XX t(14;21)

21

Normal

Balanced
translocation
carrier

Unbalanced

Unbalanced

Fig. 5.1 Formation of reciprocal and Robertsonian translocations together with a simplified illustration of possible pregnancy outcomes. Predicting the relative probabilities of these different pregnancy outcomes is more complicated than the diagram suggests and risks of abnormality vary greatly with different translocations.

inversion, does not encompass the centromere and balanced carriers have a very low risk for having an abnormal fetus because recombination within the inversion loop will, as a rule, produce such a severe chromosome imbalance that the conceptus is non-viable.

The precise reproductive risks associated with different translocations, inversions and other structural chromosome abnormalities generally depend upon a number of factors. If ascertainment of the balanced rearrangement

37

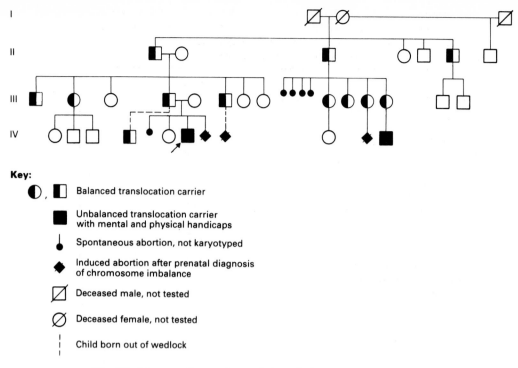

I

II

III

IV

Key:

◑, ◧   Balanced translocation carrier

■   Unbalanced translocation carrier
with mental and physical handicaps

⬤   Spontaneous abortion, not karyotyped

◆   Induced abortion after prenatal diagnosis
of chromosome imbalance

⬚   Deceased male, not tested

⊘   Deceased female, not tested

⋮   Child born out of wedlock

Fig. 5.2 A large pedigree where a balanced chromosome rearrangement is segregating. Chromosomally unbalanced gametes have been generated and caused the birth of two disabled children in generation IV. Prenatal diagnosis has prevented the birth of three affected fetuses.

was through the birth of a chromosomally abnormal child then the risk of another abnormal child is likely to be higher than if the rearrangement was ascertained through a past history of miscarriages. If the chromosome rearrangement is such that the predicted chromosome imbalance resulting from abnormal segregation at meiosis is small, then the risk of an abnormal child is higher because a larger degree of genetic imbalance is more likely to cause spontaneous abortion. Balanced rearrangements which would give rise to imbalance of certain chromosome segments (including segments of chromosomes 9, 13, 18 and 21) carry a higher risk for producing abnormal offspring. Summary estimates of risks in different situations are given in Table 5.1. A practical point is that some small or subtle rearrangements may be difficult for the laboratory to detect, so close liaison between clinical and laboratory staff is required when advising families with chromosome rearrangements about the reliability of prenatal diagnosis.

Parent with child affected by chromosome aneuploidy syndrome

If a woman has had a previous child affected by trisomy 21 Down syndrome or a previous prenatal diagnosis of trisomy 21 Down syndrome, then a considerable body of empiric data indicates that her risk of a second

Table 5.1 Approximate risks for chromosome abnormality when one parent carries a balanced chromosome rearrangement. More precise estimates are available for carriers of particular reciprocal translocations which are based upon the family history and predicted cytogenetic imbalances resulting from the particular translocation

Type of rearrangement present in carrier parent	Risk of unbalanced pregnancy (%)
Balanced reciprocal translocation carrier	
Ascertained through miscarriage or by chance	≤5
Ascertained after birth of an affected child	≥20
Balanced Robertsonian translocation carrier	
D/D translocation, (commonly 13/14) either parent	1
D/21 translocation, (commonly 14/21) maternal	15
D/21 translocation, (commonly 14/21) paternal	5
21/21 translocation — either parent	100
Pericentric inversion carrier	
Either parent, no previous recombinant offspring	1–3
Small distal segments on inverted chromosome and/or previous liveborn recombinant offspring	5–10
Paracentric inversion carrier	Low

affected pregnancy is increased about twentyfold to between 0.5% and 4% depending upon her maternal age at the time of a subsequent delivery. For most women the risk is between 1% and 2% but the precise figure is also dependent upon whether the risk of a Down syndrome birth (lower) or Down syndrome fetus (higher) is considered and whether the possibility of other chromosome abnormality syndromes occurring is included. Risk variations are, however, small and usually do not influence a couple's decision whether to undergo prenatal diagnosis in subsequent pregnancies.

Empiric data on risks in pregnancies subsequent to the birth of a child with any other maternal age-related aneuploidy syndrome are scanty but trisomy 13, trisomy 18, 47,XXX syndrome and 47,XXY may be regarded as conferring a maximum increased recurrence risk of about 1–2% for any age-related aneuploidy syndrome including trisomy 21. In contrast, couples who have had an infant or fetus with either Turner syndrome (45,X) or 47,XYY syndrome do not appear to have an increased risk for chromosomal abnormality in subsequent pregnancies. This is consistent with the observation that incidences of these two disorders do not show a parental age effect.

Past history of pregnancy loss

In about 5% of couples who suffer recurrent abortions, one partner will carry a balanced chromosome rearrangement which is the likely cause of the abortions through the generation of unbalanced gametes. Recurrent abortion is therefore an indication for karyotyping the parents but not for offering prenatal diagnosis in subsequent pregnancies unless a cytogenetic rearrangement has already been diagnosed in one parent.

Although the vast majority of chromosomally abnormal spontaneous abortions have a non-recurring abnormality, when counselling an individual patient the obstetrician may feel uncertain since very few early abortions are karyotyped. Hook (1992) has reassuringly estimated that the excess risk of trisomy 21 or other viable autosomal trisomy in pregnancies of karyotypically normal parents who have suffered recurring abortions of *unknown* karyotype, is less than 0.5%. It is not clear whether pregnancies with *proven* trisomy 13, 18 or 21 which abort spontaneously confer the same increased risk of recurrent chromosome abnormality as there would have been had an affected infant been born.

Parent with autosomal imbalance or mental handicap

Imbalance of autosomal material is usually associated with severe or moderate mental handicap. However, mild intellectual impairment has been documented in individuals with a number of different chromosome abnormality syndromes. Genetic counselling in general and prenatal diagnosis counselling in particular may be very difficult when one or both parents have significant intellectual disability which may be transmitted to their children. As a rule, the obstetrician should offer referral for investigation and counselling to all couples where one or both partners have unexplained mental disability. Where there is an apparently known cause for a patient's disability, the obstetrician should seek written confirmation of this along with a clear account of any possible genetic implications. In the specific case of pregnancy in a woman with trisomy 21 Down syndrome, the risk that her offspring will have trisomy 21 is high, perhaps just less than 50%, and there may even be an additional risk of handicap in the chromosomally normal offspring because of genetic factors from the paternal side (if he is mentally disabled). In males with Down syndrome, fertility is exceptional.

Parent with sex chromosome imbalance

Infertility is the norm in 45,X Turner syndrome but a small proportion of affected females ovulate spontaneously, especially during teenage years, and pregnancies are documented. Experience also suggests that nearly all men with 47,XXY Klinefelter syndrome are infertile but, in contrast, men with 47,XYY and women with 47,XXX are likely to be undiagnosed, fertile and have chromosomally normal offspring. If pregnancy occurs when one partner is known to be affected by either 47,XYY or 47,XXX it is usual to offer genetic counselling and prenatal cytogenetic diagnosis as there is theoretically an increased (but poorly documented) chance of chromosome abnormality in offspring.

Fragile X syndrome

Conventional cytogenetic tests for at-risk women to determine carrier status are imperfect and DNA tests are preferable (see Chapter 8). First trimester prenatal diagnosis by DNA methods has also largely replaced prenatal cytogenetic analysis. Molecular genetic analysis has demonstrated that all mothers of affected boys are carriers and in affected families the size of the genetic mutation is not constant from generation to generation. Studies which seek to correlate the extent of the mutation with the severity of disability in affected males and affected females are currently in progress and may yield data important for prenatal diagnosis of this condition which displays variable expression and decreased penetrance. Genetic counselling is indicated for either a known affected family or, indeed, for any family which has a history of unexplained mental disability in male relatives.

Child with a chromosome breakage syndrome

Several rare autosomal recessive conditions including ataxia telangiectasia, Bloom syndrome, xeroderma pigmentosum and Fanconi anaemia are associated with an increased incidence of spontaneous and induced chromosome breaks and rearrangements. These conditions carry a 25% recurrence risk within sibships and at-risk couples will only be identified after the birth of an affected child. Prenatal cytogenetic diagnosis using amniocytes or cultured chorionic villus cells is possible in certain conditions but laboratory testing requires specialized expertise. Thus, the obstetrician should only undertake prenatal diagnosis after consulting with the genetics laboratory.

Positive maternal serum screening and advanced maternal age

The use of maternal serum biochemical markers in combination with maternal age data to compute an individual mother's risk for carrying a fetus with Down syndrome is discussed in detail in Chapter 3. Present practice in this area is evolving rapidly and different tests and protocols currently exist within different regions of the UK. For genetic counselling purposes, it is still useful to have access to data on maternal age risks of chromosomal abnormality and again it should be noted that these risks vary according to gestational age at the time of prenatal testing (Table 5.2).

An interesting consequence of newly developed serum screening programmes for Down syndrome is that they may be associated with increased uptake of diagnostic chromosome testing compared with the low uptake

Table 5.2 Maternal age-related risks of trisomy 21 and other chromosome abnormalities in pregnancies tested during first trimester, second trimester and term. These risks are derived from rates given in Hook (1992) and are rounded for genetic counselling purposes

Maternal age (years)	First trimester All abnormalities	Second trimester		Term	
		Trisomy 21	All abnormalities	Trisomy 21	All abnormalities
33	—	1/415	1/210	1/625	1/310
34	—	1/335	1/150	1/500	1/250
35	1/115	1/250	1/130	1/385	1/200
36	1/85	1/190	1/105	1/295	1/165
37	1/65	1/150	1/85	1/225	1/130
38	1/50	1/105	1/65	1/175	1/105
39	1/40	1/90	1/55	1/135	1/80
40	1/30	1/70	1/40	1/105	1/65
41	1/20	1/55	1/30	1/80	1/50
42	1/15	1/40	1/25	1/65	1/40
43	1/13	1/30	1/20	1/50	1/30
44	1/10	1/25	1/15	1/40	1/25
45	1/18	1/20	1/12	1/30	1/20

rate when maternal age was the only guide to risk. Increased uptake of diagnostic testing means that other conditions, including Klinefelter syndrome and triple X syndrome, are also increasingly diagnosed in the prenatal period. The lesson for genetic counselling is that women who undergo a diagnostic test for Down syndrome should always be informed of the possibility that other cytogenetic abnormality syndromes, some less severe and some more severe than Down syndrome, will be detected.

Abnormal ultrasound scan

Many studies have demonstrated that there is a high incidence of fetal chromosome abnormalities amongst fetuses with ultrasonographically visualized malformation and the incidence is particularly high (*circa* 30%) when multiple abnormalities are present (see Table 4.1). Thus, antenatal screening by ultrasound in the second trimester for major fetal malformation and, in the first trimester, for certain minor abnormalities such as nuchal thickening, could result in the detection of a significant proportion of chromosomally abnormal fetuses even in the absence of a biochemical maternal serum screening programme.

The cytogenetically abnormal fetus — genetic counselling guidelines

When confronted with an abnormal cytogenetic report, parents will inquire about the consequences for an affected child. The obstetrician often requires expert advice to answer parents' questions and, except in the case of commoner chromosomal syndromes such as trisomy for chromosome 21, 13 or 18, referral to the genetic counselling clinic is usually appropriate.

NUMERICAL ABNORMALITIES

Trisomy 21 Down syndrome

This is the commonest serious chromosome abnormality syndrome. The risk of occurrence rises as mother's age increases (see Table 5.2). In 90−95% of cases the extra chromosome derives from an accidental, non-disjunction event during oogenesis. The outlook for Down syndrome infants has greatly improved in recent years and their life expectancy is presently around 60 years. Nevertheless, moderate mental impairment is the rule and in adult life most affected individuals will remain dependent upon others. The neuropathological signs of Alzheimer's disease are commonly identified in brains of adults with Down syndrome. Congenital heart defects are present in 40% of Down syndrome individuals and the commonest severe lesion, an atrio-ventricular canal defect, may be a valuable prenatal ultrasonographic marker as may duodenal atresia since approximately 20% of infants with that congenital malformation have Down syndrome. Parents usually request pregnancy termination following second trimester prenatal diagnosis of Down syndrome but in the rare instances when an affected pregnancy continues, parents should be told that *in utero* mortality is as high as 30%.

Down syndrome mosaicism, that is the presence of chromosomally normal and abnormal cell lines in the same individual, is present in about 1% of cases. Although there is an overall tendency for individuals with mosaicism and a cytogenetically normal cell line to be less severely affected, in an individual case the phenotype can be as severe as that present in non-mosaic Down syndrome. Thus, prognostication on the basis of the percentage of abnormal cells sampled from amniotic fluid, fetal blood or both, is quite unwise.

In 4% of cases, Down syndrome is due to a translocation involving chromosome 21, which causes a clinical phenotype indistinguishable from trisomy 21 Down syndrome. The important genetic distinction is that in translocation Down syndrome the additional chromosome 21 is attached to another chromosome, commonly chromosome 13 or 14. Thus, an affected individual has the normal diploid number (46) of chromosomes. If the parents of an affected person are cytogenetically normal, as happens in 55% of instances, then the translocation is presumed to have arisen *de novo* and the parents and other family members can be reassured that the recurrence risk is very low. The recurrence risk for the parents is not negligible, however, because of the possibility of gonadal mosaicism in either parent and therefore it is not unreasonable to offer chromosomally normal parents prenatal diagnosis in subsequent pregnancies. In 45% of instances one parent carries a balanced form of the translocation, having 45 chromosomes in total, and there is a substantial recurrence risk (see Table 5.1) in future pregnancies. Formal genetic counselling is indicated since other, outwardly normal family members may also carry the translocation and have a substantial risk for having an affected child.

Trisomy 18 (Edwards' syndrome)

Between 1 in 3000 and 1 in 12 000 newborns are affected by this condition which causes a recognizable pattern of dysmorphic features and congenital abnormalities. The condition is increasingly diagnosed in prenatal life after an ultrasound scan reveals suspicious signs: intrauterine growth retardation associated with any combination of neural tube defect, exomphalos, congenital heart defect and polyhydramnios (often due to oesophageal atresia). Trisomy 18 is the commonest cytogenetic syndrome in pregnancies where there are several ultrasonographically detectable fetal abnormalities. A significant proportion of affected fetuses may be detected prenatally by virtue of an elevated maternal serum α-fetoprotein (AFP) level resulting from either an open neural tube defect or an abdominal wall defect. Recently, it has been confirmed that very low levels of maternal serum human chorionic gonadotrophin (hCG) may indicate that the fetus has trisomy 18 and other biochemical indicators are presently being assessed (see Chapter 3). Usually, an affected infant dies within days or weeks of birth; median survival is 6 days (Goldstein and Nielsen, 1988) but 2.5% survive to age 6 months and experience suggests that parents should always be forewarned about the remote possibility of prolonged survival. Surviving infants always show profound physical and mental retardation. A 1% recurrence risk for any serious chromosomal abnormality after an affected pregnancy is usually given but actual data in support of this are scanty. It is customary to offer parents of an affected fetus prenatal diagnosis in subsequent pregnancies.

Trisomy 13 (Patau syndrome)

Estimates of the birth prevalence of this disorder vary between 1 in 5000 and 1 in 30 000 newborn infants. Like trisomy 18, it can be diagnosed clinically through causing a recognizable pattern of dysmorphisms and malformations. Microcephaly with holoprosencephaly, microphthalmia, bilateral cleft lip and palate, congenital heart defect and polydactyly are typical findings. Scalp defects or abdominal wall defects may occur and lead to elevation of maternal serum AFP in the second trimester. Trisomy 13 is a rare cause of the so-called prune belly syndrome (see Chapter 14) which might be diagnosed by a fetal anomaly scan early in the second trimester. Usually, trisomy 13 infants succumb shortly after birth, median survival of affected infants being 2.5 days in one study (Goldstein and Nielsen, 1988). However, as in trisomy 18, a small number of infants have prolonged survival and profoundly disabled adults have been reported. A 1% recurrence risk for serious chromosomal abnormality in pregnancies subsequent to an affected one is usually given but again data to support this figure are scanty. Rarely, the affected fetus has translocation trisomy 13 and in such cases it is vital to karyotype the parents to exclude the possibility that one parent carries a balanced translocation. A rare autosomal recessive condition called pseudo-trisomy 13 has also been delineated (Cohen and Gorlin, 1991) and especially in view of its high recurrence risk, this particular diagnosis should be considered if cytogenetic confirmation is not forthcoming in a typically affected case.

Supernumerary marker chromosome

This term applies to any unidentified, small chromosome which is present in addition to the normal complement of 46 chromosomes. Frequently, carriers of such markers are mosaic with an additional normal cell line (presumably as a result of a tendency for such markers to be lost during mitosis). After a marker is detected in the fetus, both parents should have urgent blood cytogenetic studies performed; if the marker chromosome was inherited from one parent and if that parent is clinically normal, then the fetus is presumed not to be at increased risk of disability even though there is a remote possibility that a mosaic carrier parent who is phenotypically normal could have a clinically affected child who carries the same marker. In contrast, if the marker in the fetus has arisen *de novo*, there may be a considerable risk of mental disability or congenital abnormality in the fetus. Estimation of the precise risk of abnormality in any particular case is difficult and partly depends upon the size and staining properties of the marker including whether chromosomal satellites are present. The commonest identified marker is called an inverted duplication of chromosome 15 but even this precise identification gives no more than a guide to the genetic risk which is dependent upon the quantity of euchromatin or active genetic material between the centromeres. Recently, molecular cytogenetic studies employing the non-radioactive *in situ* hybridization technique have been used to identify marker chromosomes and this development may permit refinement of the estimated risk of phenotypic abnormality (Callen *et al.*, 1992). Detailed ultrasound screening for fetal malformation may, if positive, indicate a definitely affected fetus but the absence of visible defect does not guarantee normality; in this situation an overall empiric risk of 10% for handicap in a child with a *de novo* marker is appropriate in the light of the best available data (Warburton, 1991). This figure should also be given if the marker is present in a proportion of cells only. The recurrence risk after a pregnancy with a *de novo* marker chromosome is likely to be very low but since a parent could conceivably have low-grade mosaicism which is undetected and since such markers are more frequent in pregnancies of older mothers, it is reasonable to offer prenatal diagnosis to provide reassurance.

*Sex chromosome aneuploidy syndromes — 45,X; 47,XXX;
47,XXY; 47,XYY*

In total, these conditions occur in about 1 in 250 amniocenteses and they are therefore more frequent than the common autosomal aneuploidy syndromes including Down syndrome. Yet, a recent survey noted that many parents of affected children were not told of the possibility of sex chromosome aneuploidy in the counselling they had received prior to undergoing prenatal cytogenetic diagnosis (Robinson *et al.*, 1992). Nowadays, many parents choose to continue their pregnancy after prenatal diagnosis of sex chromosome aneuploidy because modern studies (e.g. Ratcliffe *et al.*, 1986) of affected children ascertained by neonatal cytogenetic surveys have revealed that clinical consequences of sex chromosome imbalance are often very mild. In contrast, previous studies based upon populations of children with phenotypic abnormalities who were diagnosed after hospital referral, gave an excessively pessimistic view of these syndromes. The majority of affected individuals function quite satisfactorily within society even though many affected children do have problems with learning and behaviour. Given up-to-date counselling following second trimester prenatal diagnosis of sex chromosome aneuploidy, about 50% or more of couples will elect to continue with their affected pregnancy.

45,X Turner syndrome. It is estimated that 1% of all conceptions are 45,X and 98% of these will spontaneously abort since only 1 in 2500 female births have Turner syndrome. Most abortions occur in the first trimester and the embryo is represented by a fragment of macerated tissue at the end of a well developed cord; 5% of embryos abort in the second trimester and ultrasound findings include large nuchal cystic hygromata and generalized oedema, however, these ultrasonographic signs are not specific, being commonly present in fetuses with trisomy 21 and other autosomal aneuploidies. In 80% of cases the paternal X chromosome is lost but a correlation between the phenotype (early abortion or liveborn infant) and the parental origin of the solitary X has not been established (Lorda-Sanchez *et al.*, 1992). There is a suggestion that mosaicism with a normal cell line is commoner in pregnancies which continue to term. Newborn infants with Turner syndrome may be completely unremarkable or have a few physical signs such as a short broad neck, pedal oedema and nail dysplasia. Congenital heart defect is present in 10–15% and affected newborn infants should be carefully examined to exclude coarctation of the aorta. Growth in childhood is deficient but modern treatment with synthetic human growth hormone prevents disabling short stature. Affected girls usually have atrophic ovaries and require hormone replacement therapy from mid-childhood but a small percentage have spontaneous pubertal development, ovulate and may even conceive. Recently, infertility in Turner syndrome has been successfully treated with egg donation and embryo transplant. Normal intelligence is the rule in Turner syndrome but mild–moderate intellectual impairment may be commoner in some cytogenetic variants of the condition such as 45,X/46,X ring(X) mosaicism. A small proportion of women with Turner syndrome have low grade mosaicism for Y chromosome derived DNA sequences and in these cases extirpation of streak gonads is recommended because of an increased risk (about 20%) that malignancy may develop. If parents of an affected fetus elect to continue with their pregnancy, the booklet produced by the Restricted Growth Association in the UK, which gives a clear account of the syndrome in affected children and adults, can be very helpful.

47,XXX. One in 1000 females have this chromosome constitution but those affected usually have no physical signs except slightly taller stature than average. Prospectively gathered data indicate that children are at a significantly increased risk of mild to moderate intellectual impairment and behavioural disturbance with over 50% requiring remedial teaching at school. However, some affected women have above average intelligence. Despite the common, associated cognitive problems in many but not all children with 47,XXX, diagnosis in childhood is rare since physical appearance is normal. Problems inconsistently associated with affected adults are menstrual irregularity, infertility, premature ovarian failure and increased risk of miscarriage. Overall, about 25% of reported, affected women have had some sort of ovarian dysfunction but despite this, fertility is the rule and the risk of aneuploidy amongst offspring of 47,XXX women appears to be low.

47,XYY. This disorder affects 1 in 1000 newborn males. Early reports of an 'XYY syndrome' described affected males resident in prison or psychiatric hospital diagnosed during cytogenetic surveys of the occupants of these institutions. It would therefore have been surprising if such affected males did not have serious psychiatric illness or a criminal tendency. In contrast, follow-up studies on affected infants diagnosed at birth or through prenatal screening have shown that they are not unusually violent or sociopathic (Ratcliffe *et al.* 1991). Average height is increased by about 6 cm and some individuals are exceptionally tall. Delay in speech development may be present and there is increased susceptibility to behaviour problems during early school years, however, such problems appear to be surmountable with appropriate teaching. Measured intelligence quotients are, on average, 10–15 points below those expected from family attainments but some affected individuals are of superior intelligence. In adult life there are no clinical stigmata and fertility is not usually impaired. It is reasonable to offer partners of known cases prenatal cytogenetic diagnosis even though there is little evidence to support the notion that offspring are more likely to have an abnormal number of sex chromosomes.

47,XXY (Klinefelter syndrome). This affects 1 in 1000 males and is usually diagnosed in adulthood because of infertility due to azoospermia. Some cases are diagnosed in childhood on account of learning difficulties and behaviour problems. Boys with this condition are not at increased risk for severe mental disability but, as with XYY, measured intelligence quotients of affected boys are some 10–15 points below those expected from family attainments. Again, some affected males may have above average intelligence. Physicians may diagnose the condition in early adulthood because of gynaecomastia (30% of cases) and hypogonadism. Surgery is rarely required for the former problem and the latter is commonly treated with testosterone. This karyotype is not known to predispose to abnormal sexual orientation and most affected males function satisfactorily within society.

Sex chromosome mosaicism. A large number of mosaic karyotypes have been described, many involving additional structural abnormalities of the X and Y chromosomes; the commonest occurring karyotypes are 45,X/46,XX and 45,X/46,XY. Data on cases ascertained through prenatal diagnosis indicate that 85% of girls with 45,X/46,XX are phenotypically normal. If the 45,X cell line predominates then there is likely to be an increased risk of miscarriage after prenatal diagnosis in affected pregnancies. Of infants born after prenatal diagnosis of 45,X/46,XY mosaicism, 90% have a normal male phenotye (Hsu, 1989). However, longer follow-up of cases discovered through prenatal diagnosis is required to determine if fertility is impaired in affected men and women. There is some anecdotal evidence that women with 46,XX/47,XXX mosaicism and 45,X/46,XX mosaicism have a greater likelihood of suffering multiple miscarriages, but the overall conclusion is that the prognosis for infants diagnosed prenatally is considerably more favourable than it would appear from clinical reports of cases diagnosed in postnatal life due to presentation with genital hypoplasia or ambiguity.

STRUCTURAL ABNORMALITIES

A very large number of diverse structural abnormalities have been described in the literature. These include translocations, deletions, duplications and inversions of chromosome material. As discussed above, inversions and translocations may be balanced or unbalanced. Unbalanced karyotypes often arise at meiosis through genetic recombination in the gametes of clinically normal balanced carriers. Prediction of phenotypic abnormality which is due to a particular unbalanced karyotype requires extensive knowledge of the literature and thorough appreciation of possible pitfalls.

De novo, *unbalanced structural abnormality in the fetus*

In about 1 in 2000 amniocenteses the fetal karyotype is abnormal because of an unbalanced structural abnormality which has arisen *de novo* because both parents have normal karyotypes. *De novo* translocation Down syndrome is one example in this category but any chromosome or combination of chromosomes may have deletion or duplication of chromosome material. Clinically recognized, rare syndromes are Wolf–Hirschhorn syndrome (4p−) and Cri du Chat syndrome (5p−). If autosomal imbalance occurs then likely clinical effects are mental disability and congenital malformation, however, pitfalls exist for the unwary counsellor; for example, Fig. 5.3 shows the pedigree of an unusual family where autosomal imbalance has

49

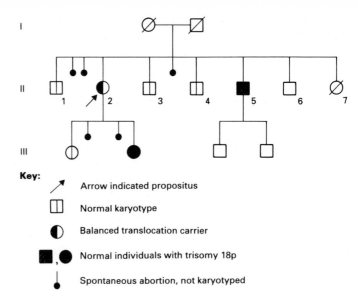

Key:

↗   Arrow indicated propositus

▯   Normal karyotype

◑   Balanced translocation carrier

■,●   Normal individuals with trisomy 18p

●   Spontaneous abortion, not karyotyped

Fig. 5.3 The propositus, II 2, carries a balanced reciprocal translocation detected after two miscarriages. She was counselled that her karyotype could predispose to the birth of a disabled child due to chromosome imbalance and prenatal diagnosis was offered. In a subsequent pregnancy CVS revealed an abnormal fetal karyotype with trisomy for chromosome 18p. Simultaneously, 18p trisomy was identified in II 5, a normal brother of the propositus. The propositus thus elected to continue with her pregnancy and she gave birth to a healthy female infant, III 2, with 18p trisomy.

not caused disability. If sex chromosome imbalance is present then the risk of severe mental or physical disability is much less: specialist advice should be sought in order to provide the parents with detailed genetic counselling information. The recurrence risk for a *de novo* abnormality is very low but not negligible because of the possibilities of gonadal mosaicism or non-paternity. Thus, some couples opt for reassurance which is provided by normal prenatal chromosomal analysis in future pregnancies.

*Unbalanced structural abnormality in fetus —
balanced structural abnormality in parent*

Prenatal diagnosis may be preceded by genetic counselling when the parent is a known balanced carrier and usually a prior decision is made to terminate an affected pregnancy. Occasionally, prenatal diagnosis is performed for another reason and subsequent cytogenetic studies show the abnormal fetal karyotype is derived from a balanced rearrangement in a healthy parent. Most pregnancies so diagnosed are terminated but parents suffer a double blow when they learn of the high recurrence risk in their future pregnancies. In an individual case any prediction in respect of expected clinical abnormality is guided by information on comparable cases in the medical literature. If the patient's family history reveals that other affected individuals have been born, then the severity of their handicap might provide the best indication of problems to be expected in a liveborn, affected infant. Referral for genetic counselling is clearly important if the family or at-risk relatives have not previously been counselled.

Inherited unbalanced structural abnormality in parent and fetus

Parents with autosomal imbalance rarely reproduce since they are usually affected by significant mental disability. However, several affected children have been born to mildly affected parents. The genetic counselling issues are clear in that there is a high recurrence risk and prenatal cytogenetic diagnosis is possible. However, communication with the parents may be difficult because of impaired understanding of risks and procedures. As a general rule, affected infants are similar to their affected parents but the possibility of the same chromosomal abnormality causing differing degrees of disability in affected parent and child cannot be discounted.

De novo *balanced structural abnormality —*
translocations and inversions

A balanced rearrangement is identified in the fetus but not in either parent in 1 in 2000 amniocenteses. Although carriers of balanced rearrangements are usually clinically normal, several studies have documented an excess of apparently balanced rearrangements amongst mentally retarded individuals and it has been suggested that disability in these patients is caused by sub-microscopic genetic damage at the sites of chromosome breakpoints. Current data suggest that when a *de novo* balanced chromosome rearrangement is detected prenatally there is 6–10% chance of congenital malformation and/or mental disability. A special case is the *de novo* Robertsonian (centric fusion) translocation where the risk of abnormality is considerably lower. In practice, a risk of disability of up to 10% is sufficient to sway some couples who then opt for pregnancy termination after unexpected prenatal diagnosis of a balanced rearrangement. In the future, better data on the risk of congenital abnormality in children with balanced *de novo* abnormalities will emerge from prospective studies which are following the progress of infants born after prenatal diagnosis. The recurrence risk for couples with a previously affected pregnancy is again very low (<1%) since both parents have, by definition, normal karyotypes.

Inherited balanced structural abnormality

This is diagnosed either after planned prenatal diagnosis because one parent is already known to be a balanced carrier, or perhaps when prenatal diagnosis is carried out for another indication and the fetus is found to carry a balanced rearrangement which is subsequently shown to have been transmitted by a normal parent. In either situation the risk of fetal abnormality is not increased since the presumably healthy parent carries the same rearrangement. Newly diagnosed families should be referred for genetic counselling since there will be a risk of fetal abnormality in their future pregnancies and since other relatives may be balanced carriers and so be at increased risk of having disabled children with chromosome imbalance.

Cryptic translocations and microdeletion syndromes

These terms refer to different classes of very small chromosome aberrations which are at or beyond the resolution limit of conventional cytogenetic techniques. Cryptic translocations are structural rearrangements which cannot be visualized by light microscopic examination of conventionally stained chromosomes. Such translocations have serious familial implications and cause considerable problems in genetic counselling and prenatal diagnosis. Figure 5.4 illustrates the pedigree of a family with a cryptic translocation which was suspected on the basis of the clinical and genetic history but was not demonstrable until a new molecular cytogenetic technique known as FISH (fluorescence *in situ* hybridization) was developed; this replaced conventional, high resolution cytogenetic banding studies which were normal in this family. The pedigree illustrates many relatives

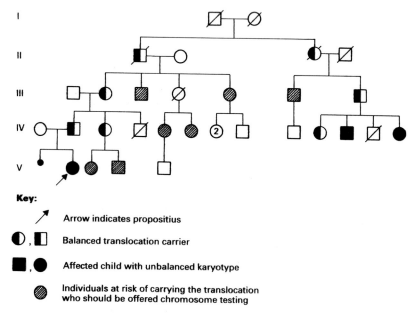

Key:

↗ Arrow indicates propositius

◐ , ◨ Balanced translocation carrier

■ , ● Affected child with unbalanced karyotype

◕ Individuals at risk of carrying the translocation who should be offered chromosome testing

Fig. 5.4 Conventional chromosome studies gave repeatedly normal results in this family but chromosome examination employing the fluorescence *in situ* hybridization technique revealed a cryptic 4/11 translocation which caused chromosome imbalance in three relatives affected by mental disability and a similar pattern of dysmorphism. An autosomal recessive syndrome was the initial, erroneous diagnosis for affected siblings in generation IV. Only after the birth of the propositus was it appreciated that other family members were at risk of having an affected child.

who have substantial risk of being carriers of this particular cryptic translocation and who, until the advent of FISH, could not be offered a definitive carrier test or prenatal diagnosis.

A number of different microdeletion syndromes and their chromosomal locations are known. Examples include Prader—Willi syndrome and Angelman syndrome (both 15q11—13), DiGeorge syndrome and velo-cardio-facial syndrome (both 22q11), Wilms tumour-aniridia syndrome (11p13), Langer—Giedion syndrome (8q23) and Miller—Dieker syndrome (17p13). The obstetrician is unlikely to be familiar with these rare disorders which are increasingly diagnosed by the application of new molecular cytogenetic and recombinant DNA techniques. Rarely, affected individuals have a family history of affected relatives. Prader—Willi syndrome has a birth incidence somewhere between 1 in 10 000 and 1 in 25 000. This condition can present to the obstetrician with polyhydramnios associated with poor fetal swallowing and poor fetal movements but without major malformation (another genetic disorder which should be considered in this situation is myotonic dystrophy inherited by the fetus from an affected mother). DiGeorge syndrome and velo-cardio-facial syndrome were previously considered quite distinct on clinical grounds, but molecular genetic studies have revealed they have a chromosome 22q11 abnormality in common. Both conditions are sometimes familial and are associated with a congenital heart defect; in fact, these two rare conditions exemplify the importance of obtaining a detailed family history from the parents of a fetus with a heart defect or indeed with any malformation which is detected antenatally. The remaining conditions mentioned above are very unlikely to be diagnosed antenatally in the absence of prior suspicion because routine prenatal cytogenetic analysis, carried out to exclude another condition such as Down syndrome, will not provide a sufficiently high quality chromosome preparation to permit detection of a microdeletion syndrome.

MOSAICISM

Mosaicism is the presence of two or more cell lines each with different chromosome complements. Usually, a karyotypically normal cell line co-exists with one or more abnormal cell lines but sometimes neither cell line is normal as in the case of 45,X/47,XXX mosaicism. If mosaicism is detected at amniocentesis or after chorionic villus sampling (CVS), then very difficult diagnostic and counselling problems may ensue. Genetic counselling is complicated in two respects: (1) there may be uncertainty about the phenotype since different tissues quite possibly contain differing proportions of abnormal cells or even none at all; and (2) complex technical issues often need to be addressed such as the distinction between 'true mosaicism,' which is likely to be present *in vivo*, and 'pseudomosaicism,' which is presumed to have arisen in one or more cells in the laboratory during the process of cell culture. Also, in relation to CVS, there is the problem of 'confined' mosaicism where the abnormal cell line is present *in vivo* but is confined to extra-fetal tissues, such as the placenta, where it does not have the same clinical significance as fetal mosaicism. Generally, in prenatal diagnosis the interpretive problems posed by mosaicism fall into one or more of the following areas:

1. The abnormal cell line exists in a small proportion of cells

Low level, true mosaicism will occasionally go undetected because the cytogeneticist usually analyses a limited number of cells derived from a single sample. Obviously, the smaller the percentage of abnormal cells the less chance they have of being detected and the smaller the risk of adverse clinical effect, but there is a danger of false reassurance because in an individual fetus the proportion of abnormal cells present in many tissues including the central nervous system is actually unknown. Therefore, it is perilous to infer that a low proportion of abnormal cells in a prenatal diagnostic sample predicts a mild clinical phenotype.

2. The abnormal cell line is present in some fetal tissues but not in others

Mosaicism confined to some tissues is well recognized in clinical cytogenetics. Amniotic fluid cells are thought to be derived from different sources including fetal skin, bronchopulmonary tract and fetal urine. Multiple sources of origin will increase the likelihood of a good correlation between positive cytogenetic findings and the presence of fetal abnormality. In contrast, cytogenetic analysis of a single tissue, such as fetal blood, will sometimes reveal only a normal cell line even in a clinically abnormal fetus. For example, tetrasomy 12p and diploid–triploid mosaicism are two well-recognized conditions where the abnormal cells are only readily identified amongst fibroblasts derived from a skin biopsy. That mosaicism can never be ruled out should always be remembered before undertaking a second invasive prenatal test in an attempt to clarify an earlier unusual or ambiguous result.

3. True mosaicism and pseudomosaicism

In large surveys of prenatal cytogenetic diagnosis the combined frequencies of true chromosome mosaicism and pseudomosaicism have ranged from approximately 3–7%.

True mosaicism is chromosome mosaicism which is regarded as existing *in vivo*. It is defined as the presence of abnormal cells in at least two out of three culture flasks or colonies independently established from the original amniotic fluid sample and it is present in 0.3% of amniocenteses. If discovered antenatally it is usually assumed to have clinical consequences conferring a risk of mental disability and malformation if imbalance of autosomes is present. A possible difficult exception is trisomy 20 mosaicism present in amniotic fluid. Trisomy 20 mosaicism is one of the commonest autosomal trisomy mosaic results present in amniotic fluid cells but it has yet to be confirmed in a fetal blood sample or in a postnatal blood sample. Trisomy 20 cells have been identified in fibroblasts from a liveborn infant (Brothman *et al.*, 1992) but the evidence that they cause clinical abnormality is not strong hence the good chance of a normal pregnancy outcome after this prenatal diagnosis.

Pseudomosaicism, that is, the detection of a single chromosomally abnormal cell (Level I pseudomosaicism), or the detection of several cells with the same abnormality in a single flask or colony (Level II pseudomosaicism), is more frequently encountered and is assumed to have arisen *in vitro*. Exceptionally, apparent pseudomosaicism actually reflects true mosaicism in the fetus and hence pseudomosaic results provide strong (but not absolute) reassurance.

4. Mosaicism in CVS including confined placental mosaicism

Obstetricians who regularly perform CVS will be aware of instances where the chromosome result proved difficult to interpret. In total, about 1.5% of all test results are classed by the laboratory as 'problem cases', and these mostly involve mosaic chromosome abnormalities including structural and numerical abnormalities of sex chromosomes and autosomes. Chromosome mosaicism occurs both in 'direct' preparations of spontaneously dividing cells derived from the outer surface of the villus (cytotrophoblast) and amongst cultured cells derived from the mesenchymal core of the villus. Less frequently, mosaicism occurs in both direct and cultured preparations, this result can reflect either true fetal mosaicism or so-called confined placental mosaicism where the embryo is chromosomally normal but the placenta has a chromosomally abnormal cell line (Kalousek and Dill, 1983). Certain chromosomal abnormalities including trisomies for 2, 7, 8 and sex chromosome abnormalities are more likely to be confined to the placenta and do not have any adverse effect on the fetus (Wang *et al.*, 1993). However, Kalousek (1990) suggested that the presence of an abnormal cell line in the placenta can cause growth retardation of a chromosomally normal fetus whereas, in contrast, a normal cell line in the placenta may help ensure viability of a fully trisomic fetus. Somewhat reassuringly, a recent follow-up investigation, with identification of control pregnancies for comparison, failed to find an increased incidence of pregnancy loss, congenital malformation or developmental delay in infants born after confined chorionic mosaicism was diagnosed (Fryburg *et al.*, 1993). Less reassuring, in the same paper, was the discussion of two cases where true mosaicism for trisomy 5 was confirmed indicating that mosaicism for so-called non-viable trisomies could conceivably have a phenotypic effect in liveborn infants.

5. Investigation of mosaicism and counselling guidelines

Chorionic villus sampling. The incidence of false positive results after CVS is minimized by performing chromosome analysis on both the direct cyto-trophoblast preparation and also chorionic stromal cells which become established in long-term culture and are embryologically closer to the embryo proper. If mosaicism is detected in direct preparations of spontaneously dividing cytotrophoblast cells, the clinician should wait for the result of chromosome analysis on cultured cells. The discovery of mosaicism for structural chromosome rearrangements is most likely artefactual and mosaicism for non-viable trisomies can also be artefactual or confined to the placenta. Mosaicism in both directly analysed and cultured CVS cells could be present in the fetus or confined to the placenta and in problematic cases, subsequent chromosome studies on amniotic fluid cells and fetal blood cells together with detailed ultrasound examination of the fetus may provide the couple with sufficient reassurance to continue the pregnancy, if normal results are obtained. If, on the other hand, abnormal cells are detected in these secondary investigations then the likelihood of fetal abnormality rises considerably and the option of pregnancy termination should be discussed.

Amniotic fluid. When a mosaic chromosome result is observed in two flasks or culture vessels it should be considered a true reflection of the fetal karyotype and the genetics literature should be searched for reports of cases with the same karyotypic abnormality. Detailed ultrasound examination of the fetus might provide evidence of malformation, but a normal scan appearance should not be regarded as evidence that the fetus is unaffected. Fetal blood sampling might clarify the likely significance of an ambiguously abnormal karyotype result, but it should be recalled that some cytogenetic problems are not expressed in fetal blood. Since both mosaicism itself and also its potential adverse clinical effect can almost never be 'ruled out', there is frequently uncertainty and very difficult genetic counselling dilemmas may ensue.

FURTHER READING

The following monograph and chapters in major textbooks are particularly recommended:

Gardener, R.J.M. and Sutherland, G.R. (1989) *Chromosome Abnormalities and Genetic*

Counselling. Oxford monographs on medical genetics No. 17. Oxford University Press, Oxford.

Hook, E.B. (1992) Prevalence, risks and recurrence, in *Prenatal diagnosis and screening* (eds D.J.H. Brock, C.H. Rodeck and M.A. Ferguson-Smith), Churchill Livingstone, Edinburgh, pp. 351−92.

Hsu, L.Y.F. (1992) Prenatal diagnosis of chromosomal abnormalities through amniocentesis. In *Genetic Disorders and the fetus. Diagnosis, Prevention and Treatment*. Johns Hopkins University Press, Baltimore and London, pp. 155−210.

REFERENCES

Brothman, A.R., Rehberg, K., Storto, P.D., Phillips, S.E. and Mosby, R.T. (1992) Confirmation of true mosaic trisomy 20 in a phenotypically normal liveborn male. *Clinical Genetics*, **42**, 47−49.

Callen, D.F., Eyre, H., Yip, M-Y., Freemantle, J. and Haan, E. (1992) Molecular cytogenetic and clinical studies of 42 patients with marker chromosomes. *American Journal of Medical Genetics*, **43**, 709−15.

Cohen, M.M. and Gorlin, R.J. (1991) Pseudo-trisomy 13 syndrome. *American Journal of Medical Genetics*, **39**, 332−35.

Fryburg, J.S., Dimaio, M.S., Yang-Fen, T.L. and Mahoney, M.J. (1993) Follow-up of pregnancies complicated by placental mosaicism diagnosed by chorionic villus sampling. *Prenatal diagnosis*, **13**, 481−494.

Goldstein, H. and Neilsen, K.G. (1988) Rates and survival of individuals with trisomy 13 and trisomy 18. Data from a 10-year period in Denmark. *Clinical Genetics*, **34**, 366−72.

Hsu, L.Y.F. (1989) Prenatal diagnosis of 45,X/46,XY mosaicism — a review and update. *Prenatal Diagnosis*, **9**, 31−48.

Kalousek, D.K. (1990) Confined placental mosaicism and intrauterine development. *Pediatric Pathology*, **10**, 69−77.

Kalousek, D.K. and Dill, F.J. (1983) Chromosome mosaicism confined to the placenta in human conceptions. *Science*, **221**, 665−67.

Lorda-Sanchez, I., Binkert, F., Maechler, M. and Schinzel, A. (1992) Molecular study of 45,X conceptuses: correlation with clinical findings. *American Journal of Medical Genetics*, **42**, 487−90.

Pellestor, F. (1991) Frequency and distribution of aneuploidy in human female gametes. *Human Genetics*, **86**, 283−88.

Ratcliffe, S.G., Butler, G.E. and Jones, M. (1991) Children and young adults with sex chromosome aneuploidy, in *Birth Defects: Original Article Series 26* (eds. Evans, J.A., Hamerton, J.L., Robinson A.), pp. 1−44.

Ratcliffe, S.G., Murray, L. and Teague, P. (1986) Edinburgh study of growth and development in children with sex chromosome abnormalities III. *Prospective studies on children with sex chromosome aneuploidy* (ed. S.G. Ratcliffe and N. Paul), Alan R. Liss, New York, pp. 23−72.

Robinson, A., Bender, B. and Linden, M.G. (1992) Prognosis of prenatally diagnosed children with sex chromosome aneuploidy. *American Journal of Medical Genetics*, **44**, 365−68.

Wang, B.B.T., Rubin, C.H. and Williams, J. (1993) Mosaicism in chorionic villus sampling: an analysis of incidence and chromosomes involved in 2612 consecutive cases. *Prenatal Diagnosis*, **13**, 179−90.

Warburton, D. (1991) De novo balanced chromosome rearrangements and extra marker chromosomes identified at prenatal diagnosis: clinical significance and distribution of breakpoints. *American Journal of Human Genetics*, **49**, 995−1013.

Zenzes, M.T., Wang, P. and Casper, R.F. (1992) Chromosome status of untransferred (spare) embryos and probability of pregnancy after in-vitro fertilisation. *Lancet*, **340**, 391−94.

Chapter 6
Biochemical Diagnosis of Inborn Errors of Metabolism

D. A. AITKEN

The basic biochemical defect has been identified as an absent or defective enzyme or non-enzymatic protein in over 300 different inborn errors of metabolism (IEM) (McKusick, 1992). Although the majority of IEM are rare, collectively they are about twice as frequent as the chromosomal disorders and some may be present at very high frequency in certain ethnic groups (e.g. Tay−Sachs disease in Ashkenazi Jews). A classification scheme indicating the approximate number of disorders in each group and the population incidence of some of the more common disorders is presented in Table 6.1. Comprehensive reviews of the clinical, biochemical and genetic features of the IEM can be found in Scriver *et al.* (1989), Benson and Fensom (1985) and Galjaard (1980).

In most cases, because of the mainly recessive mode of inheritance of IEM, there will be no family history of the condition before the birth of an affected child but a high risk of recurrence in any future pregnancy. Many IEM are associated with significant morbidity or mortality in affected individuals and effective treatment is available for very few. Prenatal diagnosis and selective termination of affected pregnancies is therefore usually the only means to prevent the birth of an affected child in at-risk families.

Over 100 different IEM have been diagnosed prenatally (see Appendix) and substantial experience of several hundred diagnoses accumulated for some specific disorders such as: Tay−Sachs disease; cystic fibrosis; mucopolysaccharidoses types I and II; glycogenosis type II; Krabbe's disease; metachromatic leucodystrophy; cystinosis; and maple syrup urine disease (Galjaard, 1987). For most of the others, however, experience is limited by their low incidence to a few dozen cases or less. Initially, biochemical investigation of cultured amniotic fluid cells in the second trimester was the established method of prenatal diagnosis but analyses of enzymes, proteins and metabolites in a variety of other tissues including chorionic villi, fetal blood, fetal liver and cell-free amniotic fluid have extended the scope and timing of prenatal investigations.

DIAGNOSIS IN THE INDEX CASE

Because of their mainly recessive mode of inheritance, most IEM occur in

58

Table 6.1 Variety and incidence of metabolic disorders

Disorder (No. of types)	Approx. incidence 100 000 births	Ethnic group
Carbohydrate metabolism (24)	18	Caucasian
Glycogen storage diseases (14)		
e.g. von Gierke	1.0	
Others		
e.g. Galactosaemia	2.0	
Amino acid metabolism (30)	>40	Caucasian
Urea cycle defects		
e.g. Citrullinaemia	1.4	
Sulphur amino acid defects		
e.g. Homocystinuria	0.3	
Aromatic amino acid defects		
e.g. Phenylketonuria	2−25	Caucasian
Branched chain amino acid defects		
e.g. Maple syrup urine disease	1.0	
Organic acid metabolism (30)	16	
e.g. Methylmalonic acidaemia	5−10	
Lysosomal storage disorders (30)	11	
Mucopolysaccharidoses (11)	8	European
e.g. Hunter's syndrome	1	
Sphingolipidoses (8)		
e.g. Gaucher disease	1−2	Caucasian
	150	Ashkenazi Jews
Tay−Sachs disease	0.3	Caucasian
	30	Ashkenazi Jews
Mucolipidoses (3)		
e.g. I-cell disease	0.1	
Glycoproteinoses (4)		
e.g. Sialdosis	0.1	
Purine and pyrimidine metabolism (10)	7.0	
e.g. Lesch−Nyhan syndrome	5.0	Caucasian
Adenosine deaminase deficiency	0.1	Caucasian
Lipoprotein and lipid metabolism (17)	>200	
e.g. Familial hypercholesterolaemia	200	Panethnic
Porphyrin and haem metabolism (12)	11	
e.g. Acute intermittent porphyria	10	North American
Peroxisomal disorders (14)	7.4	
e.g. Zellweger syndrome	1−2	European
Membrane transport (16)	80	
e.g. Cystic fibrosis	50	Caucasian
Cystinuria	14	
Metal metabolism (3)	3.0	
e.g. Menkes disease	2.0	

(Continued)

Table 6.1 (*Cont.*)

Disorder (No. of types)	Approx. incidence 100 000 births	Ethnic group
Steroid hormone metabolism (15)	60	
e.g. Congenital adrenal hyperplasia	1.5−7	Caucasian
	60−200	Eskimos
Steroid sulphatase deficiency	10	Caucasian
Miscellaneous		
e.g. Hypophosphatasia	1.0	
Oculocutaneous albinism (6)	5.0	Caucasian
	10	US blacks
Ehlers−Danlos syndromes (10)	17	

children of parents who have no previous family history of the condition. Establishing a primary diagnosis may prove to be both a difficult and protracted process. However, demonstration of a specific enzyme or protein defect in the index case is mandatory if prenatal diagnosis is to be undertaken with confidence in any future pregnancy. A clinical diagnosis is not sufficient as certain disorders which appear clinically identical, for example, Sanfilippo A disease (Heparan *N* sulphatase deficiency) and Sanfillippo B disease (*N* acetyl α glucosaminidase deficiency), are clinically indistinguishable yet are the result of different enzyme deficiencies.

The specific enzyme defects in the majority of IEM listed in the Appendix can be demonstrated in erythrocytes or leucocytes (prepared from freshly collected anticoagulated blood) or in cultured fibroblasts derived from a skin biopsy. Blood is likely to provide the most rapid diagnosis since no culture period is required prior to analysis. However, fibroblasts have other advantages. They provide a permanent source of material independent of patient survival on which a series of biochemical tests may be performed to establish a diagnosis. They are also available as a reference culture (stored frozen in the laboratory liquid nitrogen cell bank) which can be reconstituted and assayed in parallel with tissue or cultured material from the fetus in any future prenatal investigation. In some cases significant residual enzyme activity may be present in *in vitro* cultures from affected individuals which give rise to difficulties in interpretation at prenatal diagnosis and in this instance control material from the index case is vital. Skin fibroblast cultures from the carrier parents may also be valuable for defining the intermediate enzyme levels which might be expected in a heterozygous fetus. However, extreme caution must be exercised when comparing enzyme activities in cultured fibroblasts with activities in tissues of fetal origin since the overall level of activity may be very different in the different cell types.

GENETIC COUNSELLING

Once a diagnosis has been established in the index case the prospects for, and desirability of, any future prenatal diagnosis can be discussed with the parents. Not all IEM are severe enough to justify selective termination of affected pregnancies and a small number may be regarded as treatable. On the other hand, for the majority of metabolic disorders with a poor prognosis, couples may be deterred from embarking on a further pregnancy when the high risk of recurrence is explained. Others will wish to have prenatal diagnosis and the option of termination of an affected fetus. Factors which need to be discussed are the risks to the fetus of the diagnostic procedures, the stage of pregnancy at which the test can be carried out, the time scale required to provide a diagnosis and the reliability of the tests.

DIAGNOSIS OF IEM

While the majority of the disorders listed in the Appendix can be diagnosed with a high degree of reliability, all prenatal testing is vulnerable to errors. Apart from the risks to the fetus imposed by the invasive procedures required to obtain fetal material (see Chapter 17), the parents should be made aware of the technical limitations of the prenatal test. For analyses requiring cultured amniotic fluid or chorionic villus cells there is the inevitable delay associated with cell culture and up to 4 weeks or more may be required to accumulate sufficient cells for analysis. Also, failure of cell growth or contamination may affect around 1% of cultures in even the most experienced laboratories. Contamination of growing cells by mycoplasma may provide a source of enzyme activity (e.g. for purine metabolic disorders) which may conceal a deficiency in the amniotic fluid cells. Cultures should be screened and confirmed mycoplasma-free before their use for prenatal diagnosis. The risks of misinterpretation of analytical results can be minimized by a thorough knowledge of the disorder, through detailed study of the index case and acquisition of the necessary controls. However, in some instances inadequate samples (either in amount or purity) will be collected and this is the most likely cause of failure to obtain a result, or of errors in interpretation.

SCREENING FOR CARRIERS OF IEM

For disorders in which carriers may be identified with a high degree of confidence, testing may be extended to other family members and their spouses to establish their carrier status although, because of the low frequency in the general population of most IEM with an autosomal recessive mode of inheritance, the risk to non-consanguineous couples is likely to be low. An exceptional situation exists in the case of Tay−Sachs

61

disease. Because of the high carrier frequency in Ashkenazi Jews, carrier screening can be offered to all couples of Jewish origin. In contrast, in X-linked conditions such as Hunter's syndrome and the Lesch–Nyhan syndrome, other female relatives are at substantial risk of being carriers and need genetic counselling. However, for most IEM, in the absence of definitive carrier testing by mutation analysis, biochemical methods may not provide clear information on carrier status and couples may remain uncertain of the risks on which to base a decision on prenatal testing.

PRENATAL DIAGNOSIS

Generally, prenatal diagnosis of IEM does not fall within the category of routine laboratory testing and usually, particularly for some of the rarer disorders, the services of a specialized laboratory will have to be enlisted. Because of the individual rarity of most IEM and their collective variety, no single laboratory is able to provide a diagnostic service for all the biochemical disorders listed in the Appendix. It is important that the laboratory performing the enzymatic analysis has experience in the assay of cells from affected cases as well as up-to-date information on normal ranges, heterozygote levels and residual activities in the appropriate tissue at the appropriate stage of gestation. Ideally, the laboratory will already have been involved with the diagnosis of the index case of the family, and will have stored material for use as analytical controls.

Choice of tissues

As a general rule, when an enzyme defect can be demonstrated in skin fibroblast cultures from an affected individual, the same defect will be expressed in amniotic fluid cell cultures obtained from an affected pregnancy, a rule which also applies (with certain precautions) to the expression of IEM in chorionic villi. The established method of prenatal diagnosis of metabolic disorders has been by identification of a specific enzyme defect in cultured amniotic fluid cells obtained by amniocentesis in the second trimester. However, the advantages of first trimester diagnosis offered by chorionic villus sampling (CVS) have displaced amniocentesis as the automatic choice. When the defect is not expressed in amniotic fluid cultures or chorionic villi, fetal blood or fetal tissue (e.g. liver) may be an alternative source of diagnostic material.

Cultured amniotic fluid cells

With the exception of cystic fibrosis (see below), around 15 weeks' gestation is the optimum time for amniocentesis for prenatal diagnosis of metabolic disorders. At this stage an adequate volume (20 ml) of amniotic fluid containing sufficient viable cells can be obtained. Although there is a trend towards earlier amniocentesis, smaller volume samples will generally be obtained at this stage with lower numbers of viable cells and this may result in longer culture times. Microtechniques of enzyme assay which require only a few hundred cells and therefore shorter culture times have been applied successfully in a few specialized centres (Galjaard, 1980) but this approach has been largely displaced by earlier sampling offered by CVS. The potentially more rapid approach using uncultured amniotic fluid cells is unreliable.

Amniotic fluid supernatant

Clearly if a metabolic disorder can be diagnosed using amniotic fluid supernatant, the lengthy delays involved in cell culture are avoided. However, the concentration profiles of soluble proteins in amniotic fluid vary widely at different gestations and the majority have a maternal origin and are therefore inappropriate for prenatal diagnosis of fetal metabolic disease. A few proteins are of fetal origin or have a fetal component and have been exploited as indicators of fetal abnormality. Most of these investigations have been carried out in the second trimester and caution should be exercised in the use of amniotic fluid obtained at earlier gestations until more experience is accumulated for such samples.

Reliable diagnoses have been made using enzyme analysis of amniotic fluid. Iduronate sulphatase activity is deficient in amniotic fluid from pregnancies in which the fetus has mucopolysaccharidosis II (Hunter's syndrome) and elevated levels of multiple lysosomal enzymes are found in liquor from pregnancies with mucolipidosis II (I-cell disease). Significantly reduced activities of a number of amniotic fluid microvillar enzymes (e.g. γ-glutamyltranspeptidase, intestinal alkaline phosphatase) are found in pregnancies in which the fetus has cystic fibrosis with secondary meconium ileus (Brock *et al.*, 1988). The sensitivity and specificity of this method of prenatal diagnosis of cystic fibrosis approaches 95% in couples with a previously affected child if amniocentesis is performed at 17−18 weeks' gestation. However, the prenatal diagnosis of cystic fibrosis has been generally superseded by DNA analysis which has the advantages of earlier diagnosis and greater accuracy (see Chapter 8).

An approach which is finding increasing application for prenatal diagnosis of IEM using amniotic fluid supernatant is the analysis of metabolites which characterize the metabolic block. At least 14 different amino- and organic acid disorders can be reliably prenatally diagnosed using stable isotope dilution gas chromatography−mass spectrometry with selected ion monitoring (Jakobs *et al.*, 1990).

Other IEM can also be prenatally diagnosed by metabolite assay. Congenital adrenal hyperplasia can be diagnosed by measurement of amniotic fluid 17α-hydroxy progesterone (Hughes *et al.*, 1987) and the characteristic patterns of glycosaminoglycan accumulation in amniotic fluid revealed by two-dimensional electrophoresis can provide a rapid differential diagnosis of the mucopolysaccharidoses (Mossman and Patrick, 1982) although the latter should always be confirmed by analysis of the specific enzyme defect in cultured amniotic fluid cells.

Chorionic villus sampling

Direct biochemical analysis can be carried out using trophoblastic tissue obtained transcervically as early as 8 weeks' gestation and with the development of transabdominal CVS, the gestational range for sampling extends into the second and third trimesters. Since the first reports in 1982 of the presence of enzyme activity in uncultured villi, the use of CVS for biochemical analysis of metabolic disorders has expanded rapidly. Over 65 different IEM have been investigated biochemically in the first trimester and experience is expanding rapidly for some of the more common disorders confirming the reliability of this approach.

The successful use of chorionic villi for prenatal diagnosis depends on obtaining samples of adequate size uncontaminated with blood or maternal decidua. Careful selection of characteristic villi by microdissection is required to exclude maternal contamination which may lead to mistaken diagnoses. About 30 mg (wet weight) tissue is required to provide sufficient material for direct study, establishment of villi cultures and for chromosome analysis. Ten milligrams of tissue should be regarded as the minimum which can be used for reliable direct biochemical analysis and while diagnostic assays may be attempted on smaller quantities for some conditions, the scope for rigorous selection of villi is correspondingly reduced. If there are doubts concerning the quality of the sample, amniocentesis is indicated to check the result; this is a possibility which must be raised during counselling. Interpretation of assay results depends on an adequate knowledge of the ranges of activity expected in cultured and uncultured CVS in homozygous affected, heterozygous and normal tissues and on potential confounding factors (see Table 6.2). Certain enzymes have very low levels of expression in uncultured chorionic villi but show markedly increased activity in cultured chorionic villi thus offering a more reliable approach to diagnosis. In the case of Hurler's syndrome (mucopolysaccharidosis type I), small amounts of maternal contamination may lead to false negative diagnoses as there is a significantly greater level of α-iduronidase activity in maternal decidua than in uncultured CVS from normal pregnancies (Fowler *et al.*, 1989). Affected fetuses have also been correctly diagnosed using cultured villi in cases of argininosuccinic aciduria (argininosuccinate lyase activity) and metachromatic leucodystrophy (aryl sulphatase A deficiency) after the results obtained following direct analysis of uncultured villi had been interpreted as normal (Galjaard, 1987). In contrast, the culture dependent variations in α-glucosidase activity (Pompe disease, glucogenosis type II) make direct assay of villi more reliable.

Table 6.2 Potential pitfalls in use of chorionic villus samples

Disorder	Enzyme deficiency	Problem
Hurler's syndrome	α-L-iduronidase	Low level of expression
Sialidosis	Neuraminidase	Low level of expression
Homocystinuria	Cystathione β synthetase	Low level of expression
Niemann–Pick disease	Sphingomyelinase	Low level of expression
I-cell disease	Multiple lysosomal enzymes	Low levels of expression
Metachromatic leucodystrophy	Aryl sulphatase A	Isoenzyme interference by Aryl sulphatase C
Maroteaux–Lamy disease	Aryl sulphatase B	Isoenzyme interference by Aryl sulphatase C

Chorionic villus sampling may also be exploited for prenatal diagnosis using metabolite analysis. Prenatal diagnosis of cystinosis has been achieved by expeditious analysis of the cystine content in fresh chorionic villi. However, as free cystine is rapidly lost even on frozen storage, a more reliable approach to diagnosis of cystinosis is to grow up villi in ^{35}S-cystine and measure the retention of the labelled metabolite (Patrick *et al.*, 1987).

It would seem prudent for all prenatal diagnoses using CVS that, where sufficient material can be obtained, activity should be measured both directly and after a period in culture. While the majority of diagnoses reported to date have been made correctly by direct analysis of villi, the activities of most enzymes are higher in cultured villi and better discrimination may be possible between normal, carrier and residual activities.

Fetal blood

By 18 weeks' gestation, pure fetal blood samples may be obtained by cordocentesis (see Chapter 17) and many IEM which have expression in red cells, white cells or plasma, become accessible to prenatal diagnosis. Although sampling is at an advanced stage of pregnancy, diagnoses can usually be made within 24 hours as no cell culture is required. Prenatal diagnosis of adenosine deaminase deficiency and severe combined immuno-deficiency is possible by enzyme analysis of fetal red cells (Simmonds *et al.*, 1983) with the added advantage that lymphocyte transformation following mitogenic stimulation can also be used as an index of cell-mediated immunity.

Other fetal tissues

The development of methods for sampling fetal tissues such as skin or liver has opened the possibility of the biochemical prenatal diagnosis of IEM in which the basic biochemical defect is not expressed in more readily accessible tissues (see Appendix). Several liver-specific enzyme deficiencies of the urea cycle have been diagnosed using fetal liver biopsies at 18–20 weeks' gestation, for example, ornithine carbamyl transferase deficiency (Rodeck *et al.*, 1982), although the increasing availability of specific gene probes for DNA analysis of CVS will eventually make this approach obsolete.

TRANSPORT OF SAMPLES

Access to the specialized analyses necessary for the prenatal diagnosis of many IEM will often require the transport of fetal material to a distant laboratory. Where such arrangements are necessary, the advice of the diagnostic laboratory on the type of sample and the conditions of shipment should be sought before the sample is obtained.

For assays requiring amniotic fluid cells, either the whole sample is dispatched, securely packed at ambient temperature by the most rapid transit means available, or the local cell culture laboratory first establishes growing cultures of amniotic fluid cells and following subculture sends one or two small flasks of growing cells. The former route is likely to yield a more rapid result but risks total loss of sample through mishandling or delay. The latter approach may take longer since the original subculture will have to be re-established in the diagnostic laboratory under the same conditions as the control cell lines before the material can be reliably assayed. However, the existence of an on-going culture at the referring centre means that more material is immediately available as a safeguard against loss in transit.

For direct analysis of CVS, most enzymes are stable for at least 24 hours at ambient temperature in freshly collected villi in culture medium. The samples must not be frozen or enzyme activity will be lost to the transport medium. As with amniotic fluid, establishing cultures at source offers a more secure method of providing material for analysis elsewhere but incurs delay in diagnosis. However, as previously indicated, confirmation of the direct assay result in cultured villi is desirable in any case, and ideal samples are those which are large enough to provide both options.

Fetal blood collected in anticoagulant may be transported satisfactorily at ambient temperature, but tissue samples (e.g. liver) should be wrapped in foil to prevent desiccation, shock frozen in liquid nitrogen immediately on collection and transported in a deep frozen state (on dry ice).

CONFIRMATION OF DIAGNOSIS

Continuing evaluation of prenatal diagnostic tests is essential to establish their sensitivity and specificity and this requires follow-up of the outcome of every case. Where an abnormal fetus is predicted and the pregnancy terminated, assay of the basic protein defect in appropriate fetal tissues is required to confirm the prenatal diagnosis. *Post mortem* fetal cultures are also an important source of analytical controls for prenatal diagnosis in a future pregnancy.

When the prenatal diagnosis indicates an unaffected pregnancy, or carrier status in the fetus, adequate assessment and follow-up is required to confirm that the infant is clinically unaffected. Collection of cord blood in anticoagulant at delivery is a useful source of material for confirmatory enzyme assays, but it should be noted that for certain metabolite assays, abnormal levels may not have accumulated in the fetal circulation at birth and a later sample may be required to confidently exclude a false negative prenatal diagnostic result.

REFERENCES

Benson, P.F. and Fensom, A.H. (1985) *Genetic Biochemical Disorders*, Oxford University Press, Oxford.

Brock, D.J.H., Clarke, H.A.K. and Barron, L. (1988) Prenatal diagnosis of cystic fibrosis by microvillar enzyme assay of a sequence of 258 pregnancies. *Human Genetics*, 78, 271−75.

Fowler, B., Giles, L., Cooper, A. and Sardharwalla, I.B. (1989) Chorionic villus sampling: diagnostic uses and limitations of enzyme assays. *Journal of Inherited Metabolic Disease*, 12, Supp 1, 105−17.

Galjaard, H. (1980) *Genetic Metabolic Disease. Early Diagnosis and Prenatal Analysis*, Elsevier, Amsterdam.

Galjaard, H. (1987) Fetal diagnosis of inborn errors of metabolism. *Fetal Diagnosis of Genetic Defects* (ed. C.M. Rodeck), Baillière Tindall, London, pp. 547−67.

Hughes, I.A., Dyas, J., Riad-Fahmy, D. and Laurence, K.M. (1987) Prenatal diagnosis of congenital adrenal hyperplasia: reliability of amniotic fluid steroid analysis. *Journal of Medical Genetics*, 24, 344−47.

Jakobs, C., Ten Brink, H.J. and Stellaard, F. (1990) Prenatal diagnosis of inherited metabolic disorders by quantitation of characteristic metabolites in amniotic fluid: facts and future. *Prenatal Diagnosis*, 10, 265−71.

McKusick, V.A. (1992) *Mendelian Inheritance in Man* 10th edn, The Johns Hopkins University Press, Baltimore, 2320 pp.

Mossman, J. and Patrick, A.D. (1982) Prenatal diagnosis of mucopolysaccharidoses by two-dimensional electrophoresis of amniotic fluid glycosaminoglycans. *Prenatal Diagnosis*, 2, 169−76.

Patrick, A.D., Young, E.P., Mossman, J., Warren, R., Keaney, L. and Rodeck, C.H. (1987) First trimester diagnosis of cystinosis using intact chorionic villi. *Prenatal Diagnosis*, 7, 71−74.

Rodeck, C.H., Patrick, A.D. and Pembrey, M.E. (1982) Fetal liver biopsy for prenatal diagnosis of ornithine carbamyl transferase deficiency. *Lancet*, ii, 297−99.

Scriver, C.R., Beaudet, A.L., Sly, W.S. and Valle, D. (1989) *The Metabolic Basis of Inherited Disease* 6th edn, McGraw-Hill.

Simmonds, H.A., Fairbanks, L.D., Webster, D.R., Rodeck, C.H., Linch, D.C. and Levinsky, R.J. (1983) Rapid prenatal diagnosis of adenosine deaminase deficiency and other purine disorders using fetal blood. *Bioscience Reports*, 3, 31−38.

Chapter 7
Haematological Disorders

E. A. LETSKY

Haematological disorders which affect the fetus may be inherited or acquired. They include red cell, white cell, platelet and coagulation abnormalities. Prenatal diagnosis of an affected pregnancy may be indicated for conditions where *in utero* treatment is available or if the disorder will result in a life-limiting or serious disease. Only the most frequent genetic and acquired disorders are discussed here. The Appendix contains references to rarer problems.

DISORDERS AFFECTING RED CELLS

Haemoglobinopathies

The genetic disorders of the synthesis or structure of haemoglobin are the commonest single gene diseases in the world population. They present a vast public health problem concentrated in the populations of the eastern Mediterranean, Middle East, parts of India, southeast Asia, Africa and the West Indies.

Following the influx of immigrants from these parts of the world, obstetricians in the UK are encountering women with genetic defects of haemoglobin seldom seen in the indigenous population. They are made up of two main groups: (1) inherited abnormalities of the synthesis of the globin chains of haemoglobin — the thalassaemias; and (2) the structural haemoglobin variants.

Under normal circumstances the carrier states for the most important of these haemoglobinopathies, β-thalassaemia and sickle cell haemoglobin are symptomless with no direct effect on the quality of life or life expectancy. Prenatal diagnosis of the fetus at risk of the serious homozygous defects is now possible and such a pregnancy at risk has to be identified early enough for the relevant procedures to be planned in advance.

Alpha and β-thalassaemias and sickle cell anaemia are all inherited as autosomal recessive traits. Pregnancies at risk can be identified either by a history of a previously affected child or by screening both parents for carrier status (Fig. 7.1).

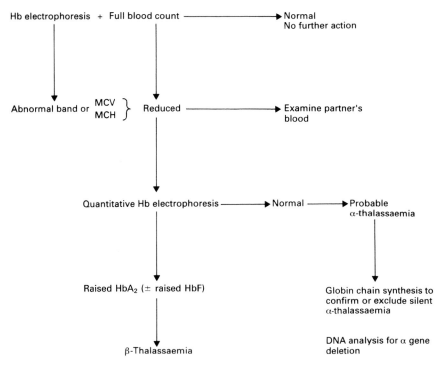

Fig. 7.1 Screening for haemoglobinopathies. MCH, mean corpuscular haemoglobin;
MCV, mean corpuscular volume.

Thalassaemia syndromes

Beta-thalassaemia. Normal β chain synthesis depends on two genes, one
inherited from each parent on chromosome 11. There are two main varieties
of β-thalassaemia, β^0- and β^+-thalassaemia, depending on an absence or
reduced output of β globin chain synthesis respectively. These may result
from small deletions of β globin gene or, more frequently, from point
mutations. The homozygous state for the β-thalassaemias are usually characterized by a transfusion dependent anaemia from the age of 6−12 months
(when adult haemoglobin (HbA) normally becomes predominant). With
adequate transfusions children with this condition enjoy a good quality life
until the second or third decade when, without iron dilution therapy, they
will succumb to the effects of iron overload. The heterozygous states for
β^0- and β^+-thalassaemia are characterized by hypochromic red cells, mild
anaemia, reduced mean corpuscular volume (MCV) and mean corpuscular
haemoglobin (MCH) values (Table 7.1) and an elevated level of HbA_2 (see
Fig. 7.1).

Alpha-thalassaemias. These conditions result from variable inability to produce α chains which are common to the three normal human haemoglobins:
HbA ($\alpha_2\beta_2$), HbA_2 ($\alpha_2\delta_2$) and HbF ($\alpha_2\gamma_2$). In the fetus, a deficiency of α

Table 7.1 Red cell indices in Iron deficiency and β-thalassaemia

		Normal range	Iron deficiency	Beta-thalassaemia heterozygotes
$\dfrac{\text{PCV}}{\text{RBC}}$	MCV	75−99 fl	Reduced	Markedly reduced
$\dfrac{\text{Hb}}{\text{RBC}}$	MCH	27−31 pg	Reduced	Markedly reduced
$\dfrac{\text{Hb}}{\text{PCV}}$	MCHC	32−36 g/dl	Reduced	Normal or slightly reduced

chains results in an excess of γ chains of fetal haemoglobin (HbF) which forms γ_4 molecules called 'Hb Barts'. In adult life a relative excess of the β chains of HbA leads to the production of tetramers β_4 termed 'HbH'. Normal α chain synthesis depends on four genes — two linked α globin genes inherited from each parent and located on chromosome 16. Alpha-thalassaemias fall into two groups α^0 and α^+. The α^0-thalassaemias result from deletions of both linked α globin genes on chromosome 16. The α^+-thalassaemias result from the loss of one of the linked pair of α globin genes. This usually results from a deletion but can also occur if there is a mutation which inactivates the α gene. The α-thalassaemias occur widely in the Mediterranean population, the Middle East, India and throughout southeast Asia where the frequency is extremely high.

There are two important clinical forms of α-thalassaemia, the Hb Barts hydrops syndrome and HbH disease. In Hb Barts hydrops syndrome, the homozygous state for α^0-thalassaemia is characterized by fetal death *in utero* or neonatal death within a few hours of delivery. The clinical picture is of severe anaemia with hydrops and massive placental hypertrophy. Pregnancy can be associated with severe maternal hypertension and protein-uria — the so-called mirror syndrome.

HbH disease, a moderately severe haemolytic anaemia, usually results from the inheritance of both α^0- and α^+-thalassaemia determinants (i.e. a single functional α-globin gene is present in the patient). It varies widely in severity but the anaemia is not usually transfusion-dependent and life expectancy is normal.

A major difficulty is the laboratory detection of the various carrier states for α-thalassaemia. Most carriers of α^0-thalassaemia trait have red cell indices with a low MCH and MCV (as for β-thalassaemia trait, see Table 7.1) but no increase in HbA_2. Carriers of α^+ trait will have only mild red cell changes and their red cell indices will usually fall within the normal range. The picture is further complicated by the fact that homo-zygous α^+-thalassaemia (one ineffective α gene on each chromosome) is phenotypically indistinguishable from α^0-thalassaemia trait.

Delta/beta-thalassaemias. These are much less common than the α- and β-thalassaemias and are usually associated with milder clinical disorders. The homozygous states for δ/β-thalassaemias which result from deletion of the δ and β genes are much milder than homozygous β-thalassaemia because of increased HbF production.

Heterozygotes for δ/β-thalassaemia have thalassaemic red cell indices and normal HbA$_2$ levels but unusually high levels of HbF in the 5−20% range.

HbE thalassaemia. One other thalassaemic syndrome is of importance in prenatal diagnosis and screening programmes. The haemoglobin variant HbE is particularly common in individuals of Indian or southeast Asian origin. In its homozygous form it gives rise to a mild anaemia. Women with HbE trait have red cells with low MCV and MCH, (i.e. thalassaemic indices). However, in combination with β-thalassaemia trait, HbE thalassaemia gives rise to a severe thalassaemic disorder which in some cases is as severe as transfusion dependent homozygous β-thalassaemia. Couples at risk should be identified and offered prenatal diagnosis.

Thalassaemia syndromes — screening for heterozygotes in the antenatal period. Although it used to be recommended that an MCV of less than 70 fl and/or MCH of less than 25 pg were indicators for further study, experience has shown that these levels are too low. The cut-off values now recommended are 80 fl and 27 pg respectively. This may entail a number of unnecessary investigations but it is important in populations where both α- and β-thalassaemia are common (e.g. in Cyprus and India).

HbA$_2$ is overall an extremely reliable method of distinguishing the carrier state of β-thalassaemia syndromes. Occasionally the value falls in a 'grey' area and globin chain synthesis studies may have to be carried out, but if the partner's blood is normal on investigation there is no urgency for these studies (see Fig. 7.1).

HbF estimation is not necessary when screening for β-thalassaemias but may be useful in individuals with frank thalassaemic red cell indices and normal A$_2$ values before embarking on complex studies which would not be necessary if δ/β-thalassaemia is identified with raised HbF values.

Haemoglobin variants

Over 250 structural variants of the globin chains of normal human haemoglobins have been described, but the most important by far, both numerically and clinically, is sickle cell haemoglobin (HbS).

Sickle syndromes. The sickling disorders include the heterozygous state for HbS, sickle cell trait (HbAS), homozygous sickle cell disease (HbSS),

71

compound heterozygotes for haemoglobin variants, the most important of which is sickle cell haemoglobin C disease (HbSC), and sickle cell thalassaemia. Although these disorders are more commonly seen in black people of African origin, they can be seen in Saudi Arabians, Indians and people from the eastern Mediterranean.

The characteristic feature of HbSS is the occurrence of periods of health punctuated by periods of crisis. Between 3 and 6 months of age, when normal HbA production usually becomes predominant, a chronic haemolytic anaemia develops, the haemoglobin level lying between 6 and 9 g/dl. Even if the haemoglobin is in the lower part of the range, symptoms due to anaemia are surprisingly few because of the low affinity of HbS for oxygen: oxygen delivery to the tissues is therefore facilitated. The acute episodes due to intravascular sickling are of far greater practical importance since they cause vascular occlusion resulting in tissue infarction. The affected part is painful and the clinical manifestations are extremely variable, depending on the site at which sickling takes place. Sickling crises are often precipitated by infection and may be exacerbated by any accompanying dehydration. The majority of deaths are because of massive sickling following an acute infection.

Sickle cell haemoglobin C disease is a milder variant of HbSS with normal or near normal levels of haemoglobin. One of the dangers of this condition is that, owing to its mildness, neither the woman nor her obstetrician may be aware of its presence. These women are at risk of massive, sometimes fatal, sickling crises during pregnancy, particularly in the puerperium. It is therefore vital that the abnormality is detected, preferably before pregnancy, so that the appropriate precautions can be taken. Clinical manifestations of the doubly heterozygous condition, sickle cell β-thalassaemia, are usually indistinguishable from HbSS. Those who make detectable amounts of HbA are usually less severely affected but are still at risk from sickling crises during pregnancy.

Sickle cell trait results in no detectable abnormality under normal circumstances, although it is easily diagnosed by specific investigations including haemoglobin electrophoresis (see below). Affected subjects are not anaemic even under the additional stress of pregnancy, unless there are additional complications, and sickling crises occur only in situations of extreme hypoxia, dehydration and acidosis.

Detection of HbS. Any test designed to screen for the presence of HbS should detect not only sickle cell disease but also distinguish HbSC, HbS thalassaemia and sickle cell trait. The classic sickling test, in which the red cell is suspended in a reducing agent, is difficult to interpret, and may occasionally give false negative results. Furthermore, it is time-consuming and its usefulness is limited when diagnosis is urgent. A proprietary product, Sickledex, is available that overcomes these drawbacks; it detects HbS by precipitation of deoxygenated HbS. It is rapid, reliable and does not give false negatives, but definitive diagnosis of the particular sickle cell syndrome involved requires haemoglobin electrophoresis and sometimes, in the case of sickle cell thalassaemia, family studies. Screening early in pregnancy, when there is no absolute urgency, is probably better carried out by performing haemoglobin electrophoresis (see below). The sickling test will then only have to be carried out on blood from those women who have an abnormal band in the S region by conventional electrophoresis in order to distinguish it from HbD, which has a similar electrophoretic mobility.

Screening for haemoglobinopathy

Unfortunately, at the moment, screening procedures are often not carried out until the woman is pregnant. In most cases this means that early prenatal diagnosis by DNA analysis of a chorionic villus sample is not possible. Selection for screening in a busy antenatal clinic may be more time-consuming than it is worth and, to be efficient, should involve detailed documentation of a woman's heritage before excluding her from testing. For this reason it is often easier to screen the whole clinic population. This involves examination of red cell indices, (see Table 7.1) haemoglobin electrophoresis, and, where indicated, quantitation of HbA_2 on every sample of blood taken at booking (see Fig. 7.1). If a haemoglobin variant or thalassaemic indices are found, the partner is requested to attend so that his blood can also be examined. This protocol allows the chances of a serious haemoglobin defect in the fetus to be assessed early in pregnancy and the parents to be advised of the potential hazards. Prenatal diagnosis by fetal blood sampling or transabdominal chorionic villus sampling can then be offered.

Implications for the future

Now that first trimester fetal diagnosis is becoming possible for an increasing number of serious haemoglobinopathies, and as the technique becomes available in more centres over the world, screening procedures should be extended beyond the antenatal clinic. It has been suggested that education and counselling should be directed at three points in people's lives, namely at school, at marriage and at family planning clinics. The information given should include details of where blood testing can be carried out and advice on when this should be done, although it should probably be left to the individual in possession of the information to request the test. This will involve education of the medical practitioners caring for these communities.

Haemolytic disease of the newborn (HDN) — allo-immune haemolysis

Although any paternally derived fetal red cell antigen which the mother lacks may provoke a maternal antibody response, the numbers of babies affected by severe HDN has fallen dramatically since the introduction of anti-D prophylaxis in the late 1960s. The problem persists, however, as a result of:

failure to identify the woman at risk and to give anti-D post delivery

administration of insufficient anti-D post delivery if unusually large feto-maternal bleed is not identified

antenatal sensitization — in centres where antenatal prophylaxis is not routine (1% of D-negative pregnant women)

sensitization after invasive procedures (e.g. amniocentesis, or chorionic villus sampling) if anti-D is not given.

In addition, there is a rising proportion of women with immunoglobulin G (IgG) allo-immune antibodies other than anti-D. Although there is an extensive list of these, the only important ones, in terms of serious HDN in the fetus warranting prenatal diagnosis, are anti-c and anti-Kell (see below).

Most peripheral centres will only see one or two women at risk per year. It is therefore essential that any women at risk, once identified, should at least be drawn to the attention of an expert referral centre so that collective experience may be applied to her case. The aim is to prevent hydrops *in utero* and to time delivery so that the infant has the optimum chance of survival. Death of the fetus from severe anaemia may be prevented by transfusion of compatible adult donor cells from as early as 18 weeks' gestation. The dangerous breakdown products of haemoglobin are cleared from the fetal circulation transplacentally by the maternal liver. Some bilirubin enters the amniotic fluid and gives a crude estimate of the severity of haemolysis in limited circumstances.

Screening for haemolytic disease of the fetus

Management of the unsensitized pregnancy. All pregnant women should have their ABO blood group and Rhesus (D) type determined at their booking visit. The serum should be screened for atypical antibodies. Women who are Rh(D) positive and who have no atypical antibodies should have their blood checked again at 30−34 weeks. Such screening is not only relevant to the fetus but is also important should maternal transfusion be required. Unsensitized Rh(D) negative mothers should have their blood checked at 28 weeks and again at 34 weeks.

Management of the sensitized pregnancy. Women who have irregular antibodies at booking should be retested at monthly intervals to determine the rise in antibody titre. The paternal phenotype should be determined to establish whether the antibody could react with a paternally derived red cell antigen. Frequently the maternal antibody is either the result of a previous transfusion (e.g. anti-Kell) or naturally occurring (e.g. anti-E).

Haemolytic disease due to anti-D. Anti-D is still the most important antibody with very few exceptions both in terms of numbers affected and severity of haemolysis. Detection of maternal anti-D antibody alerts to the possibility of haemolytic disease in the fetus but does not indicate whether the fetus is Rh(D) positive, or how severe the anaemia is. A single quantitation is of little value. However, repeated estimations showing a rising concentration usually (but not always) indicate that the fetus is affected by HDN but give no indication of severity of the disease process. Whilst there is some dispute over the critical antibody level to be taken, a value of 4 iu/ml or greater indicates that there will be a need to undertake amniocentesis or fetal blood sampling at some time during pregnancy to evaluate the extent of the haemolytic process.

The use of amniocentesis in the management of HDN has become controversial although it remains useful in the majority of cases. The measurement of the amniotic fluid optical density at 450 nm by spectrophotometry provides an indication of the concentration of bilirubin and hence the extent of the fetal red cell haemolysis. Certainly, results prior to 27 weeks of pregnancy must be interpreted with caution as it is possible to obtain a normal result even when the fetus is severely anaemic. Whitfield's action line (Fig. 7.2) superimposed on Liley's zones of severity of fetal haemolysis based on amniotic fluid bilirubin estimations gives guidelines for appropriate management related to gestation, i.e. intrauterine transfusion or delivery and exchange transfusion if indicated. Those cases with previous, severely affected pregnancies prior to 24 weeks will understandably require evaluation by early fetal blood sampling and should be referred to a specialist centre preferably during the first trimester.

When there is a history of severe disease and the partner is heterozygous, early determination of the fetal blood group will allow the option of terminating the Rh(D) positive pregnancies. Fetal blood group determination has been achieved by DNA analysis of chorionic villus samples or, preferably, from amniotic fluid fibroblasts (Bennett *et al.*, 1993). A recent advance has been the successful rhesus grouping of the fetus in Rh negative mothers using PCR amplification of Rh(D) sequences from fetal cells in the maternal peripheral blood (Lo *et al.*, 1993).

The improved treatment of a severely affected fetus is a result of gaining access to the fetal circulation and enabling intravascular transfusion (IVT) under ultrasound guidance. Transfusions can be commenced as early as 18 weeks' gestation in the most severe cases but the procedural-related fetal losses are much higher between 18 and 22 weeks than later in gestation and this early period is avoided if possible. Fetal losses after 22 weeks are about 2% per transfusion, usually related to tamponade or other haemodynamic disturbances (see Chapter 17).

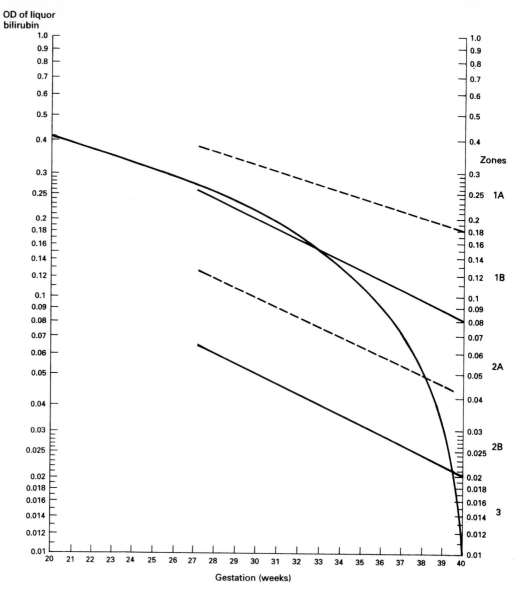

Fig. 7.2 Chart showing the Whitfield curved action line extrapolated to 20 weeks. Note Liley's zones which commence at 27 weeks.

Intravascular transfusion ensures immediate correction of fetal anaemia and is particularly valuable in hydrops, when intraperitoneal transfusion (IPT) is often ineffective due to slow absorption. Reversal of hydrops has now been observed many times following IVT, whereas IPT may, in such cases, lead to fetal death. However, IPT is very effective in the absence of hydrops and it may also be used in combination with IVT to increase, by the slower absorption of blood given intraperitoneally, the interval between transfusions (up to 4–5 weeks) and also reducing the total number of invasive procedures per pregnancy (Nicolini and Rodeck,

1988). Postnatally, neonates usually do well, but paediatricians must be warned to monitor the baby's haemoglobin carefully as profound anaemia may develop for up to 3 months of age.

Antibodies other than anti-D. IgG antibodies may be identified in maternal serum antenatally but only two (anti-c and anti-Kell) warrant investigation. Both can cause severe fetal anaemia and investigations and management are along standard lines. However, anti-Kell is particularly unusual and amniotic fluid analysis gives unhelpful results. This is probably because the antibody may cause suppression of fetal erythropoiesis as well as haemolysis. Management of the potentially affected pregnancy should be with a combination of early fetal blood sampling for Kell grouping and assessment of anaemia and regular ultrasound evaluations for the development of ascites.

When other antibodies are involved, like anti-E, anti-Duffy and anti-Kidd, the risk of fetal anaemia will usually be slight although regard to the past history remains important. In any case paediatricians should be alerted and the cord blood of all infants born to mothers with these antibodies should be grouped and a direct antiglobulin test (Coombs) performed. The neonate should be assessed for the development of jaundice within the first 48 hours of life.

It is vitally important to refer couples at risk early in pregnancy, or even before pregnancy is embarked upon in certain cases, so that appropriate measures can be taken and strategy planned, taking advantage of all the exciting recent developments to give an optimal chance of a good outcome.

DISORDERS OF PLATELETS

Fetal thrombocytopenia and functional platelet disorders arise from a diverse list of causes both genetic and acquired. In normal circumstances the fetal platelet count is within the adult range $(150-350 \times 10^9/l)$ by 20 weeks' gestation. Low platelet counts from this gestation onwards performed on fetal cord blood samples are therefore significant. Some genetic thrombocytopenia syndromes are associated with skeletal and other abnormalities, for example, TAR (thrombocytopenia with absent radii) and ultrasound examination will aid in their prenatal diagnosis.

Maternal thrombocytopenia (platelet count $< 150 \times 10^9/l$) is a relatively common finding (7–8%), especially in the third trimester. However, the frequency of mild thrombocytopenia (4%) in the babies born to such mothers is similar to that of those born to mothers with normal platelet counts.

Pathological thrombocytopenia in pregnancy may arise from underproduction, increased destruction or sequestration in an enlarged spleen.

The various causes have been well reviewed (Pillai, 1993).

The most frequent and controversial diagnostic and management problems for the obstetrician arise from the immune fetal thrombocytopenias — both auto-immune and allo-immune.

Auto-immune thrombocytopenia (ITP)

There are two clinical forms of ITP — acute and chronic. Chronic ITP, unlike the acute self-limiting ITP, which usually occurs in children, is particularly common in young women in reproductive years. It is the most frequent immune disorder complicating pregnancy but it may be confused with incidental thrombocytopenia of pregnancy. Auto-immune thrombocytopenia in pregnancy, therefore, often presents diagnostic and management problems that involve both the mother and fetus.

Pathogenesis of ITP

The platelet associated IgG antibody can cross the placenta and cause thrombocytopenia in the fetus and neonate. Unfortunately there are no indirect tests on the maternal blood or clues from the maternal history which can predict with certainty the platelet count of the newborn at delivery, although trends can be shown. Thrombocytopenia in the fetus caused by maternal ITP is not associated with spontaneous fetal haemorrhage, unlike that caused by allo-immune thrombocytopenia. The greatest hazard for the fetus with significant thrombocytopenia caused by maternal ITP is thought to be intracranial haemorrhage arising from trauma at delivery.

It is not widely appreciated that the nadir of the platelet count in the neonate affected by maternal ITP occurs 2–4 days after delivery, in spite of static or falling platelet antibody levels. This is thought to be due to the establishment of the neonatal splenic circulation which will remove the IgG coated platelets more efficiently. The platelet count usually rises to normal within the first month of life, but occasionally thrombocytopenia persists for 12–16 weeks.

Presentation. Occasionally, mothers have an acute clinical onset with petechiae, purpura and mucus membrane bleeding. Very occasionally, there may be no previous history and evidence of a normal platelet count in early pregnancy. These patients will need urgent therapy to bring the platelet count to safe haemostatic levels.

The majority of women with presumed ITP in pregnancy are identified because of a routine blood count during the antenatal period. They have no history of haemostatic incompetence and, apart from the isolated low platelet count, they are otherwise well.

Management of ITP in pregnancy

Management of the mother. The most important decision to make is whether the pregnant woman needs any treatment at all. Many patients have significant thrombocytopenia (platelet count less than 100×10^9/l) but no evidence of an *in vivo* haemostatic disorder. In general, the platelet count must be less than 50×10^9/l for capillary bleeding and purpura to occur.

There is no need to treat any asymptomatic women with platelet counts above 50×10^9/l and a normal bleeding time. However, the maternal platelet count should be monitored regularly and signs of haemostatic impairment looked for. The platelet count will show a downward trend during pregnancy, with a nadir in the third trimester, and active treatment may have to be instituted to achieve a safe haemostatic concentration of platelets for delivery at term. The incidence of antepartum haemorrhage is not increased in maternal ITP but there is a small increased risk of postpartum haemorrhagic complications from surgical incisions such as episiotomy and from soft tissue lacerations.

Treatment to raise the platelet count is required in the antenatal period in a woman with bruising or petechiae; bleeding from mucus membranes may be life threatening and demands urgent treatment with platelet transfusions, intravenous IgG and occasionally emergency splenectomy.

The real dilemma in the pregnant woman with true ITP is that nearly all patients have chronic disease. The hazard for the mother who is monitored carefully and in whom appropriate measures have been taken is negligible; most of her management is orientated towards what are thought to be optimal conditions for the delivery of the fetus who, in turn, may or may not be thrombocytopenic.

Corticosteroids are a satisfactory short-term therapy but are unacceptable as long-term support unless the maintenance dose is very small. The recent use of monomeric polyvalent human IgG has proved efficacious and has altered the management options dramatically. Used in the original recommended doses of 0.4 g/kg daily for 5 days by intravenous infusion, a persistent and predictable response was obtained in more than 80% of reported cases. Recently introduced alternative dosage regimens are easier to manage and involve less total dosage of this costly therapy. A typical dose is 1 g/kg over 8 hours on one day. This dose will raise the platelet count to normal or safe levels in approximately half of the patients. In those in whom the platelet count does not rise, a similar dose can be repeated 2 days later. The advantages of this treatment are that it is safe, has very few side effects and the response to therapy is more rapid than with steroids. The response usually occurs within 48 hours and is maintained for 2–3 weeks. The main disadvantage is that it is very expensive and seldom produces a cure of the ITP.

There is no doubt about the value of IgG in selected cases of severe symptomatic thrombocytopenia where a rapid response is required, but its indiscriminate use in all cases with significant thrombocytopenia would have to be shown to dramatically improve both maternal and fetal outcome to justify the high cost.

Assessment of the fetal platelet count. The literature from 1950−83 suggested an overall incidence of neonatal thrombocytopenia of 52%, with significant morbidity in 12% of births. The incidence increased to 70% if maternal platelet counts were less than 100×10^9/l at term.

A report by Samuels *et al.* (1990) suggested an 11% incidence of thrombocytopenia in the offspring of women with ITP, but two important factors emerged. A negative history of ITP before pregnancy or the absence of detectable platelet-associated IgG in the index pregnancy in those with a history, made the risk of severe thrombocytopenia in the fetus at term negligible.

Some investigators have suggested that maternal splenectomy increases the probability of neonatal thrombocytopenia but, in fact, it is only in those women with splenectomy and persistent thrombocytopenia (less than 100×10^9/l) that the risk of neonatal thrombocytopenia is increased (Burrows and Kelton, 1992). What has become clear over the years is that analysis of the older literature gave an exaggerated incidence of neonatal thrombocytopenia and of the morbidity and mortality arising from it. However, it is still impossible to predict the fetal platelet count in any individual case (Kaplan *et al.*, 1990) and to plan the mode of delivery based on these maternal parameters is not logical or sensible.

Fetal blood sampling. A method for direct measurement of the fetal platelet count in scalp blood obtained transcervically prior to or early in labour has been described (Ayromlooi, 1978). It is suggested that caesarean section be performed in all cases where the fetal platelet count is less than 50×10^9/l. This approach is more logical than a decision about the mode of delivery made on the basis of maternal platelet count, concentration of IgG or splenectomy status, but it is not without risk of significant haemorrhage in the truly thrombocytopenic fetus: it often gives false positive results and demands urgent action to be taken on the results. Furthermore, the cervix must be sufficiently dilated to allow the fetal scalp to be sampled and the uterine contraction to achieve this may have caused the fetus to descend so far in the birth canal that caesarean section is technically difficult and also traumatic for the fetus.

The only way a reliable fetal platelet count can be obtained so that a decision concerning the optimal mode of delivery can be taken is by cordocentesis. It should be performed at 37−38 weeks' gestation, when the transfer of IgG increases; an earlier sample may give a higher fetal platelet count than one taken nearer term. It is important to ensure that the blood is placed in EDTA anticoagulant and not heparin, which tends to cause platelet clumping and will falsely lower the count. There is a risk associated with the sampling but, in skilled hands, this is no more than 1%. However, given the low probability of identifying a problem and the risk of associated complications *in utero*, cordocentesis cannot be justified in all ITP pregnancies.

Intrauterine fetal blood sampling should only be recommended for: (1) women who enter pregnancy with a history of ITP together with currently identifiable platelet associated IgG antibodies or; (2) women who have to be treated for ITP during the index pregnancy.

Neonatal platelet count. After birth the platelet count will continue to fall for 2−5 days. If the cord platelet count shows severe thrombocytopenia and especially if there is evidence of skin or mucus membrane bleeding, measures can be taken to prevent this predicted fall. Intravenous hydrocortisone and platelet transfusion have been used with success in the neonate but the recommended therapy nowadays should be intravenous IgG because of its relative safety and the rapidity with which a response is observed. Platelet transfusion should be reserved for those neonates with hazardous levels of thrombocytopenia in the cord blood and given in combination with intravenous IgG.

Allo-immune thrombocytopenia (AIT) (Levine and Berkowitz, 1991)

Fetal allo-immune thrombocytopenia is a syndrome that develops as a result of maternal sensitization to fetal platelet antigens. The antibody, usually Hpa[1] (formerly known as Pla[1]), is directed specifically against a paternally derived antigen which the mother lacks (cf. Rh(D) haemolytic disease).

The mother is not thrombocytopenic herself but the fetus is and, in addition, its platelets have altered function. The platelet-specific antibody attaches to the membrane of the Hpa[1] binding site and interferes with the function of the glycoprotein IIb-IIIa ligand binding sites thus impairing platelet aggregation. The affected thrombocytopenic fetus is at risk of spontaneous intracranial haemorrhage from early in gestation unlike the fetus affected by maternal ITP.

It is obvious that the fetus at risk must be identified early in gestation if measures are to be taken to prevent intrauterine intracranial haemorrhage occurring but this is not easy. In the vast majority of cases, a fetus at risk is identified because of a previously affected sibling. Hpa[1] is the most common antigen associated with AIT. The antigen is present in 97−98% of the population. Two alleles are present, Hpa[1] and Hpa[2], and 69% of the population are homozygous for Hpa[1], the stronger sensitizing antigen.

The immune response of the Hpa[1] negative mother seems to be determined in part by genes of the histocompatibility complex, and antibody formation appears to be confined to those with HLA-B8 and HLA DR3 antigens. Unlike Rh disease, first pregnancies may be affected. Subsequent affected pregnancies will be of similar or increased severity and the recurrence rate is estimated to be between 75 and 90%.

The monitoring of severity of the disease process differs greatly from Rh haemolytic disease. The absence of antibodies does not guarantee a normal fetal platelet count although women with identifiable antibodies are at risk of producing a fetus with thrombocytopenia. Rises in titre and concentration of antibody do not correlate with severity.

To identify all women at risk of developing platelet allo-antibodies by platelet (Hpa[1]) grouping and HLA typing of all pregnant women is not cost-effective or feasible at the moment, but the appropriate investigations should be carried out on all female relatives of women known to have had a baby affected by this disorder.

The incidence of neonatal AIT has been estimated to be 1 in 5000 births although more recent studies give a higher frequency of 1 in 2–3000 births. Not all cases necessarily have severe manifestation.

Management of AIT

Management protocols are currently at an evolutionary stage. Some involve fetal blood sampling early in gestation, but preferably after 22 weeks, when the risk of the procedure is reduced. In the identified affected fetus, subsequent management is controversial. Weekly maternal IgG infusion (1 g/kg) with or without prednisone has been used in the successful management of pregnancies at risk of AIT (Lynch *et al.*, 1992). This has not been the universal experience, however. Others recommend weekly Hpa[1] negative platelet infusions until fetal lung maturity is achieved. All protocols involve frequent ultrasound examinations to check that no intracranial bleeds have occurred. Mode of delivery will be determined by maturity, fetal platelet count and obstetric indications.

The use of maternal platelet infusions to the fetus or neonate should be discouraged. Unless they are repeatedly washed, the infused anti-Hpa[1] antibody has a much longer half life than the platelets themselves. Repeated washing of platelets also reduces their function. Moreover, suitably prepared platelets from accredited donors provided by the regional Blood Transfusion Service are more effective and probably much safer. Post-delivery, the disease is usually self-limiting within a few weeks. If therapy is required, Hpa compatible platelets are the treatment of choice. The aim of all controversial antenatal management is to deliver a relatively mature infant who has not suffered intracranial haemorrhage antenatally or during delivery.

Allo-immune thrombocytopenia can be a devastating fetal disease and it should be excluded in all cases of fetal intracranial haemorrhage, un-explained porencephaly and neonatal thrombocytopenia.

Unlike ITP, and because of the risk of spontaneous intrauterine fetal haemorrhage, early fetal blood sampling may be indicated and a mother with this potential problem should be referred early in pregnancy to an expert fetal medicine unit for investigation and management, although delivery of a treated infant may still take place at the centre of referral (see Chapter 17).

WHITE CELL DISORDERS

Immunodeficiency disorders

These are a complex group of relatively rare inherited disorders which present with recurrent infection and failure to thrive. Multiple defects have been defined involving granulocytes, T and B lymphocytes and immuno-globulin production of all classes. It is essential that a precise identification of the disorder is made in order for prenatal diagnosis to be carried out appropriately.

The family in whom such a defect may be present must be referred to a centre with a special interest in this group of defects. Inheritance is usually either as an X-linked recessive or autosomal recessive trait.

Prenatal diagnosis of the severe and untreatable varieties may involve biochemical, haematological or DNA studies depending on the particular syndrome involved (see Appendix).

COAGULATION DISORDERS

The most important hereditary coagulation disorders are the X-linked haemophilias due to the deficiency of plasma Factor VIII coagulant protein (VIIIC) and Christmas Disease which results from deficiency of Factor IXC — known as haemophilia A and B respectively.

Haemophilia is a relatively uncommon disease. In the UK there are between 3000 and 4000 cases and 1 in 25 000 of the population has the disease in a severe form. The ratio of haemophilia A to Christmas Disease is in the region of 5 : 1. Affected males within the same family have similar residual levels of coagulation Factor activity (<1% severe, 1−5% moderate, >6% mild). Antenatal screening for these conditions will be largely restricted to families in which there is a history of the disease. It is usually indicated if a woman wishes to undergo prenatal diagnosis to determine whether her male fetus has the disease.

Female carriers of haemophilia have on average 50% of the normal mean level of the coagulation factor involved, but because of the wide range of normal and variability of lyonization of the X chromosome, carriers often have levels within the normal range. As far as Haemophilia A is concerned, it is sometimes possible to improve discrimination by measuring the level of von Willebrand factor (vWF), the autosomally coded carrier protein for Factor VIII. Carriers, unlike the normal population, have lower levels of VIIIC than vWF (reduced VIIIC:vWF ratio) — but firm diagnosis of carrier status is still not possible in around 15% of cases.

In recent years specialist centres managing these diseases are turning to DNA technology for diagnosis. The Factor VIII and IX genes have been isolated and sequenced and many of the mutations that underlie haemophilia and Christmas Disease have been determined. They may result from point mutations or deletions involving these genes. In addition, many restriction fragment length polymorphisms (RFLPs) have been found both within and in the flanking regions of these genes (Peake *et al.*, 1993). The specialist studies involved can be undertaken by the regional haemophilia centre in collaboration with the regional genetics centre.

In identified female carriers, prenatal diagnosis can be offered in the majority of cases by DNA analysis of chorionic villus samples. In the few families where DNA analysis is not currently informative, assay of plasma Factor VIIIC or Factor IXC in a fetal blood sample taken from 18 week's gestation onwards will provide an accurate but late prenatal diagnosis.

REFERENCES AND FURTHER READING

General

Hann, I.M., Gibson, B.E.S. and Letsky, E.A. (1991) *Fetal and Neonatal Haematology.* Baillière Tindall, London.
Weatherall, D.J. (1991) *The New Genetics and Clinical Practice.* 3rd edn, Oxford University Press, Oxford.

Haemoglobinopathies

Letsky, E.A. (1991) Haemoglobinopathies. In *Perinatal Haematological Problems* (ed. T.L. Turner), John Wiley and Sons Ltd., Chichester, pp. 65–83.

Haemolytic disease of the newborn

Bennett, P.R., Le Van Kim, C., Colin, Y. *et al.* (1993) Prenatal determination of fetal RhD genotype by DNA amplification following chorion villus biopsy or amnio-centesis. *New England Journal of Medicine,* **329,** 607–10.
Bowell, P.J., Allen, D.L. and Entwhistle, C.C. (1986) Blood group antibody screening tests during pregnancy. *British Journal of Obstetrics and Gynaecology,* **93,** 1038–43.
Lo, Y.M.D., Bowell, P.J., Selinger, M. *et al.* (1993) Prenatal determination of fetal RhD status by analysis of peripheral blood of rhesus negative mothers. *Lancet,* **341,** 1147–48.
Nicolaides, K.H., Rodeck, C.H., Mibashan, R.S. and Kemp, J.R. (1986) Have Liley

charts outlived their usefulness? *American Journal of Obstetrics and Gynaecology,*
155, 90−94.

Nicolini, U. and Rodeck, C.H. (1988) A proposed scheme for planning intrauterine
transfusion in patients with severe Rh-immunization. *Journal of Obstetrics and
Gynecology,* **9**, 162−63.

Rodeck, C.H. and Letsky, E.A. (1989) How the management of erythroblastosis fetalis
has changed. *British Journal of Obstetrics and Gynaecology,* **96**, 759−63.

Vaughan, J.I., Warwick, R., Letsky, E.A., Nicolini, U., Rodeck, C.H. and Fisk, N.M.
(1994) Erythropoietic suppression in fetal anemia because of Kell alloimmunization.
American Journal of Obstetrics and Gynecology, **171**, 247−52.

Platelet disorders

Ayromlooi, J. (1978) A new approach to the management of immunologic thrombocytopenic purpura in pregnancy. *American Journal of Obstetrics and Gynecology,*
130, 235−36.

Burrows, R.F. and Kelton, J.G. (1990) Thrombocytopenia at delivery: A prospective
survey of 6,715 deliveries. *American Journal of Obstetrics and Gynecology,* **162**,
731−34.

Burrows, R.F. and Kelton, J.G. (1992) Thrombocytopenia during pregnancy. In *Haemostasis and Thrombosis in Obstetrics and Gynaecology* (eds. I.A. Greer, A.G.G.
Turpie and C.D. Forbes), Chapman and Hall, London, pp. 407−29.

Hegde, U.M. (1985) Immune thrombocytopenia in pregnancy and the newborn. *British
Journal of Obstetrics and Gynaecology,* **92**, 657−59.

Kaplan, C., Daffos, F., Forestier, F. *et al.* (1990) Fetal platelet counts in thrombocytopenic pregnancy. *Lancet,* **336**, 979−82.

Levine, A.B. and Berkowitz, R.L. (1991) Neonatal alloimmune thrombocytopenia.
Seminars in Perinatology, **15**, 35−40.

Lynch, L., Bussel, J.B., McFarland, J.G. *et al.* (1992) Antenatal treatment of alloimmune
thrombocytopenia. *Obstetrics and Gynecology,* **80**, 67−71.

Pillai, M. (1993) Platelets and pregnancy. *British Journal of Obstetrics and Gynaecology,*
100, 201−204.

Samuels, P., Bussel, J.B., Braitman, L.E. *et al.* (1990) Estimation of the risk of thrombocytopenia in the offspring of pregnant women with presumed immune thrombocytopenic purpura. *New England Journal of Medicine,* **323**, 229−35.

White cell disorders

Kinnan, C., Jones, A.M. and Levinsky, R.J. (1992) Immunodeficiency diseases. In
Prenatal Diagnosis & Screening (eds. J.H. Brock, C.H. Rodeck and M.A. Ferguson-
Smith), Churchill Livingstone, Edinburgh, pp. 491−502.

Lau, Y.L. and Levinsky, R.J. (1988) Prenatal diagnosis and carrier detection in primary
immunodeficiency disorders. *Archives of Disease in Childhood,* **63**, 758−64.

Coagulation disorders

Peake, I.R., Lillicrap, D.P., Boulyjenkov, V. *et al.* (1993) Report of a joint WHO/WFH
meeting on the control of haemophilia: carrier detection and prenatal diagnosis.
Blood Coagulation and Fibrinolysis, **4**, 313−44.

Chapter 8
Prenatal Diagnosis of Single Gene Disorders by DNA Analysis

J. M. CONNOR

Single gene (mendelian) disorders are caused by faults in one or both members of a pair of genes on the autosomes or sex chromosomes. These conditions are mostly uncommon but are numerous and collectively affect at least 1% of livebirths (Table 8.1). The single gene disorders often carry high recurrence risks within a family and this, coupled with the limitations of therapy at the present time, means that prenatal diagnosis with selective termination of pregnancy is an important option for couples at risk.

Each structural gene is responsible for encoding a protein product which in turn, by acting as a structural component, enzyme or carrier molecule, effects the gene's function. Prenatal diagnosis of single gene disorders may therefore be accomplished by direct demonstration of the gene mutation, by indirect gene tracking, by demonstration of a reduced or faulty protein product (see Chapter 6) or, in some instances, by the effect on the fetus (e.g. ultrasound imaging in single gene disorders associated with congenital malformations).

Direct demonstration of gene mutations and indirect mutant gene tracking have become possible with advances in recombinant DNA technology. After outlining the normal organization of DNA and range of human molecular pathology, this chapter will focus on the clinical applications of this technology. Those requiring further scientific detail are referred to the further reading list.

ORGANIZATION OF DNA

Each chromosome is believed to consist of a single molecule of coiled and condensed DNA which has two strands held together by obligatory base pairing between nitrogenous bases such that adenine (A) always pairs with thymine (T) and guanine (G) always pairs with cytosine (C). Hence the parallel strands are complementary to one another and if one strand reads ATGA the complementary strand must read TACT. Lengths of DNA are measured in terms of the number of base pairs (bp) with 1000 bp in a kilobase (kb) and 1000 kb in a megabase (Mb). The total length of human DNA in each gamete, which contains an estimated 100 000 genes, is 3000 million base pairs (3000 Mb). The genes vary widely in size, from small genes such as α-globin (850 bp) to enormous genes such as dystrophin

Table 8.1 Examples of single gene disorders where there is a demand for prenatal diagnosis

Autosomal dominant traits
Adult polycystic kidney disease, familial polyposis coli, Huntington disease, myotonic dystrophy, neurofibromatosis types I and II, tuberous sclerosis, von Willebrand disease (homozygotes)

Autosomal recessive traits
Alpha-thalassaemia, β-thalassaemia, cystic fibrosis, mucopolysaccharidoses (several types), sickle cell disease, recessive mental disability (multiple subtypes), spinal muscular atrophy (types I–III), Tay–Sachs disease

X-linked recessive traits
Duchenne muscular dystrophy, fragile X syndrome, haemophilias A and B, X-linked mental disability (multiple subtypes)

(2.4 Mb). The average size is about 15 kb and thus the genes account for only 1500 Mb or one-half of the total DNA. The intergenic DNA between adjacent genes is involved in functional regulation or has no known function.

Each gene codes for a protein whose amino acid sequence is determined by the combination of each set of three base pairs (or triplet). First the DNA is transcribed to messenger ribonucleic acid (mRNA), then it is modified by splicing to remove areas corresponding to non-coding gene sequences (called introns or intervening sequences) and finally it is translated to protein by the ribosomes. Single gene disorders can be caused by faults in any of these stages (Fig. 8.1) and most conditions show a diversity of molecular lesions (heterogeneity of molecular pathology).

MOLECULAR PATHOLOGY

Normally DNA replication at mitosis or meiosis is completely accurate but errors or mutations can occur. These mutations are broadly divisible into length mutations with gain or loss of genetic material and point mutations with alteration of the genetic code but no gain or loss of genetic material. Length mutations include deletions, duplications, insertions and trinucleotide amplifications. Deletions of DNA can range from 1 bp to many megabases. Deletions involving one or more structural genes may extend to several megabases and may (if over 4 Mb) be visible by conventional cytogenetic methods. Removal of all of a gene directly prevents transcription but smaller deletions of more or less than three or a multiple of three base pairs can be equally serious by altering the reading frame of mRNA (frame shift mutations, Table 8.2).

These length mutations are normally stably inherited but unstable

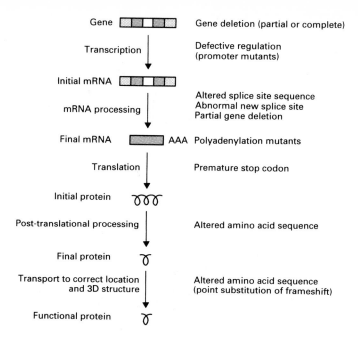

Fig. 8.1 Possible faults in protein biosynthesis.

length mutations have been observed in some genes (e.g. fragile X syndrome and myotonic dystrophy). In these conditions the gene normally contains a repeated trinucleotide sequence and the length mutation represents an expansion of this repeated sequence beyond the upper limit of normal.

In a point mutation a single nucleotide base is replaced by a different nucleotide base. This may (25%) lead to no change in the amino acid coded by the triplet (e.g. CAG and CAA both code for glutamine) or may result in the substitution of a different amino acid (70%, missense mutations) or alteration to a chain terminator (5%, see Table 8.2).

Mutations can be described using a standardized nomenclature which is based upon the type of mutation, the amino acid short code and the amino acid position within the protein (Table 8.3).

As indicated in Table 8.3, multiple mutations can cause cystic fibrosis (with over 300 now described). This variety or heterogeneity of molecular pathology, including both length and point mutations, is encountered for most single gene disorders and has important implications for mutational analysis. Sickle cell anaemia is an exception as all patients have an identical point mutation with substitution of A for T at nucleotide 17 and hence substitution of valine for glutamic acid at amino acid position 6 in the β globin chain (E6V).

DNA POLYMORPHISMS

Many, but not all, mutations in protein-coding DNA result in an altered

Table 8.2 Examples of DNA mutation

DNA base sequence	mRNA sequence	Amino acid sequence	Comment
CAA TTC CGA CGA	GUU AAG GCU GCU	Val-Lys-Ala-Ala	Normal sequence
CAA TTT CGA CGA	GUU AAA GCU GCU	Val-Lys-Ala-Ala	Point mutation with unchanged AA sequence
CAA CTC CGA CGA	GUU GAG GCU GCU	Val-Glu-Ala-Ala	Point mutation with AA substitution (missense mutation)
CAA ATC CGA CGA	GUU UAG GCU GCU	Val-stop	Point mutation with premature chain termination (nonsense mutation)
CAA–TCC GAC GA	GUU AGG CUG CU	Val-Arg-Leu	Base deletion with frame shift (nonsense mutation)
CAA TTT CCG ACG A	GUU AAA GGC UGC	Val-Lys-Gly-Cys	Base insertion with frame shift (nonsense mutation)

Table 8.3 Examples of mutations which can cause cystic fibrosis

Name	Mutation	Consequence
ΔF508	3 bp deletion nt 1652−1655 in exon 10	Deletion of phenylalanine at codon 508
G542X	G→T at nt 1756 in exon 11	Glycine to stop at codon 542
G551D	G→A at nt 1784 in exon 11	Glycine to aspartic acid at codon 551
W128X	G→A at nt 3978 in exon 20	Tryptophan to stop at codon 1282
3905insT	Insertion of T after nt 3905 in exon 20	Frame shift
621+1G→T	G→T at nt 1 from 5′ junction of intron 4	Splice mutation
1717−1G→A	G→A at nt 1 from 3′ junction of intron 10	Splice mutation

nt, nucleotide.

protein which may or may not cause disease. In contrast, mutations in non-protein coding DNA (intervening sequences and intergenic DNA) usually do not cause disease. Many of these mutations, (intra- and extra-genic) which are not associated with disease, are found at relatively high frequencies within the population and by definition if 1 in 50 or more have the variant it is called a DNA polymorphism.

Length or point mutations can be involved in DNA polymorphisms. The length polymorphisms are usually associated with multiple repeats of a dinucleotide or tetranucleotide (microsatellite repeats), or larger repeat unit (commonly 10−15 bp, minisatellite repeats). Dinucleotide repeats, especially CA and CT, are very frequent with an estimated total of 50 000 dispersed throughout the genome. This abundance, coupled with the fact that most (about 70%) individuals generate different sized fragments (i.e. heterozygous) from each member of a chromosome pair, has meant that this type of polymorphism is very useful for tracking mutant genes within affected families and for gene mapping studies.

Polymorphisms due to point mutations occur every 200−500 bp and as only two alternative sequences (normal and altered) are found, most individuals have identical sequences (homozygous) on their paired chromosomes and relatively few (up to 35%) are heterozygous. This type of polymorphism is usually demonstrated by loss (or gain) of a cutting site for a DNA cleavage enzyme (restriction enzyme) and thus they are usually called restriction fragment length polymorphisms (RFLPs).

All of these DNA polymorphisms are normally stably inherited and will cosegregate with neighbouring genes. This cosegregation is known as *linkage* and it allows mutant genes to be tracked within families.

NUCLEIC ACID ANALYSIS

DNA can be extracted from any nucleated tissue and lymphocytes from a 10 ml venous blood sample (EDTA anticoagulated) should yield about 300 μg of DNA which is sufficient for many DNA analyses. Each milligram (wet weight) of chorionic villus tissue yields about 1 μg of DNA and the size of the chorionic villus sample required depends upon the type of DNA analysis (see below). Spun cells from an amniotic fluid sample may yield sufficient DNA for a polymerase chain reaction (PCR) analysis (see below) but otherwise culture is generally required. In consequence chorionic villus sampling (CVS) is generally chosen if prenatal diagnosis by DNA analysis is to be undertaken. The CVS sample needs to be transported without undue delay in sterile culture medium. At postmortem, a sample of spleen can be taken into a dry sterile tube or snap-frozen in liquid nitrogen and stored at −20°C pending DNA extraction.

DNA probes are labelled (radioactive or non-radioactive) sections of DNA from tens of base pairs to several kilobases in size which are used to identify fragments with a complementary sequence amongst a mixture of DNA fragments. The probe and target DNA are first rendered single-stranded (by heating or exposure to alkali) and complementary fragments hybridize to form labelled double-stranded DNA fragments which can be visualized. For visualization, a large number of labelled hybrid DNA fragments need to be formed and this is achieved either by starting with a relatively large amount of target DNA (Southern analysis) or by selectively amplifying the target sequence(s) from an initial tiny sample of DNA (polymerase chain reaction analysis, PCR analysis). In general, Southern analysis utilizes 5−10 μg of DNA for each analysis and takes 5−7 days to produce a result. In Southern analysis the target DNA is fragmented with an appropriate restriction enzyme, separated according to fragment size by gel electrophoresis and then transferred to a DNA binding filter. The appropriate DNA probe will then identify the complementary sequence(s) and the labelled hybrid molecules are identified by autoradiography (for radiolabelled probes, Fig. 8.2).

Each PCR reaction needs target DNA, a pair of primers which are complementary to DNA sequences flanking the target sequence and an enzyme (Taq polymerase) which directs repeated rounds of localized DNA replication. Theoretically, amplification will increase exponentially to 2^n (where n is the number of cycles) and amplification of more than one million-fold can be routinely obtained from 30 or so cycles. This takes a couple of hours in an automated procedure. The amplified DNA segment can then be digested if required with the appropriate restriction enzyme

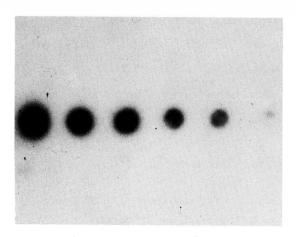

Fig. 8.2 Autoradiograph of hybridization of a probe to its complementary sequence showing a reduction in radioactive signal in proportion to the concentration of target DNA.

and the resulting fragment(s) separated according to size by gel electrophoresis and visualized directly when stained with ethidium bromide and viewed under ultraviolet light (Fig. 8.3). Direct visualization in this fashion gives white target DNA bands on a dark background as compared with autoradiography in Southern analysis which gives black target DNA bands on a light background. Each PCR analysis can start with $0.5-1\,\mu g$ of target DNA and produces a result in a matter of hours. Its speed and sensitivity are key advantages over Southern analysis but it can only be applied for DNA sequences where a flanking primer sequence is available and its extreme sensitivity means that meticulous care to avoid exogenous DNA contamination (and hence a false result) is required. As PCR analysis can use tiny starting quantities of impure genomic DNA it has proved possible to use PCR amplification to provide a DNA analysis on buccal mucosal cells from a mouth rinse, single hairs, single cells (sperm, ova, pre-implantation biopsies and fetal cells isolated from the maternal circulation), fixed pathological specimens and dried blood spots including stored neo-natal screening cards.

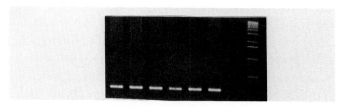

Fig. 8.3 Direct visualization of PCR amplified specific DNA fragments in six DNA samples with size controls in the right-hand lane.

DIRECT DEMONSTRATION OF MUTANT GENES

Large length mutations may be visible on cytogenetic analysis but if less than 4 Mb in size then DNA analysis is required. Southern or PCR analysis may be employed to reveal absence or a reduced size of a specific DNA fragment (Figs. 8.4 and 8.5). With appropriate modifications of technique even tiny deletions can be revealed. The single commonest mutation in cystic fibrosis is a three base pair deletion which removes the codon for phenylalanine at position 508. Figure 8.6 demonstrates a prenatal diagnosis for a couple who each carry this mutation. Trinucleotide amplifications produce a fragment larger than expected and whilst small amplifications may be demonstrable with PCR analysis, larger expansions require Southern analysis.

Point mutations can be detected by several approaches including loss or gain of a cutting site for a restriction enzyme and by allele specific oligonucleotide probes. Figure 8.7 shows an example of a point mutation, which can be detected by loss of a cutting site for a restriction enzyme. Allele specific oligonucleotide (ASO) probes are short (17−30 nucleotide) probes which have the complementary sequence to either the normal DNA or the mutant DNA at the point of interest. Under appropriate experimental conditions the presence or absence of hybridization with these probes will distinguish normal homozygotes from heterozygotes and homozygous affected individuals.

The above approaches relate to prenatal diagnosis where the mutation(s) is known in the family. A variety of approaches can be used to discover the molecular pathology within an affected family. Screening for length mutations can be performed by Southern analysis or PCR analysis with absence of specific hybridization or an altered length of the specific DNA

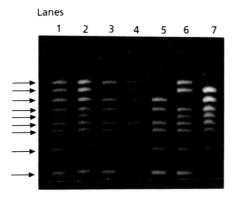

Fig. 8.4 Simultaneous PCR amplification of nine segments (arrowed) of the gene for Duchenne muscular dystrophy in seven patients (lanes 1−7). Note missing bands corresponding to deletions in lanes 3, 5, 6 and 7.

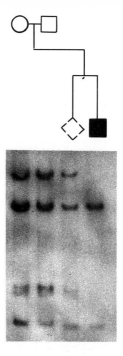

Fig. 8.5 Prenatal diagnosis in a family with Duchenne muscular dystrophy using a dystrophin cDNA probe. The affected son is deleted for two DNA fragments whereas the male fetus has a normal pattern and is hence unaffected.

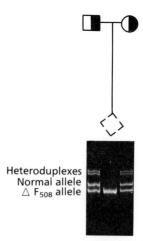

Fig. 8.6 Prenatal diagnosis for a couple who are both carriers of the ΔF_{508} cystic fibrosis mutation. Each parent is heterozygous with a faster moving band representing the mutant allele (and bands above the normal allele representing heteroduplexes). The fetus has received both mutant alleles and is thus homozygous affected.

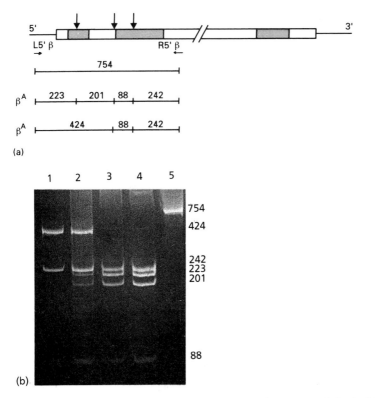

Fig. 8.7 Diagram (a) and results (b) or PCR amplification of a portion of the β globin gene and digestion with the restriction enzyme *Mst*II in a sickle cell homozygote (lane 1), a sickle cell heterozygote (lane 2) and two normal homozygotes (lanes 3 and 4). Lane 5 is a control containing amplified but undigested DNA.

fragment. Screening for point mutations is more difficult and several approaches are under evaluation. In each instance, confirmation of the suspected point mutation requires DNA sequencing to distinguish pathogenic point mutations from DNA polymorphisms (Fig. 8.8).

INDIRECT MUTANT GENE TRACKING

If the mutant gene has not been cloned or if the mutation is unknown in a family then prenatal diagnosis may still be possible by indirect mutant gene tracking using DNA polymorphisms (Figs. 8.9 and 8.10).

In both of these examples the DNA polymorphisms are used to track the mutant gene and the DNA analysis does not confirm the clinical diagnosis. This is an important advantage of direct mutation analysis which confirms the clinical diagnosis and so avoids difficulties due to *genetic heterogeneity* (where mutations in different genes result in clinically similar conditions). Indirect analysis also requires DNA samples from several family members in order to distinguish the mutant and normal

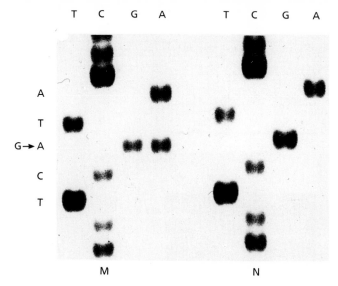

Fig. 8.8 DNA sequencing. The sequence is read from the bottom and the columns correspond to the bases thymine (T), cytosine (C), guanine (G) and adenine (A). The normal gene sequence is shown on the right whereas the patient on the left has a point mutation (G to A).

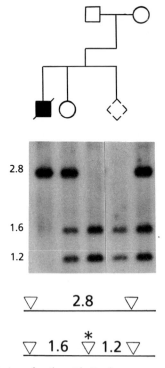

Fig. 8.9 Prenatal diagnosis in a family with Duchenne muscular dystrophy using indirect gene tracking with an intragenic RFLP (87.15/*Xmn*I). The polymorphic site (*) gives alternative alleles of 2.8 kb and 1.6 kb + 1.2 kb at this locus. The mother is a carrier on the basis of elevated creatine kinase levels and the 2.8 kb fragment indicates the mutant gene as it was inherited by the affected son. The male fetus is predicted to be unaffected as it has inherited the 1.6 kb and 1.2 kb fragments but the daughter is predicted to be a carrier as she has inherited the 2.8 kb fragment from her mother.

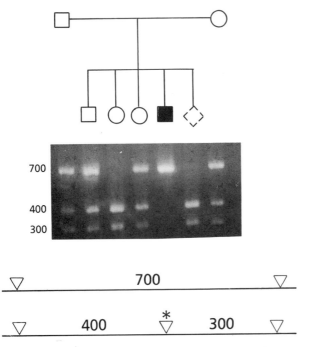

Fig. 8.10 Prenatal diagnosis in a family with cystic fibrosis using indirect gene tracking with an extragenic RFLP (XV-2c/*Taq*I). The polymorphic site (*) gives alternative alleles of 700 bp and 400 bp + 300 bp at this locus. The affected son is homozygous for the 700 bp alleles and thus his brother and younger sister are carriers (heterozygotes) whereas his older sister and the fetus are homozygous normal.

genes and may not be applicable if few samples are available or if key individuals are homozygous for the polymorphic site. This emphasizes the need to bank DNA samples from affected persons with single gene disorders even if a prenatal diagnosis is not imminent as the DNA can be stored for prolonged periods prior to analysis. Indirect gene tracking can also be hampered by non-paternity and the results are conditional on no recombination between the DNA polymorphism and the gene mutation. This error rate due to recombination increases as more distant polymorphic markers are employed and hence intragenic or tightly linked extragenic polymorphisms should be employed wherever possible. Direct mutation detection circumvents many of these difficulties but has the pre-requisites that the gene in question needs to have been cloned and the mutation(s) defined in each family.

SUMMARY OF DIAGNOSABLE SINGLE GENE DISORDERS

The first human gene (human placental lactogen) was cloned in 1977 and by 1993 over 10 000 complete or partial human gene sequences had been

Table 8.4 Commoner single gene disorders for which DNA based prenatal diagnosis is available (alphabetical order)

Condition	Direct mutation detection	Indirect mutant gene tracking
Adult polycystic kidney disease	−	+
Alpha$_1$ antitrypsin deficiency	+	+
Alpha-thalassaemia	+	+
Beta-thalassaemia	+	+
Congenital adrenal hyperplasia	+	+
Cystic fibrosis	+	+
Duchenne (and Becker) muscular dystrophy	+	+
Familial hypercholesterolaemia	+	+
Fragile X syndrome	+	+
Friedreich's ataxia	−	+
Haemophilia A	+	+
Haemophilia B	+	+
Huntington disease	+	+
Lesch−Nyhan syndrome	+	+
Myotonic dystrophy	+	+
Neurofibromatosis type I	+	+
Sickle cell disease	+	+
Spinal muscular atrophy	−	+

cloned. This represents over 10% of the estimated total number of human genes and includes many clinically important conditions where there is a demand for prenatal diagnosis.

The first prenatal diagnosis using DNA analysis (of sickle cell disease) was made in 1978 and the Appendix includes over 150 single gene disorders for which successful prenatal diagnosis by DNA analysis has been reported. Table 8.4 lists some of the commoner conditions for which prenatal DNA diagnosis is considered together with the availability of direct and/or indirect diagnosis. Other conditions are included in the Appendix and as this area is rapidly evolving it is important to check with the Regional Genetics Centre before concluding that DNA analysis cannot be offered for a condition. The Appendix also includes single gene disorders where prenatal diagnosis can be offered by biochemical analysis or by other approaches. Where more than one approach can be employed, discussion with the laboratory should help to determine the optimal strategy for each family.

FURTHER READING

Antonarakis, S.E. (1989) Diagnosis of genetic disorders at the DNA level. *New England Journal of Medicine*, **320**, 153−63.
Brock, D.J.H. (1993) *Molecular Genetics for the Clinician*, Cambridge University Press, Cambridge.

Connor, J.M. and Ferguson-Smith, M.A. (1993) *Essential Medical Genetics* 4th edn, Blackwell Scientific Publications, Oxford, 260 pp.

Cotton, R.G.H. (1989) Detection of single base changes in nucleic acids. *Biochemical Journal*, **263**, 1−10.

Eisenstein, B.I. (1990) The polymerase chain reaction. A new method using molecular genetics for medical diagnosis. *New England Journal of Medicine*, **322**, 178−83.

Miles, J.S. and Wolf, C.R. (1989) Principles of DNA cloning. *British Medical Journal*, **299**, 1019−1022.

Weatherall, D.J. (1991) *The New Genetics and Clinical Medicine* 3rd edn, Oxford University Press, Oxford.

Chapter 9
Infections

D. CARRINGTON

Although systemic maternal infections commonly lead to fetal infection, this is not invariable and the consequences for the fetus depend upon the agent and the gestation. Hence this chapter not only outlines the identification of pregnancies at risk for the commoner fetal infections but also covers the prenatal investigation and management of the infected pregnancy.

IDENTIFICATION OF AT-RISK PREGNANCIES

Pregnancies at risk of fetal infection are usually identified because of an acute maternal illness or by screening of pregnant women at particular risk (Table 9.1). Occasionally a fetal abnormality, such as hydrops, will alert the clinician to the possibility of a congenital infection at the time of an ultrasound examination. For maternal investigation a clotted blood sample (10 ml) should be sent to the virus laboratory (with a 'danger of infection' sticker if appropriate) and swabs for isolation of viruses should be transported in sterile containers containing virus transport medium.

MANAGEMENT OF THE AT-RISK PREGNANCY

Hepatitis B virus (HBV)

Early serological markers of acute HBV infection include the appearance of HBsAg, HBeAg and HBV-DNA, but these are replaced in convalescence with the detection of HBcIgM, HBeAb and HBsAb indicating immune clearance of this virus (Table 9.2).

In 5−10% of acute HBV infections, antigenaemia persists as a chronic carrier state. In certain populations (e.g. western Europe) there is a steady drop in HBsAg in the majority of cases with the eventual disappearance of HBsAg and HBeAg 5−10 years after infection. The appearance of HBeAb signals a lower infectivity state that rarely leads to perinatal infection, or chronic liver disease in the mother (Table 9.3).

Acute HBV infection in the later stages of pregnancy may result in premature delivery. If a patient is viraemic at delivery, the baby is likely to be infected perinatally. But intrauterine infection with HBV, although reported, appears to be rare. The presence of small amounts of HBsAg in

Table 9.1

CHAPTER 9
Infections

Infectious agent	Clinical clues to the at-risk pregnancy	Maternal investigations to consider
Hepatitis B virus	Acute maternal hepatitis	Early HBsAg, HBeAg and HBV-DNA. Later HBcIgM, HBeAb, and HBsAb
	Chronic carriers — previous acute hepatitis (5–10%), intravenous drug abuser, sexual contact of known carrier, prostitute, tattooed, from endemic area (Far East, India, Africa, Caribbean, Turkey, Middle East)	HBsAg, HBeAg, HBeAb, HBcAb
Herpes simplex virus	Acute or recurrent genital infection	Virus isolation from lesions. Serology of limited value
Varicella zoster virus	Varicella or herpes zoster	Virus isolation from lesions may be considered. Serology useful for susceptibility and diagnosis
Chlamydia trachomatis	Vaginal discharge or contact with nonspecific urethritis	Endocervical swabs for culture/direct examination
Treponema pallidum	Usually none	Treponema-specific serum screening tests (VDRL, TPHA, TPI, FTA-ABS)
Rubella virus	Maternal contact/ infection, rash, cervical lymphadenopathy	Rubella specific IgM and IgG
Cytomegalovirus	Usually none, occasional growth retardation	Fetal ultrasound
Toxoplasma gondii	Usually none	Sabin–Feldman toxoplasma specific IgM and dye test, fetal ultrasound
Human immunodeficiency virus	Usually asymptomatic; suspect if intravenous drug abuser, sexual contact of known carrier, prostitute, from endemic area, treated with unscreened blood products	ELISA for HIV specific antibodies. Confirmation with 'Western blot' analysis
Human parvovirus (B19)	Usually none, occasionally facial rash, arthropathy	B19 specific IgM, MSAFP, B19 probes, fetal ultrasound

cord blood is more likely to indicate maternal–fetal contamination at the time of separation of the placenta. The development of significant amounts of HBsAg and HBeAg in the infant's blood 4–12 weeks after delivery indicates perinatal infection. A chronic carrier state in the infant is the

Table 9.2 HBV markers and their significance

HBsAg	Hepatitis B surface antigen	Outercoat of virus, earliest marker of infection
HBsAb	Surface antibody	'Immune' response with future protection
HBeAg	e antigen	A marker of high infectivity in HBsAg carrier
HBeAb	e antibody	Marker of low infectivity in HBsAg carriers
HBcAg	Core antigen	Rarely measured, only found in active disease
HBcIgG	Core immunoglobin G	A permanent marker of previous exposure to HBV
HBcIgM	Core immunoglobin M	Indicator of acute infection
HBV-DNA	Deoxyribonucleic acid	An indicator of viral replication

Table 9.3 Maternal e status and risk of perinatal HBV infection in the infant (Cumulative data from literature)

e status	No. of infants	No. infected (%)	Chronic carrier child (%)
HBeAg pos	82	95.1	87.5
HBeAg ⎤ ⎬ neg HBeAb ⎦	16	25.0	12.5
HBeAb pos	32	12.5	0.0

HBV, hepatitis B virus.

usual consequence of perinatal infection, although neonatal hepatitis at 3 months of age is described.

The pregnant patient carrying the HBV marker HBsAg is not a risk to other antenatal or postnatal patients, nor does a baby born to a HBsAg positive mother pose a risk to other infants, as this agent is a serum or sexually transmitted virus. However, the patient should if possible be nursed in a sideroom in the post-partum period, with her baby in the same room, and special care should be paid to the disposal of infective discharges. In endemic areas, nursing in a sideroom is not practical but careful disposal of infected dressings/linen will still be required.

Perinatal transmission can be prevented by the use of hepatitis B vaccine and convalescent immunoglobulin (HBIg) containing large amounts of HBsAb. This immunoglobulin preparation is given at birth (or within 6 hours) as 0.3 ml HBIg/kg bodyweight as 200 iu HBsAb/ml together with 10 mg of hepatitis B vaccine (e.g. Engerix B-SK & F) if the mother is

HBsAg positive. For infants born to HBsAg and HBeAb positive mothers, a course of vaccine alone is sufficient. The vaccine programme at birth is followed by a second active immunization at 1 month and a third at 6 months of age. There is no evidence to suggest that HBsAg positive mothers present a greater risk of perinatal transmission if they breast feed rather than bottle feed their infants.

Herpes simplex virus (HSV)

Although the estimated overall risk of neonatal HSV infection is about 1 in 7500, of those delivered vaginally to mothers with primary genital HSV infection, more than 50% may develop clinical manifestations. This risk is reduced to less than 5% for the infant if maternal vaginal infection is recurrent rather than primary (perhaps due to transplacental passage of neutralizing antibody). In contrast to perinatal infection, congenital infection is rare but can result in widespread or localized vesiculation, conjunctivitis, meningoencephalitis with microcephaly or hydrocephalus, chorioretinitis, cataracts, hepatosplenomegaly and pneumonitis. Congenital infection can occur at any stage of pregnancy resulting in abortion in the first and second trimester of pregnancy, stillbirth or neonatal death.

As most problems related to maternal genital HSV infection occur around the perinatal period, direct assessment of the fetus during pregnancy is rarely justified. A past history of genital herpes should not prompt surveillance cultures as elective caesarean sections should not be undertaken for asymptomatic shedding of HSV. With clinically active primary or recurrent HSV disease of the cervix or vagina close to parturition, an elective caesarean delivery should be considered to prevent serious perinatal infection. No current antiviral drug is considered safe for use in pregnancy although teratogenicity has not been documented with systemic acyclovir treatment given in the third trimester.

At delivery, the baby of a mother known to be excreting HSV should be investigated actively. Throat, nose and eye swabs should be taken routinely for viral culture and the baby empirically treated with intravenous acyclovir at 5 mg/kg bodyweight three times daily, if the maternal infection is suspected to be primary. If the mother gives a history of previous herpetic eruptions active in pregnancy but thought to be resolved at the time of delivery, the risk of perinatal transmission is likely to be low. Swabbing of the infant and treatment on first signs of infection or first positive culture is a reasonable management strategy.

Varicella zoster virus

The risk of maternal primary varicella zoster virus (VZV) infection during pregnancy is about 1 in 7500 but reactivations in the form of herpes zoster are more frequent (about 1 in 1000 pregnancies). In general, the prognosis for either primary or secondary episodes for both mother and child is favourable. However, following primary infection there is a well-defined congenital varicella syndrome characterized by limb hypoplasia, cutaneous scars, cataracts, chorioretinitis, cerebral cortical atrophy and cerebellar hypoplasia. The CNS manifestations result in microcephaly, convulsions and mental retardation. Fortunately, this syndrome is rare, with an overall incidence of 0.6% (2.3% for infections during the first trimester). Infection late in pregnancy may result in premature labour and neonatal varicella or herpes zoster in the first year of life. Herpes zoster during pregnancy rarely leads to the congenital varicella syndrome.

Perinatal transmission to the newborn occurs when a fetus is infected during maternal viraemia within 10 days of birth and especially when the infant is born 1 day before to 4 days after the onset of maternal varicella (i.e. before maternal antibodies could reach the fetus). The infected neonate develops a widespread rash, high fever and occasionally pneumonitis and encephalitis. Overall mortality is 5%.

For a mother with a varicella or zoster contact, a previous history of infection allows immediate reassurance to be given. For those with negative or doubtful histories a blood sample should be taken without delay and analysed for VZV antibodies by a sensitive test, e.g. IFAT, ELISA or RIA. The majority will be seropositive and can be reassured. For seronegative cases human varicella zoster immunoglobulin should be given immediately and repeated if there is a re-exposure more than 3 weeks after the previous dose. However, this treatment is reserved for when exposure has been within 96 hours and more than a passing encounter. This preparation may modify and reduce the complications of varicella and may be useful in preventing congenital varicella or disseminated neonatal varicella. In established complicated maternal VZV infection intravenous acyclovir initially at 10 mg/kg body weight three times daily should be used. If the patient is receiving immunosuppressive therapy the acyclovir should be started at 15–18 mg/kg as varicella pneumonitis in these patients may be fatal.

Varicella zoster virus infection during pregnancy carries a low overall risk to the fetus and should not be viewed as grounds for termination of pregnancy.

Chlamydia trachomatis

In a mother with genital infection, perinatal transmission (likely in 25–50% of cases) may result in neonatal conjunctivitis and/or pneumonia but intrauterine infection appears to be rare unless complicated by premature rupture of the membranes. The value of screening depends on the local prevalence but if done it ought to be close to the point of delivery (36 weeks plus) when antimicrobials can be safely given and the infection terminated without reinfection before delivery. As oral tetracyclines are contraindicated in pregnancy, erythromycin 250 mg four times daily for 14 days should be given or if erythromycin is not well tolerated, amoxycillin 2 g daily may be substituted for a similar period (Alexander and Harrison, 1983). In all cases identified, a test of cure is advised together with the treatment of the sexual partner(s). For the neonate, oral erythromycin suspension 30−50 mg/kg/day in divided doses for 14 days is recommended for both conjunctivitis or pneumonia. Topical ophthalmic therapy is less effective, and is of no additional benefit when given in combination with systemic therapy.

Treponema pallidum

Congenital syphilis is becoming a rare event in the western world because of antenatal screening procedures. These tests are important as *Treponema pallidum* infection is invariably asymptomatic in pregnant women.

As congenital syphilis is preventable if the mother is adequately treated during pregnancy, routine treponemal specific serum screening tests performed at booking are standard practice (usually a lipoidal test e.g. RPR, VDRL and a specific treponemal test e.g. TPHA or ELISA). Fetal infection is most likely after the fifth month of gestation and is seen in women with early untreated or late syphilis (especially the former). Untreated pregnancies can result in spontaneous abortion (33%). An untreated mother appears to become less infectious to the fetus with each successive pregnancy and a woman with untreated congenital syphilis rarely infects her own fetus. Once adequately treated, a woman will not infect subsequent fetuses.

Penicillin is still the treatment of choice for syphilis. Daily injections of 1.2 megaunit of procaine penicillin given as 1.6 megaunit of Bicillin (a mixture of procaine and benzyl penicillin) for 10−15 days are curative. If penicillin is contraindicated, erythromycin 500 mg four times daily for 3 weeks is an alternative but the mother and baby must be carefully followed up, and the baby treated if neonatal serum is FTA IgM positive or a decline in treponemal antibodies (passively acquired from the mother) is not seen during the first 3 months after birth. In each case the advice of a specialist in sexually transmitted diseases should be sought, not only to supervise treatment, but also to arrange contact tracing.

Rubella virus

In the UK, rubella in pregnant women is seen most commonly in young primigravidae who have missed 'vaccination rounds' at school and women 30−35 years of age who left school before rubella vaccination was introduced. Of women with confirmed rubella, 95% present with a rash and the remainder have no symptoms. Nearly one-half of the fetuses will be infected (Table 9.4). In contrast, the risk of fetal involvement in subclinical rubella reinfection seem to be very low.

The clinical diagnosis of rubella is difficult as many viruses induce a rubella-like rash and serological confirmation is mandatory. Preferably, the

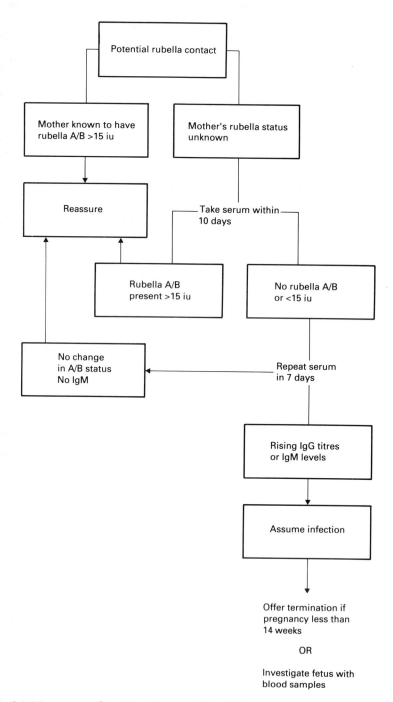

Fig. 9.1 Management flow chart for potential rubella contacts.

Table 9.4 Risk of congenital rubella defects (adapted from Miller *et al.*, 1982)

Gestation (weeks)	No. fetuses infected (%)	Overall risk of defects (% of those infected)	Main defects
<11	100	90	Multiple defects — brain, eye, heart
11–12	67	33	Deafness
13–14	67	11	Deafness
15–16	47	24	Deafness
17–36	37	0	None
>36	100	0	None

rubella status should be known prior to pregnancy with screening by single radial haemolysis (SRH) or ELISA to detect specific IgG.

A flow chart (Fig. 9.1) indicates the steps to take following a potential rubella contact. The time course for the immune response to rubella infection is shown in Fig. 9.2. If there is a delay of more than 10 days between rash and investigation, a serological rise may not be seen. Then the measurement of complement fixing antibodies (CFT) may be useful. Specific IgM tests remain positive for at least 4 weeks after the rash appears in primary infections and this is the most definitive test.

Once infection has been confirmed, the management depends largely on the state of pregnancy at the time of involvement. Table 9.4 shows the likelihood of infection and subsequent sequelae related to gestational age. It is now clear, after numerous studies, that fetal abnormalities occur no

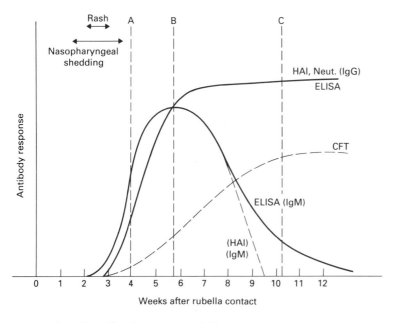

Fig. 9.2 Serological profile of a primary rubella response.

more frequently than in non-infected pregnancies if the maternal rash appears after the 17th week of gestation.

In primary infection or clinically overt reinfection before 17 weeks of pregnancy, termination should be considered. In asymptomatic reinfection the outcome is likely to be favourable and the pregnancy should be continued although it is important that arrangements are made for follow-up.

The alternative to termination is to evaluate the pregnancy further to establish whether or not the fetus has been infected. This is almost inevitable when maternal infection occurs before 11 or 12 weeks' gestation but with later infections (i.e. between 12 and 17 weeks) fetal investigation should be considered as the risk of congenital infection may be substantially reduced.

Fetal blood obtained by cordocentesis may be examined for the presence of specific IgM using sensitive assay methods. However, it appears that the fetus is not reliably immunologically competent until at least 21 weeks so sampling before that time will lead to false negative results. Amniotic fluid may be a source for isolation of the virus but a negative result may be unreliable. More recently, rubella specific probes have been used to assess chorionic tissue obtained by chorionic villus sampling and this offers hope that early identification of the infected fetus may be possible.

In spite of these developments there are still no methods which will allow the differentiation of the affected rubella fetus from one which is infected but not affected. This, and an increased effort to ensure that women are rubella immune before they become pregnant, are important aims which will help to reduce losses and damage due to this virus.

Cytomegalovirus

Congenital cytomegalovirus (CMV) is the most common congenital infection in the UK (estimated at over 400 cases per annum). Intrauterine transmission occurs in 25−50% of maternal primary CMV infections. Involvement is serious in 10% with CNS involvement (mental retardation, microcephaly, hydrocephalus), sensorineural deafness and neonatal evidence of disseminated infection (hepatosplenomegaly, petechiae). Mild or delayed sequelae may occur in a further 33%. Reactivation or reinfection, which are more frequent than primary infection, are less likely to result in an intrauterine infection.

As congenitally infected infants may be born to mothers with previous exposure to CMV (i.e. found seropositive before evidence of recurrent infection), it is clear that a state of 'immunity' following primary infection does not exist. Like herpes simplex virus, cytomegalovirus shows the property of latency and recurrences are not uncommon in pregnancy so that siblings from successive pregnancies may be infected. The risk of having a second congenitally infected child is probably low and has not been quantified. However, a second pregnancy should be delayed 6 months following a primary infection, as CMV excretion may continue at a high titre during this time. However, negative cultures will not preclude recurrence during a further pregnancy.

Serological screening of asymptomatic women for CMV antibodies to detect primary infection is discouraged. Symptomatic women infected with CMV are advised to continue with their pregnancies to term when paediatric and virological assessment should be made in the neonatal period for evidence of congenital infection. In addition to standard isolation of CMV from throat swabs and urine, taken as soon after birth as possible, the assessment of CMV specific IgM by a sensitive method, together with other non-specific markers such as total IgM level and the presence of rheumatoid factor, may further improve virological and clinical diagnosis.

As yet there are no therapies that can alter the course of CMV infection in pregnancy or prevent intrauterine infection. Neonatal sera can be negative for CMV specific IgM and cord blood sampling *in utero* may yield an unacceptable rate of false negatives if this were attempted and limit prognostic significance when applied in management decisions. The use of cloned probes to CMV may provide yet more direct evidence of fetal infection when applied to chorionic villus samples but this is likely to be of limited value as CMV infection can take place throughout pregnancy. Although live attenuated vaccines have been tested, a widespread programme of vaccination will probably require a subunit or recombinant vaccine.

Toxoplasma gondii

Acute infection is almost always asymptomatic in the pregnant woman and surveys have indicated a wide range from under 1 in 1000 (Norway, Scotland) to nearly 1 in 100 affected pregnancies (Austria, France, Germany).

Surveys suggest an overall risk of fetal infection of 5%. At least one-half of these congenitally infected fetuses will be damaged with CNS involvement (mental retardation, hydrocephalus, microcephaly, intracerebral calcification, convulsions), chorioretinitis (especially if followed up) and neonatal evidence of active infection (hepatosplenomegaly, jaundice, anaemia, pneumonitis). Only a primary infection with *Toxoplasma gondii* leads to congenital toxoplasmosis. After this primary infection there may be persistence of cysts of *T. gondii* but the development of active immunity protects the subsequent pregnancies. Infection in the first trimester is more likely to cause stillbirth or fetal damage with congenital toxoplasmosis. However, this is not exclusively so, and in high prevalence areas monthly testing of seronegatives throughout pregnancy will further reduce the incidence of congenital toxoplasmosis by selective termination of infected cases or by antimicrobial chemotherapy.

Toxoplasma surveillance aims to detect primary maternal infections in order to allow prenatal diagnosis of congenital infection. This can be accomplished by fetal blood sampling and demonstration of specific IgM. Termination of pregnancy is generally advised where the fetus shows evidence of active infection. Upon the diagnosis of maternal primary infection, therapy with pyrimethamine and a sulphonamide (or spiramycin) should be instituted pending fetal investigation as there is a significant delay period before the fetus is infected. Prophylaxis is least effective if infection is acquired late in pregnancy or if treatment is delayed.

Human immunodeficiency virus (HIV)

By March 31 1991 the Centre for Disease Control, Atlanta, USA, had reported 2963 cases of AIDS in children, 84% of which had resulted from mother to infant transmission. In the following three years the number of cases is expected to reach 9400 in the USA. Currently, in non-African countries, 70% of cases result from intravenous drug use by the mother. Transmission from mother to child is now firmly established but the relative contributions of prenatal, perinatal and postnatal routes (via breast feeding) are still unknown.

Evidence supporting *in utero* transmission is found from virus recovery from fetal and placental tissue, including *in situ* hybridization, culture from cord blood and detection of proviral sequences in blood of newborns. The ability of the virus to grow in all fetal organs has raised questions of teratogenicity (a craniofacial dysmorphic feature) but this is still unconfirmed. The development of progressive neurological manifestations in children with HIV infection (seen between 2 months and 5 years) is similarly disturbing.

It is now clear that HIV transmission between mother and fetus or infant is not inevitable as more than 50% of infants subsequently lose HIV antibody 15–18 months after birth and appear uninfected. The risk of maternal–fetal transmission is still to be accurately quantified although current data report a risk between 12.9, 25 and 50% in Europe, America and Africa respectively. Individual examples of sparing one twin have been recorded and small studies have indicated a risk of 50% (6 in 12) for an affected child in a subsequent pregnancy when the mother is positive in the first indexed pregnancy. Because of the possible delayed appearance of immunological and clinical manifestations, this figure may be an underestimate. As fetal sampling may introduce HIV from maternal contamination, attention is currently focused on the neonate born to an infected mother in an attempt to identify, at an early stage, whether or not the child is infected (see Table 9.1). Serological studies on infant serum are compromised by maternally derived HIV specific antibodies, passed on to the infant, making differentiation initially difficult as HIV specific IgM is not readily produced. Currently, the most helpful tests include monitoring the disappearance or persistence of HIV specific antibody by sensitive enzyme linked immunoassay employing recombinant or peptide antigens, HIV p24 core antigen, HIV specific IgA and sequential absolute CD4 positive cell counts. Attempts at the identification of HIV antigen in cultured neonatal blood lymphocytes have been successful and the detection of HIV proviral DNA by the polymerase chain reaction (PCR) using fetal or neonatal cells may achieve a high level of sensitivity. However, doubts over specificity (particularly maternal contamination) limits the usefulness of this potentially helpful investigation.

It is unlikely that prenatal diagnosis will be established until methods of HIV detection have been improved and more is known of the risk factors associated with HIV in pregnancy for the mother or the newborn. At present, with little to be offered from the chemotherapeutic front (azidothymidine is unlikely to be given in pregnancy), termination of pregnancy is the only method of preventing the birth of congenitally infected children. If the pregnancy is continued, breast feeding is contraindicated.

Human parvovirus B19

The commonest clinical manifestation of human parvovirus B19 infection is fifth disease or the 'slapped cheek' syndrome in children. Adults may also have an acute illness with fever and bright red cheeks but are commonly asymptomatic. This virus has a predilection for the erythroid progenitor cells and can result in aplastic anaemia in children and adults with an inherited haemolytic anaemia and in hydrops fetalis during intrauterine infection.

The frequency of human parvovirus (B19) antibodies increases with age and they are found in about 60% of unselected UK blood donors. The frequency of primary infection during pregnancy is unknown but the accumulating data suggest a 6–10% risk of an adverse fetal outcome, usually with spotaneous abortion/intrauterine death. Despite overwhelming infection seen in brain, lung, spleen and kidneys of hydropic fetuses, no conclusive evidence of congenital abnormality has been demonstrated.

The diagnosis of B19 maternal infection is usually based on the detection of B19 specific IgM in sera in those with a suggestive illness or contact. These antibodies persist for up to 18 weeks, with all sera remaining positive up to 10 weeks after onset of clinical symptoms.

During maternal B19 infection, a marker of poor fetal outcome appears to be a raised maternal serum α-fetoprotein (MSAFP) level. In these pregnancies the B19 infection is associated with a fetal aplastic crisis. The abnormal MSAFP levels appear to predate fetal ascites on ultrasonography and can thus provide a guide to fetal involvement and offer the possibility of treatment by intrauterine blood transfusion which might be considered if survivors are shown to be otherwise normal. Blood taken at cordocentesis in B19 infected fetuses has been negative for B19 specific IgM although B19 DNA probes have detected virus in blood samples taken at 21 weeks and in fetal organs following termination of pregnancy.

FURTHER READING

Hepatitis B virus

Beasley, R.P., Hwang, L.Y., Lin, C.C. *et al.* (1981) Hepatitis B immune globulin (HBIG) efficacy in the interruption of perinatal transmission of hepatitis B virus carrier state. *Lancet*, **2**, 388.

Stevens, C.E., Beasley, R.P., Tsui, J. and Lee, W.C. (1975) HBeAg and anti-HBe detection by radioimmunoassay: correlation with vertical transmission of hepatitis B virus in Taiwan. *New England Journal of Medicine*, **292**, 771.

Herpes simplex virus

Nahmias, A.J., Keyserling, H.H. and Kerrick, G. (1983) Herpes simplex. In *Infectious Diseases of the Fetus and Newborn Infant* 2nd edn (eds. J.S. Remington and J.O. Klein), WB Saunders, Philadelphia, pp. 1560–90.

Proper, C.F., Sullender, W.M., Yasukawa, L.L. *et al.* (1987) Low risk of herpes simplex virus infections in neonates exposed to the virus at the time of vaginal delivery to mothers with recurrent genital herpes simplex infections. *New England Journal of Medicine*, **316**, 240–44.

Varicella zoster virus

Paryani, S.G. and Arvin, A.M. (1986) Intrauterine infection with varicella zoster after maternal varicella. *New England Journal of Medicine*, **314**, 1542–46.

Chlamydia trachomatis

Alexander, E.R. and Harrison, H.R. (1983) Role of *Chlamydia trachomatis* in perinatal infection. *Rev. Infect. Dis.*, **5**, 713–19.

Hammerschlag, M.R., Anderka, M., Simine, D.Z. *et al.* (1979) Prospective study of maternal and infantile infection with *Chlamydia trachomatis*. *Paediatrics*, **64**, 142–47.

Treponema pallidum

Muller, F.P. (1984) *Treponema pallidum*, in *Diagnostics in Perinatal Infections* (ed. W. de Jong), Die Medizinische Verlagsgesellschaft Marburg/Lahn, Vol. 1, pp. 88–98.

Rubella

Daffos, F., Forestier, F., Grangeot-Keras, L. *et al.* (1984) Prenatal diagnosis of congenital rubella. *Lancet*, **2**, 1–3.

Miller, E., Cradock-Watson, J.E. and Pollock, T.M. (1982) Consequences of confirmed maternal rubella at successive stages of pregnancy. *Lancet*, **2**, 781–84.

Morgan-Capner, P., Hodgson, J., Hamblin, M.H. *et al.* (1985) Detection of rubella-specific IgM in subclinical rubella reinfection in pregnancy. *Lancet*, **1**, 244–46.

Cytomegalovirus

Griffiths, P.D., Stagno, S., Pass, R.F., Smith, R.J. and Alford, C.A. (1982) Congenital cytomegalovirus infection: Diagnostic and prognostic significance of the detection of specific IgM antibodies in cord serum. *Paediatrics*, **69**, 544–49.

Peckham, C.S., Chin, K.S., Coleman, J.C. *et al.* (1983) Cytomegalovirus infection in pregnancy: preliminary findings from a prospective study. *Lancet*, **1**, 1352–55.

Toxoplasma gondii

Desmonts, G., Daffos, F., Forestier, F. *et al.* (1985) Prenatal diagnosis of congenital toxoplasmosis. *Lancet*, **1**, 500–504.

Human immunodeficiency virus

Di Maria, H., Courpotin, C., Rouzioux, C. *et al.* (1986) Transplantal transmission of human immunodeficiency virus. *Lancet*, **2**, 215.

Marion, R.W., Wiznia, A.A., Hutcheon, R.G. and Rubinstein, A. (1986) Human T cell lymphotropic virus type III (HTLV III embryopathy: a new dysmorphic syndrome associated with intrauterine HTLV III infection). *American Journal of Diseases of Children*, **140**, 638–40.

Rogers, M., Ou, C.-Y., Rayfield, M. *et al.* (1989) Use of polymerase chain reaction for early detection of the provisional sequences of human immunodeficiency virus in infants born to seropositive mothers. *New England Journal of Medicine*, **320**, 1649.

Sprecher, S., Soumenhoff, G., Puissant, F. and Degueldre, M. (1986) Vertical transmission of HIV in 15 week fetus. *Lancet*, **2**, 288–89.

Human parvovirus B19

Carrington, D., Whittle, M.J., Gilmore, D.H. *et al.* (1987) Maternal serum alphafeto-protein — A marker of fetal aplastic crisis during intrauterine human parvovirus infection. *Lancet*, **1**, 433–35.

Chapter 10
Exposure to Teratogens

M. J. WHITTLE

The extent to which medications are taken during pregnancy is uncertain and although one study suggested that about 45% of women may take at least one prescribed drug (Shardein, 1985) a prospective study (Rubin *et al.*, 1986) reported that only about 10% may do so (Table 10.1). Undoubtedly the thalidomide disaster has had a considerable impact on the mother's view concerning drug ingestion during pregnancy and they are now much more likely to question the need for therapy.

Nevertheless, there are two distinct groups of patients in which concern about teratogenesis exists. The first group contains those women who have inadvertently taken preparations in early pregnancy often before they have even realized that conception has occurred. The second group, which in the author's experience, in terms of referral for advice, is numerically larger, contains women who are on long-term therapy for a recognized medical condition.

When approaching the problem of identifying a case at risk of teratogenesis three essential pieces of information are required.

Firstly, it is necessary to be aware of the critical phases in embryogenesis during which potential damage may occur. Thus from conception to about 17 days, the so-called pre-embryonic phase, the effect of teratogens is either total destruction and absorption of the conceptus or intact survival. Survival is possible because in these early stages the cells are totipotential so that the loss of some can be compensated by the remainder. Conversely, the truly embryonic phase from 18 to 55 days is the time when the developing fetus is likely to be most sensitive to potential teratogens because the tissues are differentiating rapidly and damage to them is irreparable. From 55 days to delivery the effects of drugs are either to distort normally formed structures (for example, goitre with carbimazole)

Table 10.1 Proportion of mothers reporting use of drugs in pregnancy (Rubin *et al.*, 1986)

Non-narcotic analgesia	13.0%
Antibacterials	10.0%
Antacids	7.4%
Antiemetics	5.5%
Anxiolytics	2.0%

or to produce problems by secondary mechanisms (for example, hydrocephalus with coumarins).

Secondly, the type of drug used must be accurately known and, if possible, its teratogenic potential established. Unfortunately, it is extremely difficult to be sure about the majority of agents and those few with 'certain' teratogenic effects are shown in Table 10.2. The results of animal experimentation are difficult to interpret since they cannot allow for the species differences which exist with regard to the absorption and metabolism of the drugs.

Thirdly, the potential effect of the drug on the developing fetus must be established before it is possible to determine whether or not prenatal diagnosis will be an option. The diagnosis of spina bifida or a major cardiac malformation is possible by the end of the first half of pregnancy whereas limb deformities or microcephaly may not become apparent until late pregnancy or even after delivery.

DRUGS AND TERATOGENESIS

The literature on drug effects in pregnancy is enormous and often very conflicting. This makes the distillation into a text which might be of practical value virtually impossible and indeed deserves a book in its own right. The author's approach has been to determine the type of drugs likely to be used during pregnancy, assign to them a teratogenic potential and then establish whether or not any effect might be diagnosed with high resolution ultrasound.

Table 10.3 should provide a guide but it is not exhaustive and the teratogenic potentials are a personal judgement based on the available literature and experience. In general, only human data have been used but occasionally, when the agent is considered to be a serious potential teratogen,

Table 10.2 Teratogens in man (after Shardein, 1985)

	Malformation	No. of cases
Established teratogens		
Aminopterin/methotrexate	Skull, extremities	20
Androgenic hormones	Genital	242
Thalidomide	Limbs	10 500
Coumarins	Skeleton, etc.	41
Alcohol	Central nervous system, heart, facies	600
Probable teratogens		
Ototoxic antibiotics	8th nerve	49
Cancer chemotherapy	Variable	23
Anticonvulsants	Clefts, cardiac, etc.	Uncertain
Lithium	Cardiac	13
D-Penicillamine	Connective tissue	4

Table 10.3 Drugs and their potential teratogenesis

Drug	Teratogen	Effect	Detectable	Reference
ACE inhibitors	H	Pulmonary hypoplasia, PDA renal failure	++	17
Actinomycin D	P	Neural tube defect — rabbit	++	13
Acyclovir	N			14
Alcohol	H	Microcephaly, multiple cardiac defects, facial abnormalities, growth retardation	++	5
Allopurinol	N			15
Amitriptyline	U	Various	?	4
Ampicillin	N			2
Aspirin	U	CNS, gut, talipes — rodents	+	13
Atenolol	N			2
Augmentin	N			15
Azathioprine	U		?	13
Buserelin	N			15
Busulphan	H	Cleft palate, microphthalmia	+	8
Carbamazepine	H	Spina bifida	++	16
Carbimazole	N	Goitre	+	1
Cephalosporins	N			2
Cetylpyridinum	N			15
Chlorambucil	P	CNS, clefting, renal malformation — rats	++	15
Chlordiazepoxide	N			1
Chloroquine	P	Chorioretinitis	0	1
Chlorpheniramine	N			2
Chlorpropamide	N	Poor pregnancy outcome (related to disease)	0	1
Cimetidine	N			19
Clomiphene	U	Possible increase CNS defects	++	18
Codeine	U	Respiratory malformation	0	1
Cortisone	P	Cleft lip	+	1
Coumarins	H	Hydrocephalus, nasal hypoplasia, skeletal malformations (chondrodysplasia punctata), incomplete gut rotation, IUGR	++	5
Cyclophosphamide	H	Abnormal/missing digits	+	8
Cyclosporin	U	Anencephaly, absent corpus callosum	++	6
Cytarabine	H	Multiple deformities in rodents	+	1
Danazol	L	Masculinization	0	7
Dextroamphetamine	P	Cardiac anomalies	+	1
Diazepam	U	Clefting	+	1
Diphenhydramine	N			2
Disulfiram	P	Club foot/Fetal alcohol syndrome	++	15

Table 10.3 (*Cont.*)

CHAPTER 10
*Exposure to
Teratogens*

Drug	Teratogen	Effect	Detectable	Reference
Doxorubicin	H	Multiple abnormalities in rodents	+	1
Ethambutol	N			1
Ethosuximide	U	Clefting, cardiac anomalies	+	1
Etretinate	H	see retinoic acid	++	2
Fluorouracil	H	CNS, skeletal abnormalities in rats/Radial aplasia in humans	++	1, 15
Fluphenazine	U			4
Griseofulvin	P	CNS, skeletal abnormalities in rats	+	1
Haloperidol	U		?	13
Hydrallazine	U		?	13
Idoxuridine	H	Exencephaly, polydactyly Skeletal defects — rats	++	15
Imipramine	U		?	4
Indomethacin	N	May cause premature closure of ductus arteriosus	0	2
Isoniazid	P	Non-specific reports	?	15
Isotretinol	H	see retinoic acid	++	2
Labetalol	N			19
Lithium	H	Ebstein's anomaly, other cardiac malformations	++	10
Meclofenamic acid	N			15
Meclozine	U	Clefting	+	1
Medroxy-progesterone	U	Transient clitoral hypertrophy	?	15
6-Mercaptopurine	H	Abnormal extremities in rodents — no reports in humans	?	1
Methotrexate	H	Skull and rib defects, absent digits	+	1
Methyldopa	N			1
Metronidazole	U			1
Nalidixic acid	N			15
Nifedipine	U	Minor defects in rabbits	?	15
Nortriptyline	U	Limb reductions	+	4
Oestrogens	P	Cardiac malformations, transposition, limb reductions, neural tube defects, VACTERL	++	13
Oral contraceptive	N			15
Paracetamol	N			19
Penicillamine	L	Skin/joint laxity	0	1
Phenobarbitone	U		?	15
Phenothiazines	U	Increase nonspecific malformation	?	1
Phenytoin	L	Craniofacial/limb abnormalities, clefting, growth retardation	+	5

(Continued)

Table 10.3 (*Cont.*)

Drug	Teratogen	Effect	Detectable	Reference
Pizotifen	U	Scanty data		19
Podophyllin	H	Embryonic death rather than malformation	++	15
Primidone	P	Cardiac defects, IUGR, clefting	++	3
Progesterone	L	Masculinization	0	1
Propylthiouracil	U	Goitre	+	1
Quinine	H	Hydrocephalus, heart defects, dysmelias	++	1
Retinoic acid	H	Hydrocephalus, microcephaly, microtia, heart defects, facial/limb anomalies	++	9
Rifampicin	P	Neural tube defect, clefting	++	1
Stilboestrol	H	Vaginal adenosis, male urogenital lesions	0	13
Streptomycin	L	Congenital deafness	0	1
Sulfasalazine	U	Sporadic cardiac defects, neonatal haemolysis, give folate	+	15
Sulphonamides	U	Clefting in rats	+	15
Testosterone	L	Masculinization	0	1
Tetracycline	N	Teeth staining	0	1
Tolbutamide	N	Poor pregnancy outcome (related to disease)	0	1
Trifluoperazine	U		?	4
Trimethadione	H	Microcephaly, tetralogy of Fallot, atrial and ventricular septal defects low ears, malformed hands, growth retardation	+	12
Trimethoprim	U		?	1
Valproic acid	H	Neural tube defect, tetralogy of Fallot, oral clefting, other facial abnormalities	++	11
X-rays	H	CNS, ophthalmic anomalies	+	1

PDA, patent ductus arteriosus; VACTERL, vertebral, anal, cardiac, tracheooesophageal renal and limb defects; IUGR, intrauterine growth retardation; H, high risk teratogen; L, low risk teratogen; P, possible teratogen; U, unlikely teratogen; some reports in animals/man; N, no evidence of teratogenesis; ++, prenatal diagnosis probable; +, prenatal diagnosis possible; 0, prenatal diagnosis unlikely; ?, potential for prenatal diagnosis impossible to determine.

1 Brendal, K., Duhamel, R.C. and Shepherd, T.H. (1985) Embryotoxic drugs. *Biological Research in Pregnancy*, 6, 1–54.
2 *British National Formulary*. British Medical Association and The Pharmaceutical Society of Great Britain.
3 Brodie, M.J. (1987) Epilepsy, anticonvulsants and pregnancy. In *Epilepsy in Young People* (eds. E. Ross, D. Chadwick and R. Crawford), John Wiley, Chichester, pp. 81–92.
4 Calabrese, J.R. and Gulledge, A.D. (1985) Psychotropics during pregnancy and lactation: a review. *Psychosomatics*, 26, 413–26.

5 Chernoff, G.F. and Jones, K.L. (1981) Fetal preventitive medicine; teratogens and the unborn baby. *Pediatric Annals*, **10**, 210–17.

6 Communications from the Pharmaceutical Industry.

7 Duck, S.C. and Katayama, K.P. (1981) Danazol may cause female pseudohermaphroditism. *Fertility and Sterility*, **35**, 230–31.

8 Goldman, A.S. (1980) Critical periods of prenatal insult. *Progress in Clinical Research*, **36**, 9–31.

9 Lammer, E.J., Chen, D.T., Hoar, R.M. *et al.* (1985) Retinoic acid embryopathy. *New England Journal of Medicine*, **313**, 837–41.

10 Linden, S. and Rich, C.L. (1983) The use of lithium during pregnancy and lactation. *Journal of Clinical Psychiatry*, **44**, 358–61.

11 Lindhout, D. and Schmidt, D. (1986) In utero exposure to valproate and neural tube defect. *Lancet*, **1**, 1392–3.

12 Shardein, J.L. (1985) Current status of drugs as teratogens in man. *Progress in Clinical and Biological Research*, **163C**, 181–90.

13 Tuchmann-Duplessis, H. (1984) Drugs and other xenobiotics as teratogens. *Pharmaceutical Therapeutics*, **26**, 273–344.

14 Andrews, E.B., Tilson, H.H., Hurn, B.A.L. and Cordero, J.F. (1988) Acyclovir in pregnancy registry; an observational epidemiological approach. *American Journal of Medicine*, **85**, 123–28.

15 *Catalog of teratogenic agents* (1992) 7th Edn (ed. T.H. Shepard) The Johns Hopkins University Press, Baltimore and London.

16 Rosa, F.W. (1991) S. bifida in infants of women treated with carbamazepine during pregnancy. *New England Journal of Medicine*, **324**, 674–77.

17 Brent, R.L. and Beckman, D.A. (1991) ACE inhibitors an embryopathic class of drugs with unique properties. Information for clinical teratology counsellors. *Teratology*, **43**, 543–46.

18 Mili, F., Khoury, M.J. and Lux, X. (1991) Clomiphene use and the risk of birth defect; a population based case control study. *Teratology*, **43**, 422–23.

19 ABPI datasheet compendium 1994–1995. Datapharm Publications Ltd., London.

animal evidence has been used and this has been indicated. Many of the drug effects recorded in the literature are derived from case reports alone and are often extremely difficult to interpret. There are several reasons for this, not least of which is that the dysmorphic features observed may well have nothing to do with an ingested drug. This is a particular problem with common anomalies such as cardiac defects or facial clefting. Further, some drugs may be considered to be certain teratogens but produce a constant and typical lesion very rarely. Finally, there is the problem of the influence on dysmorphogenesis of not only the drugs themselves but also the disease for which they were prescribed and other factors such as maternal age and fetal and/or maternal metabolism of the agent.

In Table 10.3 the teratogenic effects have been divided arbitrarily into five categories; it also gives some guidance concerning the potential for successful prenatal diagnosis.

The management of pregnancy at risk of teratogenesis

As mentioned earlier, the best method for managing the problem of teratogenesis is by prevention with widespread propaganda about the risks of taking medications in early pregnancy. Such a programme is the responsibility of all involved in health care and education. However, there will always be cases in which treatment in early pregnancy has occurred by accident or design and a clear management plan is necessary for these groups.

Inadvertent ingestion of agents in early pregnancy

The two most important steps are to establish exactly the gestational age at which the drug was ingested and to determine precisely the nature of the drug. In the author's experience this relatively simple exercise will allow a firm reassurance to be given to the majority of couples that their pregnancy is not at risk. When, however, it appears that a potential teratogen has been taken, its possible effects must be established and the likelihood of prenatal diagnosis determined. When the risk of teratogenesis is high and the consequences serious, but the chance of prenatal diagnosis low (a rare event), termination of pregnancy must be considered as an option.

Mothers already on medication

The problem when patients are already on treatment for a medical condition is slightly different but it is important that such couples have been fully counselled prior to the pregnancy either by their own physician or at a prepregnancy clinic. In general, the management plan for this group of patients is to discuss as realistically as possible the effects of the drug treatment, the risk of teratogenesis and the prospects for making a reliable prenatal diagnosis at a time when termination of pregnancy is still feasible. An important alternative in the prepregnancy period is to consider modifying the treatment either by reducing the dose of the current drug or by changing to a drug which has less teratogenic potential.

We believe that the team approach is vital but this demands close co-operation between physicians, family practitioners and the local prenatal diagnostic group.

REFERENCES

Rubin, P.C., Craig, G.F., Gavin, K. and Summer, D. (1986) Prospective survey of use of therapeutic drugs, alcohol and cigarettes during pregnancy. *British Medical Journal*, **292**, 81–3.
Shardein, J.L. (1985) Current status of drugs on teratogens in man. *Progress in Clinical and Biological Research*, **163C**, 181–90.

Chapter 11
Central Nervous System Malformations

A. D. CAMERON and M. B. McNAY

Central nervous system (CNS) malformations are among the commonest congenital anomalies and they account for approximately 50% of the structural abnormalities which are detected antenatally.

Although the pathogenetic mechanism is known to be failure of closure of the embryonic neural tube, the aetiology remains unknown. However, it does appear that there is a natural decline in the prevalence of the condition in high-risk areas (Omran, Stone and Mcloone, 1992). In this study, the birth prevalence of anencephaly and spina bifida dropped by 82% from 6.63 per 1000 births in 1964−68 to 1.04 per 1000 births in 1979−89. The pregnancy prevalence, which includes therapeutic terminations, declined by 46%, from 5.63 per 1000 births in 1964−68 to 3.02 per 1000 births in 1979−89. This study concluded that prenatal screening contributed just under half of the observed decline in CNS malformations and that more complex socio-economic factors are likely to play a role in the aetiology of anencephaly and spina bifida.

Central nervous system abnormalities may be isolated or associated with other malformations including several recognizable syndromes.

PRENATAL CLASSIFICATION

The structural CNS malformations which can be detected prenatally correlate well in general with the pathological diagnosis (Table 11.1).

IDENTIFICATION OF AT-RISK PREGNANCIES

As indicated in Table 11.1, several CNS malformations are inherited as either multifactorial or single gene traits. Hence a family history or previously affected child can be an important clue to an at-risk pregnancy. Polyhydramnios is common in anencephalic pregnancies and occasionally in hydrocephalus the enlarged head is suspected clinically. Several teratogens have been implicated in CNS malformations (see Table 10.3) and poorly controlled maternal diabetes mellitus is associated with an increased risk of neural tube defects. In practice, however, most affected pregnancies will not be predicted and will be identified at routine ultrasound scanning and/or by measurement of maternal serum α-fetoprotein levels (see Chapter 3).

Table 11.1 Central nervous system malformations detectable prenatally

Ultrasound diagnosis	Pathological diagnosis	Comments
Anencephaly	Same	Neural tube defects affect 3.5/1000 pregnancies in the west of Scotland, 2/1000 in southeast England, 1/1000 in USA and Canada; half anencephaly, half spina bifida. Recurrence risk 3−5% (may recur as anencephaly or spina bifida). Risk rises to 10% if two pregnancies affected
Spina bifida	Same	See general comments on neural tube defects in anencephaly entry. Hydrocephalus coexists in 80% (Arnold−Chiari malformation). Exclude trisomy 18, if additional malformations coexist
Encephalocele	Same	Usually occipital, rarely frontal. Consider Meckel syndrome (encephalocele, polydactyly, polycystic kidneys)
Iniencephaly	Same	Star-gazing posture. Open spina bifida may coexist
Hydrocephalus	Same	Isolated hydrocephalus affects 0.4/1000 pregnancies with aqueductal stenosis in one-third. May be secondary to fetal infection, occasionally (<1%) inherited as an X-linked trait (suspect if male with absence of pyramids from sections of medulla, aqueductal stenosis and characteristic hypoplastic flexed thumbs +/− a typical pedigree), more often multifactorial with an empiric recurrence risk of 4%
Microcephaly	Same	Occipito-frontal circumference more than 3 SD below expected mean. May be secondary to maternal phenylketonuria, fetal infection, chromosome abnormality, fetal alcohol syndrome or perinatal or postnatal severe insult. If cause cannot be identified, empiric recurrence risk is high (19%) reflecting several autosomal recessive traits (Tolmie *et al.*, 1987)
Holoprosencephaly	Same	Failure of development of the forebrain and associated midface, clinically varies from hypotelorism and bilateral cleft lip with an absent philtrum to absence of the nose and a single central eye. Death within 6 months is usual. Exclude trisomy 13. Empiric recurrence risk otherwise about 6%
Agenesis of the corpus callosum	Same	Patients may be asymptomatic but mental retardation, macrocephaly, microcephaly or infantile spasms occur; mostly sporadic. Rare families show autosomal or X-linked inheritance

Table 11.1 (*Cont.*)

Ultrasound diagnosis	Pathological diagnosis	Comments
Agenesis of the cerebellar vermis	Same	May be isolated or occur as a feature of Joubert syndrome (autosomal recessive-mental retardation, cerebellar ataxia, retinal colobomata)
Hydranencephaly	Same	Absent cerebral hemispheres with meninges in normal position. Low recurrence risk
Choroid plexus cysts	Same	If present with other major sonographic abnormalities, karyotyping to exclude trisomy 18. If no other ultrasound markers, follow up scan at 23 weeks and if still present offer karyotyping

Prenatal diagnosis guidelines

Normal prenatal appearances

The transverse section of a normal head has a characteristic shape and important internal landmarks (Fig. 11.1(a)) which include the midline falx, the posterior horns of the lateral ventricles, the thalamic peduncles, the septum pellucidum and the anterior horns of the lateral ventricles. The posterior fossa should contain the cerebellum. The ossification of the spine is from the three primary centres, one in the body anteriorly and one in each half of the vertebral arch posteriorly. The latter two present a 'tramline' appearance on longitudinal scan and all three centres form a circular appearance on transverse scan (Figs. 11.1(b) and (c)). It should be possible to demonstrate skin cover over the whole length of the spine both in longitudinal and transverse scan planes.

Abnormal prenatal appearances

Anencephaly. First and early second trimester diagnosis of fetal anomalies is now possible by using the high frequency transvaginal probe (Rottem *et al.*, 1989). Anencephaly is usually readily recognized by 10−12 weeks on ultrasound examination. The appearance may vary slightly but the most striking feature is the absence of the cranial vault (Figs. 11.2(a), (b) and (c)). Secondary features which may provide the first clue on scanning are the presence of polyhydramnios (even during the first trimester), extended fetal legs and prominent facial features. The exposed brain tissue may be normal or decreased in amount. Spina bifida co-exists in 20% of cases. The absence of the cranial vault makes it impossible to measure the biparietal diameter and in early pregnancy will account for a smaller than expected crown−rump length.

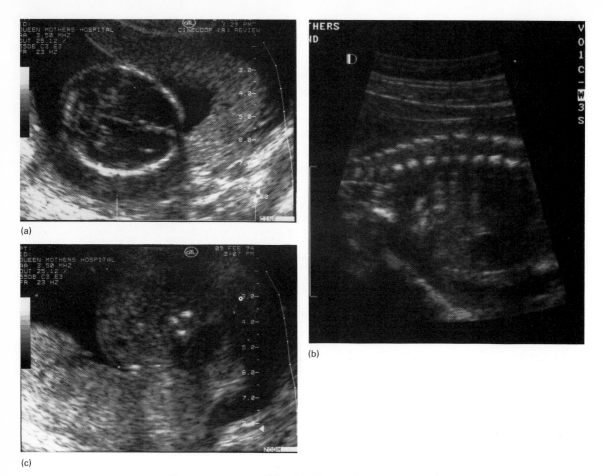

(a)

(b)

(c)

Fig. 11.1 (a) Normal head and cerebellum. (b) Normal longitudinal section of spine. (c) Transverse section of fetal spine showing ossification centres.

Spina bifida. The most severe spinal defects can be detected somewhat earlier and the least severe may not be seen until much later, especially if the lesion is small and skin covered (closed lesions comprise 20% of the total).

The anatomy of the head may provide the first clue to the presence of a spinal defect. In the transverse plane the outline of the head, which is normally oval in shape, becomes pointed anteriorly to give the lemon sign (Fig. 11.3(a)) (Nicolaides *et al.*, 1986; Penso *et al.*, 1987). This change is the result of the associated Arnold–Chiari malformation in which the cerebellum prolapses into the spinal canal and the frontal bones are drawn in. A further ultrasonic marker is the 'banana' sign which is an echo-free area anterior to the cerebellum (Fig. 11.3(b)) formed by the deformation of the cerebellum and descent of the brainstem.

Recognition of spina bifida is straightforward when a large part of the spine is involved but the detection of small defects, which can present only

124

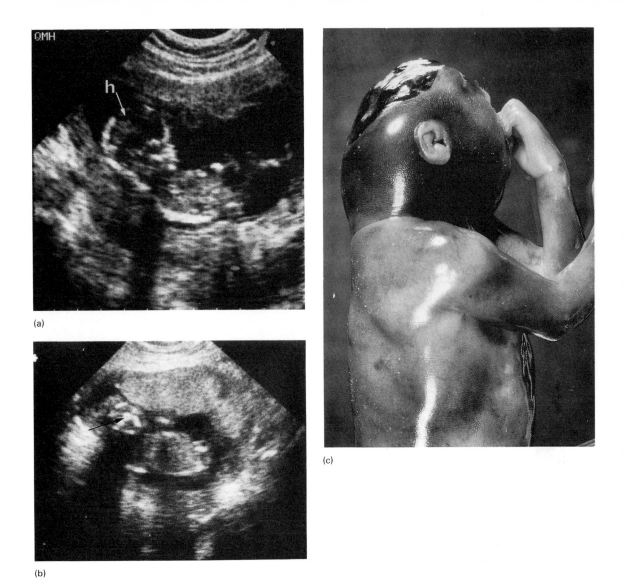

Fig. 11.2 (a) A normal fetus at 10 weeks with intact cranium, h, for comparison with Fig. 11.2b. (b) Ultrasound appearance of a 12-week anencephalic fetus — note prominent facial features. (c) Pathological appearance of anencephaly.

subtle changes on ultrasound examination, requires patience and skill and a close adherence to a routine to make sure that the whole spine has been examined. Spina bifida should not be confused with sacrococcygeal tumours which do not distort the spine. In spina bifida, deformity of the spine is seen on both longitudinal (Fig. 11.3(c)) and transverse scans (Fig. 11.3(d)). In the former, deviation from the 'tramline' occurs and on the transverse view there is a U-shaped deformity. The sac of a meningocele may be present. At present, the diagnosis of neural tube defects is best made using high resolution ultrasound and maternal serum α-fetoprotein screening,

125

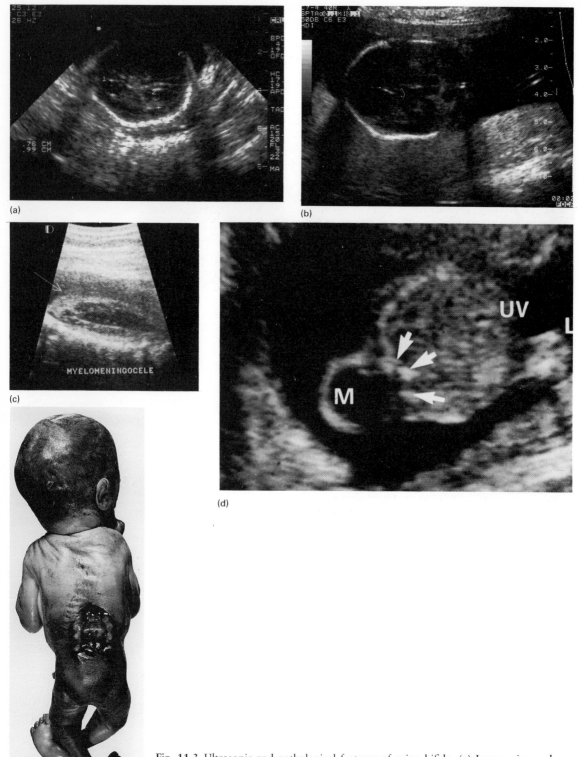

Fig. 11.3 Ultrasonic and pathological features of spina bifida. (a) Lemon sign and ventricular dilation. (b) A banana sign. (c) Large myelomeningocoele. (d) Spina bifida on transverse section scan showing: large myelomeningocoele, M; umbilical vein, UV; limb, L. (e) Pathological appearance of a thoracolumbar open spina bifida.

126

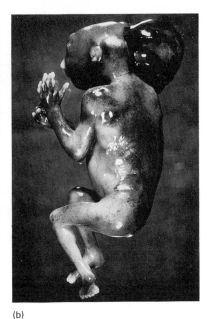

(a)

(b)

Fig. 11.4 Encephalocoele. (a) Ultrasound appearance of an 18-week fetus. Note the sac, e, contains cerebral tissue; c, cranium. (b) Pathological appearance.

thus avoiding the risks of amniocentesis (Morrow *et al.*, 1991). The pathological appearance of open spina bifida is shown in Figure 11.3(e).

Encephalocele. Encephaloceles are usually occipital but occasionally affect the frontal bones. There is a sac of varying size containing neural tissue which should be seen in continuity with the brain (Fig. 11.4(a)). The skull defect should be recognized. An encephalocele is distinguished from other soft tissue tumours at the back of the head and neck, such as cystic hygromata, by the presence of a skull defect in the former and an intact skull in the latter. Cystic hygromata tend to be mostly cystic whereas the brain tissue in an encephalocele is more solid. The value of transvaginal sonography in the discrimination of these two conditions has recently been reported (van Zalen-Sprock *et al.*, 1992). Most encephaloceles are inherited as multifactorial traits as components of the neural tube defect spectrum. In contrast, Meckel syndrome is inherited as an autosomal recessive trait (see Table 11.1).

Iniencephaly. In iniencephaly the fetus adopts the 'star-gazing' position and persistent hyperextension of the neck is readily noted. In this condition a transverse section of both head and abdomen can be seen in the one image (Fig. 11.5(a)). The pathological appearance is shown in Fig. 11.5(b).

Hydrocephalus. Hydrocephalus has a wide spectrum of appearances from the very obvious with virtually no cerebral tissue present (Fig. 11.6(a)) to

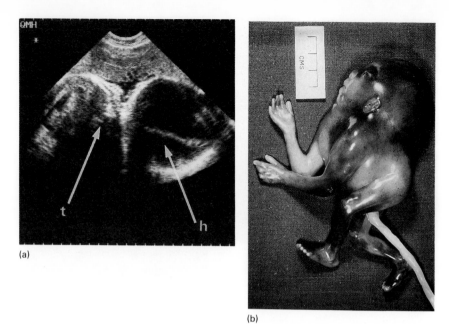

(a)

(b)

Fig. 11.5 (a) The ultrasound appearance of iniencephaly showing a transverse section of trunk, t, on the same level at the fetal head, h. There is also hydrocephalus. (b) The pathological appearance of iniencephaly.

minor degrees of ventriculomegaly which can be detected only by measurement of the width of the lateral ventricles. Assessment of the posterior horn (Fig. 11.6(b)) is considered to be the most sensitive guide to recognition of early hydrocephalus. Charts of normal ventricular:hemisphere ratios are available (Fig. 11.6(c)) (Campbell and Pearce, 1983). In general, the ventricles occupy up to 50% of the hemisphere before 20 weeks' gestation, decreasing to about 33% thereafter. Serial assessment will demonstrate progression in ventricular enlargement. In addition, the depth of the cerebral mantle may be measured, a decrease in size suggesting deterioration. It is not necessary for the head measurements, either biparietal diameter, circumference or area, to be increased for a diagnosis of hydrocephalus to be made. Head size and shape are within normal limits in the early stages of ventriculomegaly and only in extreme cases is the head clearly enlarged. Small head size with ventriculomegaly may carry a grave prognosis. Serial assessments of pregnancies at risk have revealed onset in some cases only in the third trimester or after birth.

Other cerebral malformations

Holoprosencephaly. This is a condition in which only a single large ventricle is seen, or with a small skull containing no midline echo, disorganized cerebral ventricles and prominent cerebral peduncles (Fig. 11.7). An early diagnosis of alobar holoprosencephaly at 14 weeks, employing

128

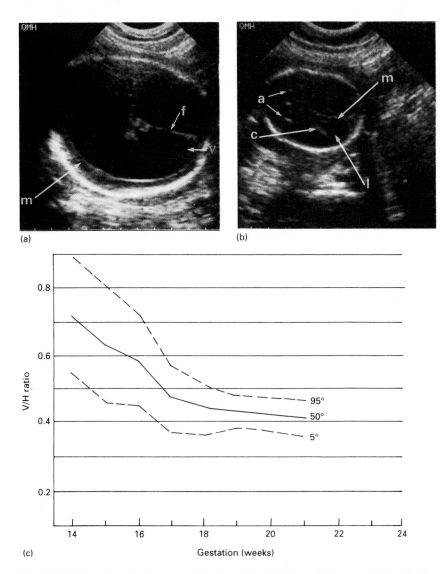

(a)

(b)

(c)

Fig. 11.6 (a) Hydrocephalus: m, cerebral mantle; f, falix cerebri; v, ventricle. (b) The appearances of a dilated posterior ventricular horn showing: c, choroid plexus; l, lateral wall; m, medial wall of posterior horn. Note that the anterior horns, a, are not displaced. (c) The normal range for ventricular : hemispheric ratios (Campbell and Pearce 1983).

transvaginal ultrasound, has been reported (Bronshtein and Wiener, 1991). The prognosis is either lethal or associated with a severe degree of mental disability whether or not the structural abnormality is associated with chromosomal defects, typically trisomy 13.

Agenesis of the corpus callosum. This is associated with an enlarged third ventricle and dilated posterior horns of the lateral ventricles. There is also increased separation of the frontal horns and bodies of the lateral ventricles,

129

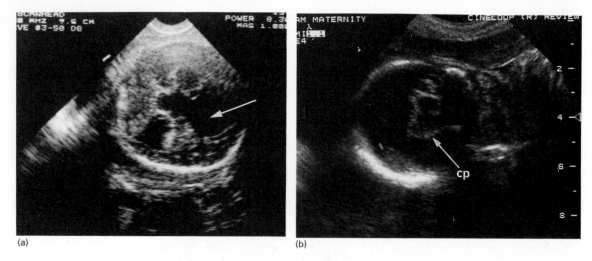

Fig. 11.7 (a) Scan showing cerebral ventricular appearances in holoprosencephaly — the fetus was at 32 weeks. (b) Prominent cerebral peduncles in a case of alobar holoprosencephaly. cp, fused cerebral peduncles.

concavity of the medial wall of the frontal horns of the lateral ventricle and absence of the cavum septum pellucidum. Antenatal diagnosis of the condition has been achieved in seven cases and a summary of these cases has been published (Bryce *et al.*, 1990). Since there is a high chance of associated cerebral anomalies, a detailed scan of the cranial and extracranial systems should be performed. If any other anomaly is detected, then the prognosis is that of the other condition, which is usually very poor. Some cases may have an autosomal recessive or sex-linked pattern of inheritance. Dandy–Walker syndrome is associated with hydrocephalus, partial or complete absence of the cerebellar vermis, posterior fossa cyst contiguous with the fourth ventricle. There is an abnormal head shape in addition to the presence of fluid filling the posterior fossa and communicating with the fourth ventricle. The Dandy–Walker syndrome is aetiologically heterogeneous with an empiric recurrence risk of 1–5% (Fig. 11.8).

Microcephaly. In microcephaly the anatomical appearance of the brain is usually normal. The diagnosis will be made only by finding abnormally small head measurements in relation to abdominal or long bone size (Fig. 11.9). The need to include measurements of several parameters of fetal size must be emphasized since the diagnosis of microcephaly would be missed if only a biparietal diameter was taken. The head/abdomen circumference can be used (Campbell and Pearce, 1983) but comparison with long bone length can be equally useful. Microcephaly is unlikely to be recognized on a single examination and inappropriate head size may not be obvious until the late second or even third trimester (Tolmie *et al.*, 1987). However, in some cases, if there is to be any chance of second trimester ultrasound

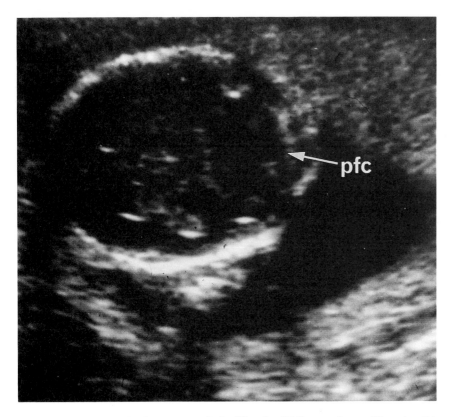

Fig. 11.8 Large posterior fossa cyst typical of Dandy–Walker syndrome. There is mild hydrocephalus. pfc, posterior fossa cyst.

diagnosis, the pregnancy must be scanned frequently from an early stage and the obstetrician should be prepared to intervene when the growth velocity fails even though measurements at this stage are within normal centiles (Tolmie, 1991).

Intracranial cysts. The appearance of cysts within the brain substance and the absence or partial absence of areas of the brain will only be appreciated by the sonographer who has a clear knowledge of the normal anatomical features of the brain throughout gestation. The differential diagnosis includes porencephalic cysts (unexplained or secondary to a dead twin) and choroid plexus cysts (Fig. 11.10). The latter are usually seen in the second trimester and in most cases resolve spontaneously by the third trimester (Ostlere *et al.*, 1989). One hundred and twenty antenatally detected choroid plexus cysts were reviewed by Bryce *et al.*, 1990, 10 of these were associated with chromosomal abnormalities (one trisomy 21 and seven trisomy 18). In each of the seven cases with trisomy 18 where a follow-up scan was performed, the cyst was noted to persist beyond 23 weeks' gestation. Choroid plexus cysts are usually small (10 mm or less) and can be unilateral

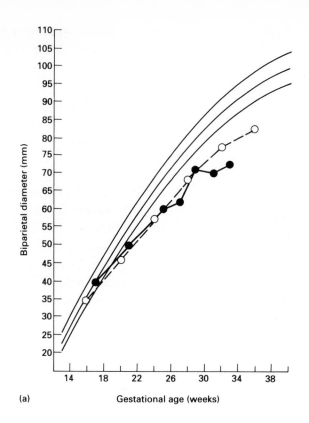

(a)

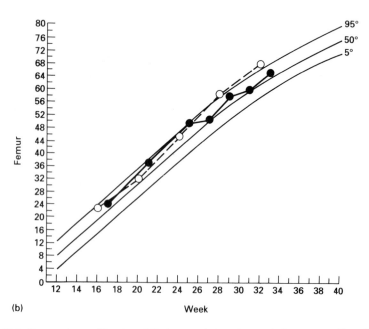

(b)

Fig. 11.9 Comparison of head and limb growth in microcephaly in two affected pregnancies. (a) Reduced change in BPD with gestational age. (b) Normal increase in femur length with gestational age.

132

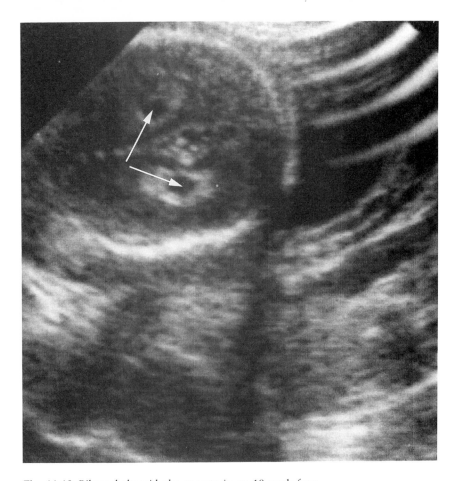

Fig. 11.10 Bilateral choroid plexus cysts in an 18-week fetus.

or bilateral; single or multiple. If the karyotype is normal they have no significant long term effects. It is recommended that if a cyst is over 10 mm in diameter or if it persists beyond 23 weeks' gestation then karyotyping should be offered, as well as detailed ultrasound, to look for other markers of trisomy 18. However, a more recent study (Howard *et al.*, 1992) concludes that the presence of choroid plexus cysts at 18–20 weeks should be an indication for a detailed ultrasound examination, and karyotyping only if dysmorphic features are present.

CNS malformations and mental retardation

Many CNS malformations are associated with mental retardation and, as indicated above, certain of these are prenatally detectable. Other causes such as chromosomal disorders (see Chapter 5), single gene disorders (see Chapters 3 and 8) and fetal infections (see Chapter 9) are also usually prenatally detectable. In the remainder, the diagnosis may be a CNS

133

malformation such as lissencephaly, which has only recently been diagnosed by ultrasound (Saltzman *et al.*, 1991), idiopathic dysmorphic syndromes (only a few of which have specific diagnostic tests) and idiopathic or unexplained mental retardation where specific prenatal diagnosis is not possible.

Lissencephaly

Defective neuronal migration during the third to fifth months can result in a smooth brain surface (lissencephaly), few broad thick gyri (pachygyria) or many small plications (polymicrogyria). These changes may co-exist in different areas of the same brain and may result in mental retardation and epilepsy with, in some cases, a characteristic EEG and computed tomography appearance. The aetiology includes several autosomal recessive traits and the Miller–Dieker syndrome due to partial deletion of the short arm of chromosome 17. The first two cases of type I lissencephaly (Miller–Dieker syndrome) have recently been reported as being detected ultrasonically (Saltzman *et al.*, 1991). For a couple with one child affected by unexplained isolated lissencephaly, the empiric recurrence risk for siblings is probably under 10%.

Idiopathic syndromes

A syndrome is a non-random concurrence of abnormalities which are aetiologically related. For many syndromes the aetiology is as yet unknown but identification is still important as it allows meaningful genetic counselling and can be a guide to prognosis. There are now several computerized databases to assist clinical geneticists in the differential diagnosis of syndromes and the largest of these contain over 1000 distinct conditions. Table 11.2 lists some of the more common of these idiopathic syndromes, which cause mental retardation, and indicates recurrence risks and, in a few, the availability of specific prenatal diagnosis.

Unexplained mental retardation

Despite the advances in techniques for investigation, about one-quarter of severe mental retardation remains unexplained (Connor and Ferguson-Smith, 1988). Genetic counselling in such families needs to use empiric (or observed) recurrence risks derived from comparable families in the medical literature (Fig. 11.11). Strictly speaking, these risks apply only to the population from which they were derived and differing criteria of study have resulted in a range of observed recurrence risks. In practice, most couples who have a child with idiopathic mental retardation have an appreciable recurrence risk, and specific prenatal diagnosis cannot be offered.

Table 11.2 Commoner idiopathic syndromes identified in mentally retarded patients. (After Connor and Ferguson-Smith 1988)

Condition	Empiric recurrence for normal parents	Specific prenatal diagnosis
Beckwith–Wiedemann syndrome	Low*	+
Coffin–Siris syndrome	Low*	−
de Lange syndrome	2–6%	(+)
Focal dermal hypoplasia (Goltz syndrome)	Negligible†	−
Happy puppet syndrome	10%	−
Hemifacial microsomia	Negligible	+
Incontinentia pigmenti	Negligible†	−
Linear sebaceous naevus syndrome	Negligible	−
Noonan syndrome	Negligible*	−
Rett syndrome	Negligible†	−
Rubinstein–Taybi syndrome	1%	−
Sotos syndrome	Negligible*	−
Sturge–Weber syndrome	Negligible	−
Williams syndrome	Negligible	−

* May be inherited as an autosomal dominant trait in some families.
† X-linked dominant inheritance with male lethality suspected.
+, Probable; −, not possible; (+), possible but uncertain.

Management

Once a fetal CNS malformation is suspected it is important that the mother is counselled accordingly and referred for a detailed anomaly scan both to confirm the suspected diagnosis and to exclude other malformations. Since CNS malformations may be secondary to chromosomal syndromes or fetal infections, fetal blood sampling for a rapid karyotype and viral studies may need to be considered in cases with good or uncertain prognosis. For certain CNS malformations such as anencephaly, hydranencephaly and holoprosencephaly, the prognosis is uniformly poor. Choroid plexus cysts may spontaneously resolve but for the remainder of prenatally detected CNS malformations the prognosis is usually uncertain. Extrapolation of potential function from anatomical appearances is fraught with difficulty and in counselling parents, one should explain the limitations of making a precise prognosis in every case. With therapy, about one-third of babies with open spina bifida survive for 5 years and of those, 85% are severely disabled; only 5% have no disability. In our experience, almost without exception, couples have chosen termination of the pregnancy when the diagnosis of anencephaly or open spina bifida is made in the second

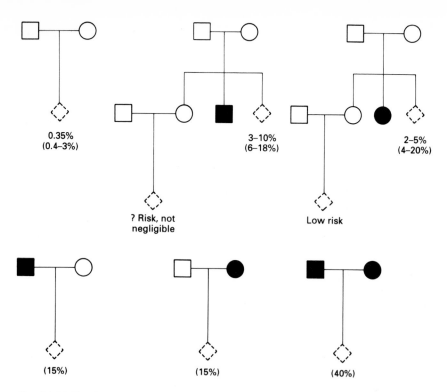

Fig. 11.11 Empiric recurrence risks are given for severe (IQ < 50) mental retardation and any degree (IQ < 70) of mental retardation (with the latter in parentheses) for various pregnancies in the absence of a specific diagnosis in the proband. (After Connor and Ferguson-Smith 1988.)

trimester. If continuation of the pregnancy is preferred, or a late diagnosis is made, serial ultrasound examinations should be performed to assess the progression of ventriculomegaly, both by measurement of the lateral ventricles and the cerebral mantle. In those cases in which pregnancy continues, delivery should be planned in a unit where the appropriate paediatric care is available. In most cases, spontaneous labour and vaginal delivery can be anticipated. Exceptions include progressive hydrocephalus when elective delivery may be indicated to allow early postnatal shunting; and extreme cases of hydrocephalus with no cerebral mantle where decompression may be necessary to facilitate vaginal delivery. Chervenak *et al.*, (1984) recommend that all cases of spina bifida should be delivered by elective caesarean section. Attempts have been made (see Chapter 17) to perform a ventriculoamniotic shunt to prevent progression of hydrocephalus (Manning *et al.*, 1986), but these efforts have met with so little success that the procedure has been abandoned.

Postnatal assessment

All couples who have had a baby with a CNS malformation should be

136

offered genetic counselling to cover the condition's recurrence risk, range of prognosis and potential for future prenatal diagnosis.

REFERENCES

Bronshtein, M. and Weiner, Z. (1991) Early transvaginal sonographic diagnosis of alobar holoprosencephaly. *Prenatal Diagnosis*, **11**, 459–62.

Bryce, F.C., Lilford, R.J. and Rodeck, C.R. (1990) Antenatal diagnosis of craniospinal defects. Chapter 1, in *Prenatal diagnosis and prognosis* (ed. R.J. Liford), Butterworth-Heinemann, Oxford.

Campbell, S. and Pearce, J.M. (1983) Ultrasound visualisation of congenital malformations. *British Medical Bulletin*, **39**, 322–31.

Chervenak, F.A., Duncan, C., Ment, L.R., Tortota, M., McClure, M. and Hobbins, J. (1984) Perinatal management of meningomyelocele. *Obstetrics and Gynecology*, **63**, 376–80.

Connor, J.M. and Ferguson-Smith, M.A. (1988) Genetic causes of mental handicap. In *Antenatal and Perinatal Causes of Handicap, Baillière's Clinical Obstetrics and Gynaecology* (eds. R. Kubli and N. Patel), Baillière Tindall, London.

Howard, R.J., Tuck, S.M., Long, J. and Thomas, V. (1992) The significance of choroid plexus cysts in fetuses at 18–20 weeks. An indication for amniocentesis? *Prenatal Diagnosis*, **12**, 685–88.

Manning, F.A., Harrison, M.R. and Rodeck, C. (1986) Catheter shunts for fetal hydrocephalus: Report of the International Fetal Surgery Registry. *New England Journal of Medicine*, **315**, 336–40.

Morrow, R.J., McNay, M.B. and Whittle, M.J. (1991) Ultrasound detection of neural tube defects in patients with elevated maternal serum alphafetoprotein. *American Journal of Obstetrics and Gynecology*, **78**, 1055–57.

Nicolaides, K.H., Campbell, S., Gabbe, S.G. and Guidetti, R. (1986) Ultrasound screening for spina bifida: cranial and cerebellar signs. *Lancet*, **2**, 72–4.

Omran, M., Stone, D.H. and McLoone, P. (1992) Pattern of decline in prevalence of anencephaly and spina bifida in a high-risk area. *Health Bulletin*, **50**(5), 407–13.

Ostlere, S.J., Irving, H.C. and Lilford, R.J. (1989) A prospective study of the incidence and significance of fetal choroid plexus cysts. *Prenatal Diagnosis*, **9**, 205–11.

Penso, C., Redline, R.W. and Benacerraf, B.R. (1987) A sonographic sign which predicts which fetuses with hydrocephalus have an associated neural tube defect. *Journal of Ultrasound Medicine*, **6**, 307–11.

Saltzman, D.H., Krauss, C.M., Goldman, J.M. and Benacerraf, B.R. (1992) Prenatal diagnosis of lissencephaly. *Prenatal Diagnosis*, **11**, 139–43.

Rottem, S., Bronshtein, M., Thaler, I. and Brandes, J.M. (1989) First trimester sonographic diagnosis of fetal anomalies. *Lancet I*, 444–45.

Tolmie, J.L. (1991) Prenatal diagnosis of microcephaly. *Prenatal Diagnosis*, **11**, 347.

Tolmie, J.L., McNay, M.B., Stephenson, J.B.P., Doyle, D. and Connor, J.M. (1987) Microcephaly: genetic counselling and antenatal diagnosis after the birth of an affected child. *American Journal of Medical Genetics*, **27**, 583–94.

van Zalen-Sprock, M.M., van Vugt, J.M.G., van der Harten, H.J. and van Geijn, H.P. (1992) Cephalocoele and cystic hygroma: diagnosis and differentiation in the first trimester of pregnancy with transvaginal sonography. Report of two cases. *International Journal of Ultrasound in Obstetrics and Gynecology*, **2**, 289–92.

Chapter 12
Gastrointestinal Tract Malformations

A. D. CAMERON and M. B. McNAY

Gastrointestinal tract malformations comprise 15% of the structural abnormalities detected antenatally. Most have characteristic appearances on ultrasound and many have a good prognosis after prompt surgical correction provided they are not components of more complex syndromes.

PRENATAL CLASSIFICATION

Table 12.1 indicates the major gastrointestinal malformations which can be identified with ultrasound and, in contrast to malformations in some other areas, there is a fairly close correlation with the pathological classification.

Identification of at-risk pregnancies

As indicated in Table 12.1, some gastrointestinal tract malformations are inherited, and thus a family history or a previously affected child can be an important clue to the at-risk pregnancy. Several teratogens may cause cleft lip and palate (see Chapter 10) but in general they are not associated with other gastrointestinal malformations. In practice, however, most affected pregnancies are not predicted and suspicion is raised by a large-for-dates uterus with polyhydramnios (intestinal atresia and most cases of diaphragmatic hernia) or by elevated maternal serum α-fetoprotein (MSAFP) (anterior abdominal wall defects).

PRENATAL DIAGNOSIS GUIDELINES

Normal prenatal appearances

Normally two fluid-filled areas are seen within the fetal abdomen — the stomach and the bladder. The stomach should be seen, in its normal position, below the heart on the left side. The anterior abdominal wall and the entrance of the cord vessels into the fetus must be carefully examined. The bowel should be examined in both longitudinal and transverse sections through the fetal abdomen. In the late third trimester the large bowel is usually apparent as sonolucent areas around the periphery of the abdominal cavity. The small bowel is usually barely distinguishable. The gall bladder may also be seen on a transverse view of the fetal abdomen.

Table 12.1 Major gastrointestinal malformations identifiable by ultrasound

Ultrasound diagnosis	Pathological diagnosis	Comments
Exomphalos/omphalocoele	Same	Affects 1/5000 pregnancies; other malformations 50%, exclude trisomy 18, Beckwith–Wiedemann syndrome (macroglossia, generalized organomegaly). Low recurrence risk if isolated (<1%)
Gastroschisis	Same	Affects 1/5000 pregnancies; may be secondary intestinal atresias. Other malformations are rare (<5%). Low recurrence risk if isolated (<1%)
Body stalk anomaly	Same anomaly	Rare; lower limbs abnormal and may be absent; very short or absent umbilical cord; may have NTD. Incompatible with independent survival. Low recurrence risk if isolated
Oesophageal atresia	Same atresia	Affects 1/3000 pregnancies; tracheo-oesophageal fistula coexists in 90%; other anomalies in over 50% including NTD and VATER association. The specific recurrence risk for oesophageal atresia is 0.6% but an unexplained threefold increase in NTD in subsequent offspring is apparent
Duodenal atresia	Same	Affects 1/10 000 pregnancies; other anomalies in over 30%, exclude trisomy 21; low recurrence risk if isolated
Jejunal atresia	Same Apple peel syndrome	Low recurrence risk Autosomal recessive trait, characteristic appearance at surgery with agenesis of the mesentery and twisting of the distal small bowel around the marginal artery
Ileal atresia	Same	Low recurrence risk
Anorectal atresia	Same	Affects 1/5000 pregnancies; may be a component of VATER syndrome; low recurrence risk if isolated
Diaphragmatic hernia	Same	Affects 1/2000 pregnancies; other anomalies in 55%. Recurrence risk under 1%. Fryns syndrome: autosomal recessive with diaphragmatic hernia, dysmorphic facies and distal digital hypoplasia

(Continued)

139

Table 12.1 (*Cont.*)

Ultrasound diagnosis	Pathological diagnosis	Comments
Meconium ileus	Cystic fibrosis Isolated meconium ileus	Autosomal recessive trait
Cleft lip/palate	Same	Affects 1/1000 pregnancies; a component of over 100 syndromes; if isolated usually inherited as a multifactorial trait with a recurrence risk of 2–5%
Intra-abdominal cysts	Choledochal cyst Ovarian cyst	Elrad *et al.* (1985) Preziosi *et al.* (1986)
Intra-abdominal calcification	Ischaemic hepatic necrosis Gallstones	Nguyen and Leonard (1986) Heijne and Ednay (1985)

NTD, neural tube defect; VATER association, vertebral, anal, cardiac, renal and radial limb anomalies.

Abnormal prenatal appearances

Exomphalos (omphalocele)

The size of an exomphalos varies from a small umbilical hernia to a large lesion containing most of the abdominal viscera. A sac should be seen in continuity with the abdominal wall and the vessels of the cord traverse the sac (Fig. 12.1(a)). The intestinal loops have normally returned to the fetal abdomen by the 12th week and a large exomphalos should be detectable from 14 to 16 weeks onwards; smaller defects may not be recognized until 18–20 weeks.

Gastroschisis

In gastroschisis there is no sac, the cord is seen separately from the defect (usually to the right) and the bowel lies free in the amniotic cavity (Fig. 12.2). Occasionally a normal umbilical cord will be mistaken for extruded fetal bowel. It is important, because of the different associations, to distinguish gastroschisis from a ruptured exomphalos (Glick *et al.*, 1985). In the latter, the remains of the sac should be evident.

Body stalk anomaly

The appearances in body stalk anomaly are grossly abnormal and there should be no difficulty in making the diagnosis.

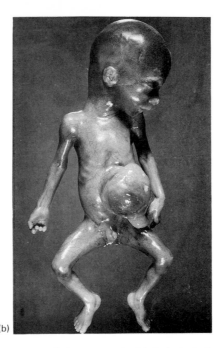

(a)

(b)

Fig. 12.1 Exomphalos. (a) Transverse section (exomphalos arrowed). (b) Pathological appearance in a fetus.

Often the surprising feature is that the fetus appears normal from the waist up but there is total disruption of the anatomy below (Fig. 12.3). Because of the degree of kyphosis and scoliosis, spina bifida may be considered as a differential diagnosis but the spine is intact though deformed.

Oesophageal atresia

Oesophageal atresia without a fistula prevents any fluid reaching the stomach although if a tracheo-oesophageal fistula (TOF) coexists fluid is seen in the stomach. Ideally, the fetus should be seen to swallow enabling the outline of the oesophagus to be identified.

Duodenal atresia

Duodenal atresia presents the classic 'double bubble' (Fig. 12.4) due to dilatation of both the stomach and the first part of the duodenum proximal to the obstruction. This appearance may only be intermittently present because of fetal vomiting.

Jejunal atresia

This presents a 'third bubble' (Fig. 12.5).

141

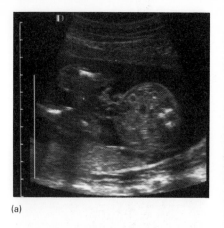

(a)

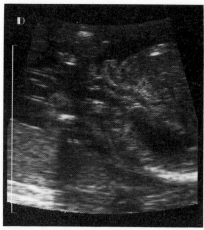

(b)

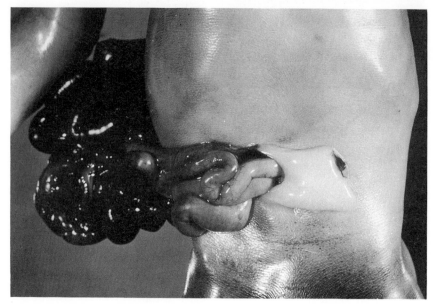

(c)

Fig. 12.2 (a) Transverse section of fetal trunk showing small bowel extending through abdominal wall defect. (b) Magnified image of 12.2(a). (c) Pathological appearance of gastroschisis in a fetus.

Lower bowel atresias

The echo patterns are less characteristic.

Meconium ileus

This is recognized as a cluster of dense echoes in the lower abdomen (Fig. 12.6(a)) (Nyberg *et al.*, 1987). In cases of cystic fibrosis, prenatal diagnosis may also be possible by DNA analysis of chorionic villi.

142

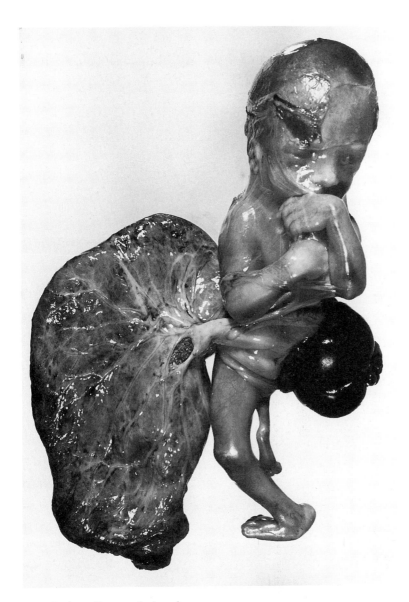

Fig. 12.3 Body stalk anomaly in a fetus.

Diaphragmatic hernia

The appearance of a diaphragmatic hernia (Fig. 12.7(a)) varies according to the size of the defect. The intact diaphragm is seen ultrasonically as an echo-free line separating the abdomen and thorax. This line either cannot be identified, or is seen only in part, when there is a defect present. The first clue is usually the finding of the stomach or bowel shadows in the chest. In severe cases the movement in the thorax of the liver during fetal 'breathing' is particularly obvious in later pregnancy. Diagnosis may not

143

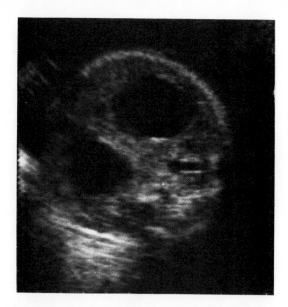

Fig. 12.4 'Double bubble' due to duodenal atresia in a fetus.

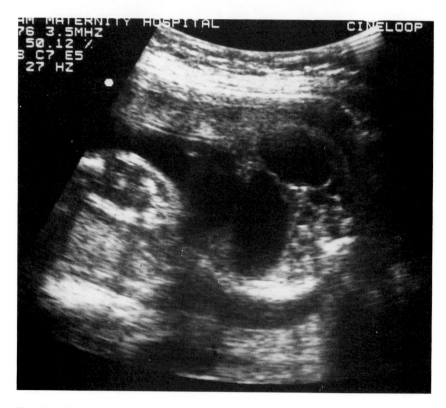

Fig. 12.5 Transverse section of a baby with jejunal atresia showing three 'bubbles'.

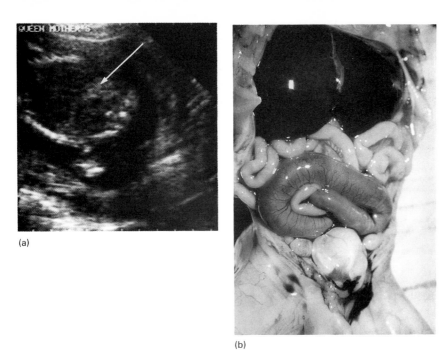

Fig. 12.6 (a) Echo dense areas of meconium plug (arrowed) in an 18-week fetus with cystic fibrosis. (b) Pathological appearance in the same fetus following termination of the pregnancy.

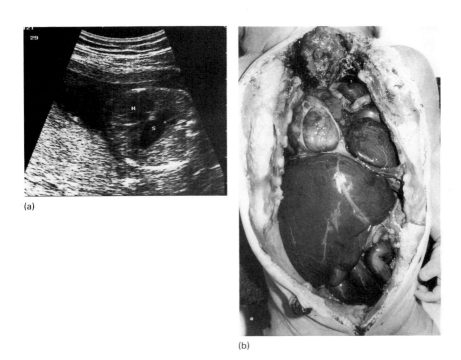

Fig. 12.7 (a) Ultrasound appearances of diaphragmatic hernia. H, heart; S, stomach. (b) Pathological appearance.

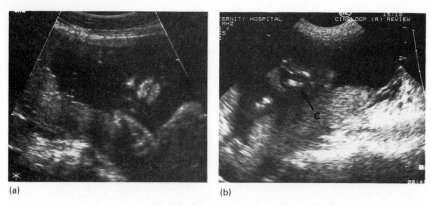

(a)   (b)

Fig. 12.8 Ultrasound appearance of fetal lips (a) normal lips. (b) large unilateral cleft. c, cleft.

be possible until after 20 weeks; differential diagnosis includes cystic adenomatoid malformation of the lung.

Cleft lip/palate

The facial features can be seen with remarkable clarity and theoretically, cleft lip could be diagnosed in all but the least severe cases from 16 weeks onwards if the time was taken to obtain the appropriate views (Seeds and Cefalo, 1983; Pilu *et al.*, 1986). Cleft palate alone is more difficult to visualize on ultrasound (Fig. 12.8).

Intra-abdominal cysts

'Cystic' areas within the fetal abdomen must be interpreted with care. They may be true cysts, portions of dilated bowel or urinary tract, or collections of fluid. Isolated cysts may occur including ovarian cysts, (Preziosi *et al.*, 1986) which may result from maternal hormone production. Cysts may reach a considerable size (Fig. 12.9) and require surgical intervention after delivery but they may regress spontaneously in the postnatal period. Cysts thought to be of mesenteric origin have been seen on ultrasound examination without any associated pathology and have regressed spontaneously prior to delivery.

Less commonly seen are choledochal cysts (Wiedman *et al.*, 1985; Elrad *et al.*, 1985) or areas which appear as cysts but are, in fact, pools of fluid collecting amongst adhesions.

Management

In all cases of gastrointestinal malformations recognized prenatally, a careful search for other structural anomalies should be performed by an

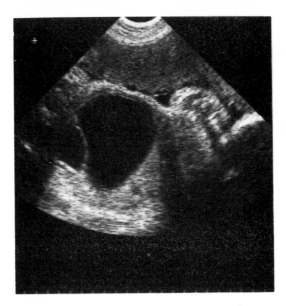

Fig. 12.9 Longitudinal section of the fetal abdomen showing a large ovarian cyst (with the normal bladder to the left).

experienced sonographer and the fetal karyotype should be obtained, preferably by fetal blood sampling for rapid results. Many of the gastro-intestinal malformations detected by ultrasound are surgically correctable and in counselling the parents the surgical prognosis for the lesion is important (see Chapter 19). Serial ultrasound examinations are made in the continuing pregnancies to assess any change in the anomaly (especially bowel obstruction in anterior abdominal wall defects), to monitor growth and development and to assess amniotic fluid volume and placental maturation (Crawford *et al.*, 1992). *In utero* surgery has been attempted for diaphragmatic hernia but the value of this approach is disputed. Termination of pregnancy may be considered in cases of body stalk anomaly and in malformations where multiple problems coexist or if the defect is large. The overall mortality for cases of diaphragmatic herniae diagnosed antenatally is 80%. Prognosis is influenced by the presence of polyhydramnios, the size of the defect (i.e. the amount of abdominal contents in the chest, displacement of the heart and alteration in the relative sizes of the right and left ventricles and the presence of other anomalies. The main cause of death in infants with diaphragmatic herniae is pulmonary hypoplasia. For babies who survive the first 48 hours of life, neonatal surgery offers a probability for survival of approximately 50% (see Chapter 19). If the parents decide to continue with the pregnancy, then there is no advantage for either abdominal or elective premature delivery.

In all other cases, continuation of the pregnancy is the likely course of action and arrangements should be made for delivery in an obstetric unit close to a paediatric centre with expert medical and surgical facilities. Treatment with extracorporeal membrane oxygenation (ECMO) may improve the prognosis for neonates with diaphragmatic herniae.

The mode of delivery in cases of exomphalos and gastroschisis has been the subject of much debate (Lenke and Hatch, 1986; Moore and Nur, 1986; Hasan and Hermansen, 1986; Kirk and Wah, 1983) and there is conflicting evidence over whether elective abdominal delivery in all cases will improve the outcome. It would seem reasonable in gastroschisis and small exomphalos, in the absence of complications, to await the spontaneous onset of labour and anticipate a vaginal delivery (Morrow *et al.*, 1993). The presence of complications or a large exomphalos, which could lead to an obstructed labour or rupture during delivery, will necessitate caesarean section. The most important feature in all cases is to make the delivery room staff and the paediatricians aware of the diagnosis. This is particularly important in cases of oesophageal atresia and diaphragmatic hernia to allow early treatment to establish the infant's airway and to prevent any attempts at oral feeding of the baby. There will be occasions when delivery at the patient's nearest maternity unit is more practical with subsequent transfer to a paediatric centre. This would be appropriate, for example, in cases of lower intestinal atresia where a delay in surgery of several hours is not life threatening.

Postnatal assessment

All couples who have had a child with a gastrointestinal malformation should be offered genetic counselling to discuss the condition's recurrence risk, range of prognosis and potential for future prenatal diagnosis.

REFERENCES

Crawford, R.A.F., Ryan, G., Wright, W.M. and Rodeck, C.H. (1992) The importance of serial biophysical assessment of fetal well-being in gastroschisis. *British Journal of Obstetrics and Gynaecology*, **99**, 899–902.

Elrad, H., Mayden, K.L., Ahart, S., Giglia, R. and Gleicher, N. (1985) Prenatal ultrasound diagnosis of choledochal cyst. *Journal of Ultrasound Medicine*, **4**, 553–55.

Glick, P.L., Harrison, M.R., Adzick, N.S., Filly, R.A., de Lorimier, A.A. and Callen, P.W. (1985) The missing link in the pathogenesis of gastroschisis. *Journal of Pediatric Surgery*, **20**, 306–309.

Hasan, S. and Hermansen, M.C. (1986) The prenatal diagnosis of ventral abdominal wall defects. *American Journal of Obstetrics and Gynecology*, **155**, 842–45.

Heijne, L. and Ednay, D. (1985) The development of fetal gallstones demonstrated by ultrasound. *Radiography*, **51**, 155–56.

Kirk, E.P. and Wah, R.M. (1983) Obstetric management of the fetus with omphalocele or gastroschisis: A review and report of one hundred and twelve cases. *American Journal of Obstetrics and Gynecology*, **146**, 512–18.

Lenke, R.R. and Hatch, E.I. (1986) Fetal gastroschisis: A preliminary report advocating the use of caesarean section. *Obstetrics and Gynecology*, **67**, 395–98.

Moore, T.C. and Nur, K. (1986) An international survey of gastroschisis and omphalocele

CHAPTER 12
*Gastrointestinal
Tract Malformations*

(490 cases). 1. Nature and distribution of additional malformations. *Paediatric Surgery International*, 1, 46−50.

Morrow, R.J., Whittle, M.J., McNay, M.B. *et al.* (1993) Prenatal diagnosis and management of anterior abdominal wall defects in the west of Scotland *Prenatal Diagnosis*, 13, 111−16.

Nguyen, D.L. and Leonard, J.C. (1986) Ischemic hepatic necrosis: a cause of fetal liver calcification. *American Journal of Radiology*, 147, 596−97.

Nyberg, D.A., Hastrup, W., Watts, H. and Mack, L.A. (1987) Dilated fetal bowel. A sonographic sign of cystic fibrosis. *Journal of Ultrasound in Medicine*, 6, 257−60.

Pilu, G., Reece, F.A., Romero, R., Bovicelli, L. and Hobbins, J.C. (1986) Prenatal diagnosis of craniofacial malformations with ultrasonography. *American Journal of Obstetrics and Gynecology*, 155, 45−50.

Preziosi, P., Fariello, G., Maiorana, A., Malena, S. and Ferro, F. (1986) Antenatal sonographic diagnosis of complicated ovarian cysts. *Journal of Clinical Ultrasound*, 14, 196−98.

Seeds, J.W. and Cefalo, R.C. (1983) Technique of early sonographic diagnosis of bilateral cleft lip and palate. *Obstetrics and Gynecology*, 62 (suppl.), 28−78.

Wiedman, M.A., Tan, A. and Martinez, C.J. (1985) Fetal sonography and neonatal scintigraphy of a choledochal cyst. *Journal of Nuclear Medicine*, 26, 893−96.

Chapter 13
Cardiovascular Malformations

M. J. WHITTLE

Structural abnormalities of the heart have a frequency of 8 per 1000 births and represent about 10% of all congenital malformations (Freed, 1984). This incidence includes both severe and more trivial abnormalities and a 6 year review suggested that 'critical' disease had an incidence of about 2 per 1000 births (Fyler *et al.*, 1980).

PRENATAL CLASSIFICATION

Most paediatric textbooks classify congenital heart disease on the basis of cyanosis which is obviously not appropriate for the fetus. From the prenatal diagnosis standpoint, conditions can be classified according to ultrasound appearance (Table 13.1).

Identification of at-risk pregnancies

The aetiology of heart disease is largely unknown except in some well-defined circumstances. About 8% of cases are associated with chromosome anomalies, such as Down syndrome, about 3% with single gene defects and about 2% with various environmental insults but in over 85% of cases there are no obvious causative factors and multifactorial inheritance is suspected.

Family and past history are a strong influence although precise risks are often quite difficult to determine since they depend upon the type of lesion. Risks also depend upon whether the parent or a sib has the cardiac anomaly (Tables 13.2 and 13.3). A recurrence is likely to be the same as the original defect in only about 50% of the cases. The risks for individual conditions are shown in Table 13.4.

Perinatal infections are a potential cause of congenital heart disease. When maternal rubella is contracted in the first trimester, a common anomaly is pulmonary arterial stenosis (50–75%) followed by patent ductus arteriosus and coarctation of the aortic isthmus.

Fetal cytomegalovirus infections have also been associated with cardiac anomalies such as atrial septal defects and mitral stenosis but on a less secure basis.

150

Table 13.1 Cardiovascular conditions classified according to ultrasound appearance

Ultrasound diagnosis	Pathological diagnosis	Comments
Abnormal four chamber view		
Ventricular septal defect	Same	Only seen if large In general good prognosis
Hypoplastic ventricles or univentricular heart	1 Hypoplastic left or right heart. Extent of hypoplasia may not correlate with ultrasound 2 Atretic valves (pulmonary, aortic, mitral)	Generally poor prognosis although some series report up to 50% survivors following surgery
Atrial septal defect (secundum)	Same	Defect exists through foramen ovale in fetus so ultrasound diagnosis not possible
Atrioventricular canal	Primum defects (endocardial cushions)	May occur with other anomalies e.g. Down syndrome. Poor prognosis
Tricuspid valve atresia	1 Tricuspid valve atresia VSD and hypoplastic right heart 2 Ebstein's anomaly — variable severity	Prognosis depends on patent foramen Prognosis in Ebstein's anomaly very variable. Associated with lithium ingestion
Cardiac tumours	Rhabdomyoma commonly	50% associated with tuberous sclerosis
Displacement of heart	1 Dextrocardia 2 Ectopia cordis	
Abnormal outflow/inflow tracts		
Narrow pulmonary artery Overriding aorta/VSD/ ventricular hypertrophy	Fallot's tetralogy	Variable severity — mild cases likely to be missed in ultrasound. Prognosis usually good
Transposition of the great vessels	Same	Extracardiac abnormalities rare. Prognosis good
Total anomalous pulmonary venous drainage (TAPVD)	Same	Unlikely to be seen unless drainage grossly distorted. Prognosis good
Coarctation of the aorta	Preductal — often associated with other anomalies Juxtaductal — often isolated anomaly	Prognosis poor — may be diagnosed by ultrasound Unlikely to be diagnosed by ultrasound unless very severe. Prognosis usually good

(Continued)

Table 13.1 *(Cont.)*

Ultrasound diagnosis	Pathological diagnosis	Comments
Disorders of rhythm		
Tachyarrhythmias	About 5–10% have structural anomalies	Rates >220 bpm Sudden onset resolution May be seen with hydrops
Bradycardias	About 40% have structural anomalies or anti-Ro/anti-La antibodies	

VSD, ventricular septal defect.

Table 13.2 Overall incidence of congenital heart disease using highest reported figures (Adapted from Harper, 1988)

	Per 1000 live births
Ventricular septal defect	5.0
Patent ductus arteriosus	1.2
Atrial septal defect	1.0
Pulmonary stenosis	0.8
Fallot's tetralogy	0.7
Endocardial cushion defect	0.7
Aortic stenosis	0.5
Transposition of the great vessels	0.4
Pulmonary atresia	0.2
Hypoplastic left heart syndrome	0.2
Coarctation of the aorta	0.15
Truncus arteriosus	0.15
Tricuspid atresia/hypoplastic right heart	0.15
Ebstein's anomaly	0.12

Table 13.3 Overall risks (%) for congenital cardiac disease (From Harper, 1988)

Population risk — all disease	1
Sibs of isolated case	2
Offspring of isolated case	3
Two sibs or parent and sib	10
More than two affected first degree relatives	50

Several drugs have been associated with cardiac malformations. Anticonvulsants such as phenytoin and phenobarbitone have been associated with an increased incidence of ventricular septal defects. Alcohol has also been linked with higher incidences of both ventricular and atrial septal defects while drugs such as lithium have been associated with Ebstein's anomaly.

152

Table 13.4 Recurrence risk (%) after an isolated abnormality in sib and parent (Adapted from Harper, 1993)

	Sib	Offspring
Ventricular septal defect	3.0	4.0
Atrial septal defect	3.0	2.5
Patent ductus arteriosus	3.0	3.0
Fallot's tetralogy	3.0	3.0
Hypoplastic left heart	2.7	—
Endocardial cushion defect	2.6	—
Aortic stenosis	2.2	3.9
Pulmonary stenosis	2.0	3.6
Coarctation of the aorta	1.8	2.7
Transposition of the great vessels	1.7	—
Pulmonary atresia	1.3	—
Truncus arteriosus	1.3	—
Tricuspid atresia	1.0	—
Ebstein's anomaly	1.0	—

Diabetes mellitus is the maternal condition most commonly associated with cardiac disorders in the fetus, ventricular septal defects being the most likely. These malformations can be minimized by careful periconceptual control of the diabetes.

Clinical presentation of isolated fetal cardiac disease is rare although a proportion of those cases in which the fetus is hydropic may present with polyhydramnios. When the cardiac anomaly is accompanied by other malformations the clinical features may relate to them. Very occasionally, fetal cardiac arrhythmias will be detected at the time of routine auscultation.

Prenatal diagnosis guidelines

The cardiovascular system is the first to function in the developing embryo and blood begins to circulate about 24 days post-conception. The construction of the heart is completed by about the eighth week and the majority of the congenital defects will be ordained by that time.

Normal prenatal appearances

In screening the fetal heart it is essential to obtain a four chamber view (DeVore, 1985) which should be seen in many cases at 16 weeks and visible in all by 18–20 weeks (Fig. 13.1).

Identification of the connections is usually best achieved between 20 and 24 weeks. At this time clear views should be obtained of the aortic arch (Fig. 13.2), pulmonary artery and ductus arteriosus (Fig. 13.3) and, in

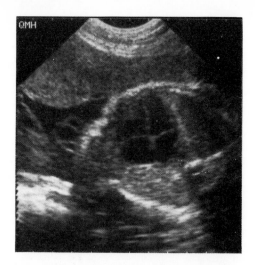

Fig. 13.1 Four chamber view of the fetal heart at 22 weeks.

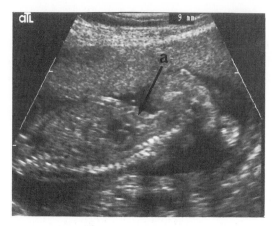

Fig. 13.2 Fetal aortic arch at 18 weeks: a, aortic arch.

addition, it should be possible to measure their calibre. The pulmonary veins can sometimes be seen draining into the left atrium.

The presence of four normal-sized chambers, an intact interventricular septum, visible atrioventricular valves which meet with the ventricular and atrial septa at the crux of the heart and a heart which occupies about one-third of the fetal chest with its apex to the left will exclude about 60% of severe cardiac conditions.

As with all ultrasound investigations, the ease with which the various cardiac structures can be seen depends not only on the skill of the operator and adequacy of the equipment but also on the body habitus of the mother and the position of the fetus within the uterus. These latter two factors are unable to be controlled although sometimes the fetus can be either

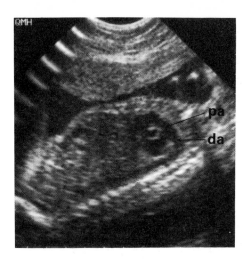

Fig. 13.3 Pulmonary artery (pa) and ductus arteriosus (da) at 18 weeks.

manoeuvered into a more favourable position or it will move spontaneously if given time. If unsatisfactory views are obtained it is imperative that a repeat scan is arranged since difficulty in scanning may be the first indication that an anomaly exists.

Abnormal prenatal appearances

The severest forms of congenital heart disease should be identifiable by ultrasound between 16 and 24 weeks (Allan *et al.*, 1986a) using either screening or diagnostic ultrasound imaging techniques. Screening all pregnancies with ultrasound is probably best achieved by including a cardiac evaluation at the time of a routine anomaly scan which in many centres is performed at about 18–20 weeks. The use of the four chamber view should identify the majority of serious anomalies. The predictive ability of this test is not clear since most of the information on diagnostic accuracy currently in the literature is derived from specialist units to which other cases are referred (Allan *et al.*, 1986a). However, some indication that the quality of referrals (and hence the pick-up rate) is improving is obtained from the observation that the proportion of affected pregnancies rose from 1 in 50 in 1980 to 1 in 12 in 1986 (Allan *et al.*, 1986a). An identification rate of about 50% for serious cardiac anomalies would probably be generally acceptable.

Conversely, the diagnosis of a case with a suspected cardiac anomaly can be very accurate when the ultrasonographer is experienced and in one study there were no false positive diagnoses and only about 10% of cases with defects were missed and most of these were described as mild cases (Allan, 1987). Interestingly, the frequency of lesions identified in the fetus by ultrasonography is fairly similar to that observed in infants (Table 13.5).

Small, although still clinically significant, ventricular septal defects may be missed and it is not possible to predict that physiological closure of the ductus arteriosus and the foramen ovale will occur at birth. Furthermore, although it may be obvious that problems such as hypoplastic left heart, transposition of the vessels and atresias of the valves will be present from the time of organogenesis, the position is less clear for conditions like preductal coarctation (Allan *et al.*, 1984b) and some forms of pulmonary atresia which may develop as a secondary effect (Allan *et al.*, 1986b). Ideas on the natural history of some cardiac defects are still developing and the importance of cardiac remodelling in response to blood flow is just being appreciated.

Colour flow Doppler can provide useful diagnostic information in cardiac disease. In essence this technique indicates whether flow is towards or away from the examining probe thus allowing the distribution of the flow to be determined. The use of this method allows very precise assessment of cardiac lesions (DeVore *et al.*, 1987) some of which may be too small to assess adequately by current techniques.

Fetal cardiac arrhythmias may present at any time but in fact the majority seem to appear after about 28 weeks (Allan, 1986). They may be

Table 13.5 Overall incidence of severe congenital heart disease found in infants (Freed, 1984) compared with that observed from fetal echocardiography (Allan *et al.*, 1984a)

	Freed 1984	Allan *et al.*, 1984a
Number	2251	72
	(%)	(%)
Ventricular septal defect	15.7	9.7
Transposition of great vessels	9.9	5.5
Fallot's tetralogy	8.9	8.3
Coarctation of the aorta	7.5	10.9
Hypoplastic left heart	7.4	5.5
Patent ductus arteriosus	6.1	—
Endocardial cushion defect	5.0	13.8
Heterotaxia	4.0	—
Pulmonary stenosis	3.3	—
Pulmonary atresia	3.1	6.8
Atrial septal defect	2.9	—
Total anomalous pulmonary drainage	2.6	—
Myocardial disease	2.6	11.1
Tricuspid atresia	2.6	2.7
Single ventricle	2.4	—
Aortic stenosis	1.9	2.7
Double outlet right ventricle	1.5	1.3
Truncus arteriosus	1.4	1.3
Other	5.6	—

discovered either because irregularity is noted on auscultation or because of the presence of clinically detectable polyhydramnios. The fetus may be hydropic. Their identification is achieved using either real-time ultrasound imaging or M-mode ultrasound.

Cardiotocography is often the initial indication that there is an abnormal fetal heart rate. In complete heart block there is a fixed bradycardia with no obvious variability. A marked tachycardia, in excess of 220 beats per minute, may be off the scale for many ante-partum monitors so that either a fixed rate is displayed, which is maximal for the instrument or, alternatively, the rate may be halved and appear to be in the normal range. It is usually impossible to determine the source of the arrhythmia using this technique.

Accurate diagnosis can only be achieved using both ultrasound imaging and M-mode techniques to demonstrate dissociation between atria and ventricles and to identify atrial flutter and fibrillation.

M-mode ultrasound allows the movement of the individual parts of the heart to be seen (Fig. 13.4). Not only can the rate of contraction of atria and ventricles be easily calculated, but the dimensions of the chambers in both systole and diastole can also be established.

Management

Once a cardiac anomaly has been suspected from a screening examination, the mother should be referred to a specialist centre for further evaluation (Fig. 13.5). There a detailed scan should be undertaken to exclude other fetal abnormalities and the nature of the cardiac anomaly should be established using both imaging and M-mode techniques. When an abnor-

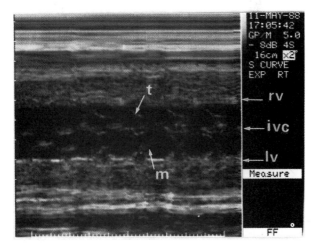

Fig. 13.4 M-mode appearance of fetal heart: right ventricular wall (rv); interventricular septum (ivc); left ventricular wall (lv); tricuspid (t) and mitral valve (m).

157

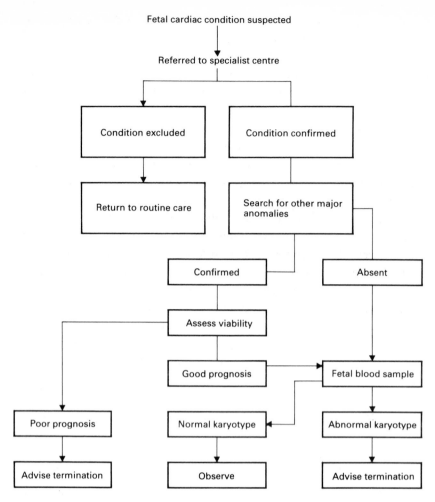

Fig. 13.5 Flow chart for management of suspected cardiac anomaly.

mality has been confirmed, when relevant, the fetal karyotype should be determined either by fetal blood sampling or by transabdominal chorionic villus sampling (CVS).

The potential for long-term survival is assessed by taking into account the severity of the cardiac lesion, the presence of other, extracardiac, anomalies and the karyotypic status. In our own practice the baby's condition will be discussed between ourselves, the parents and other specialists including a paediatric cardiologist. The prospects for survival in hypoplastic left heart are poor but, as with other cardiac lesions, they have improved over recent years. Other lesions may be remediable. If the decision, taken along with the parents' view, is to continue the pregnancy, our advice would be to monitor the pregnancy closely, watching for signs of hydrops.

If the cardiac lesion is very serious and/or is found in association with other anomalies, the outlook is very poor and in our experience many parents will opt for termination of pregnancy.

Arrhythmias present a rather different problem of management. The high incidence of anomalies associated with bradycardias makes it imperative that the heart, and the rest of the fetus as well, are carefully examined for other abnormalities. It will usually be appropriate to establish the fetal karyotype. In addition, the mother should be screened for systemic lupus erythematosus and anti-Ro/anti-La antibodies.

The tachyarrhythmias, once identified, offer the option of intrauterine treatment although the decision to undertake this depends upon the gestational age at diagnosis, the presence of associated anomalies (including karyotype) and the likelihood of cardiovascular decompensation. If the gestational age is greater than about 34 weeks and the arrhythmia is constant, immediate delivery is indicated especially if signs of decompensation exist. The prognosis for the frankly hydropic baby is rather poor although, in general, experience with this condition seems limited.

The management of fetal arrhythmias is shown in Fig. 13.6. In general the main form of treatment is with digoxin administered to the mother. The recommended dose is 0.75 mg a day although this can theoretically be titrated against the serum levels to ensure digitalization is adequate. Unfortunately, the presence of digoxin-like reacting substance makes the assay unreliable. If digoxin fails to convert the rhythm, verapamil may be used, although the mother's cardiac status must be closely monitored. The suggested dose of verapamil is 240 mg a day (Allan, 1986). Flecainide, 300 mg/day, may be more effective but maternal levels need to be carefully monitored (Allan *et al.*, 1991). Adenosine may be given by direct injection into the umbilical vein following cordocentesis.

Place and mode of delivery

When a fetal cardiac anomaly has been demonstrated and the fetus is thought to be viable, it is essential to arrange delivery in an obstetric unit attached to a high-risk neonatal department capable of resuscitating and stabilizing the baby at the time of birth. Ideally, delivery should be in a unit with neonatal cardiologists and surgeons in attendance but this is rarely possible.

The timing of delivery should be judged on obstetric grounds in most circumstances unless the cardiac status of the fetus is clearly deteriorating. Route of delivery should also be decided obstetrically except if the baby is in heart failure and is unlikely to withstand labour, under which circumstances caesarean section should be considered.

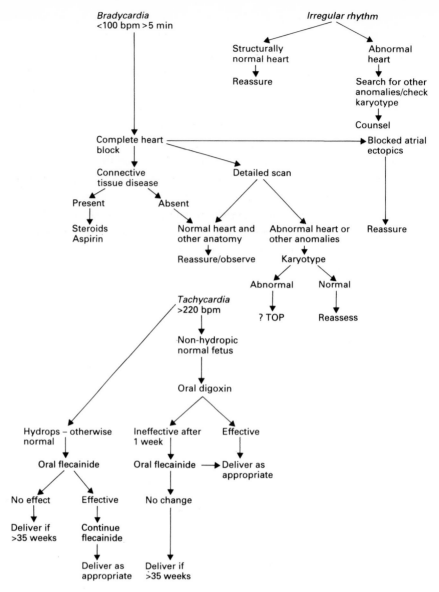

Fig. 13.6 Flow chart for the management of fetal cardiac arrythmias (Adapted from Allan, 1986).

Postnatal assessment

Although all babies will be examined fully immediately after birth and usually a few days later, those at particular risk of a cardiac defect should have, in addition, a full cardiological examination. Echocardiography should also be performed if at all possible since many serious cardiac conditions are clinically silent until the ductus arteriosus closes completely,

160

usually a few days after birth. Furthermore, fetal echocardiography may well fail to detect more minor, but still possibly significant, lesions.

After a baby has been born with a cardiac defect it is absolutely vital that the nature of the anomaly is carefully explained to the parents. It is surprising how few mothers know about their child's heart problem, particularly in cases in which the baby died. This may be for two reasons, the first relating to the difficulty of explaining a possibly complicated defect to parents who are in a highly emotional state. However, even a simple explanation will usually suffice ideally reinforced by a letter. Secondly, and more seriously, it perhaps reveals that these parents have had little discussion with their medical advisors after delivery and are simply unaware of the possible recurrence risks and, indeed, that prenatal exclusion of the most serious cardiac defects is now feasible. Ideally, the cardiologists should discuss the lesion with the parents some time after diagnosis and follow this with a letter.

REFERENCES

Allan, L.D. (1986) Arrhythmias, in *Manual of Fetal Echocardiography*, MTP Press, London, pp. 156−58.

Allan, L.D. (1987) Prenatal diagnosis of congenital heart disease. *Hospital Update*, **13**, 553−60.

Allan, L.D., Chita, S.K., Sharland, G.K., Maxwell, D., Priestly, K. (1991) Flecainide in the treatment of fetal tachycardias. *British Heart Journal*, **65**, 46−48.

Allan, L.D., Crawford, D.C., Anderson, R.H. and Tynan, M.J. (1984a) Echocardiographic and anatomical correlates in fetal congenital heart disease. *British Heart Journal*, **52**, 542−48.

Allan, L.D., Crawford, D.C. and Tynan, M. (1984b) Evolution of coarctation of the aorta in intrauterine life. *British Heart Journal*, **52**, 471−73.

Allan, L.D., Crawford, D.C., Chita, S.K. and Tynan, M.J. (1986a) Prenatal screening for congenital heart disease. *British Medical Journal*, **292**, 1717−19.

Allan, L.D., Crawford, D.C. and Tynan, M. (1986b) Pulmonary atresia in prenatal life. *Journal of the American College of Cardiology*, **8**, 1131−36.

DeVore, G.R. (1985) Prenatal diagnosis of congenital heart disease: a practical approach for the fetal ultrasonographer. *Journal of Clinical Ultrasound*, **13**, 229−5.

DeVore, G.R., Horenstein, J., Siassi, B. and Platt, L.D. (1987) Fetal echocardiography, VII. Doppler color flow mapping: a new technique for the diagnosis of congenital heart disease. *American Journal of Obstetrics and Gynecology*, **156**, 1053−64.

Freed, M.D. (1984) Congenital cardiac malformations. In *Schaffer's Diseases of the Newborn* (eds. M.E. Avery and H.W. Taeusch), W.B. Saunders, Philadelphia, pp. 243−90.

Fyler, D.C., Buckley, L.P., Hellenbrand, W.E. and Cohn, H.E. (1980) Report of New England Regional Infant Cardiac Program. *Pediatrics*, **65** (suppl.), 377−461.

Harper, P.S. (1993) *Practical Genetic Counselling* 4th edn, Butterworth-Heinemann, Oxford, pp. 34−8.

Chapter 14
Renal Tract Malformations

M. J. WHITTLE

Renal tract malformations affect about 10% of liveborn babies. They range from severe defects such as renal agenesis which are lethal to minor malformations which usually remain undiagnosed. As with other malformations they may be isolated or components of recognizable syndromes.

PRENATAL CLASSIFICATION

From a prenatal diagnosis standpoint renal tract malformations may be divided into malformations of the kidneys (agenesis, cystic disease, dysplasia) and of the collecting system (pelviureteric junction obstruction, ureterovesical obstruction/incompetence, bladder malformations, urethral obstruction). Pathological classification of some of these entities, in particular cystic renal disease, is complex and is discussed in detail elsewhere (Wigglesworth, 1984). However, whilst a precise pathological diagnosis is of importance for subsequent genetic counselling it is not possible to resolve all individual entities by their ultrasound appearance (Table 14.1).

IDENTIFICATION OF AT-RISK PREGNANCIES

As indicated in Table 14.1, some renal tract malformations are inherited and thus a family history of a previously affected child can be an important clue to the at-risk pregnancy. A few teratogens such as trimethadione, alcohol and high dose oestrogen/progestogen have been implicated in renal tract malformations. In practice, however, most affected pregnancies are not predicted and suspicion is raised by a small-for-dates uterus with oligohydramnios, polyhydramnios (in some cases of pelviureteric junction obstruction) or an abnormal appearance on a routine ultrasound scan.

Prenatal diagnosis guidelines

The presence of a renal tract malformation may not become obvious until late in pregnancy for two main reasons. Firstly, the obstructive or 'degenerative' renal changes may not appear until relatively late in pregnancy and, indeed, not until early childhood in some cases. Secondly, the urine excreted by the fetal kidneys does not become the major source of amniotic

Table 14.1 Ultrasound and pathological diagnosis of renal tract malformations

Ultrasound diagnosis	Pathological diagnosis	Comments
Unilateral absent kidney	Same	Birth incidence 1/1000
Bilateral absent kidneys	Same	Birth incidence 1/3000, recurrence risk 3−8% (Roodhooft *et al.*, 1984; Bankier *et al.*, 1985)
Cystic renal disease	Infantile polycystic disease	Autosomal recessive trait
	Adult polycystic disease	Autosomal dominant trait with occasional presentation in fetus/ neonate. Gene tracking possible (see Appendix)
	Medullary cystic disease	Autosomal recessive trait
Dysplastic kidneys	Cystic renal dysplasia	Usually sporadic, may be a feature of several syndromes including trisomy 13, trisomy 18, or Meckel syndrome
	Non-cystic renal dysplasia	As for cystic renal dysplasia. Often secondary to obstruction
Pelviureteric junction obstruction	Same	Bilateral in 20−30% (Evans, 1981)
Ureterovesical obstruction/ incompetence		Infrequently recognized *in utero* (Fitzsimmons *et al.*, 1986)
Ectopia vesicae	Same	Low recurrence risk, MSAFP may be elevated
Urethral obstruction	Urethral agenesis / Posterior urethral valves	Prune belly appearance in neonate

MSAFP, maternal serum α-fetoprotein.

fluid until 16−20 weeks so that the absence or failure of the kidneys may not become apparent, either clinically or ultrasonographically, until after that time.

Normal prenatal appearances

The fetal kidneys can usually be identified by about 16 weeks (Fig. 14.1)

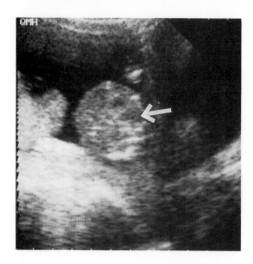

Fig. 14.1 Kidneys in a 16-week fetus — transverse section.

although this will depend on equipment, gain settings and maternal size. The internal anatomy of the kidneys should be identifiable by 18–20 weeks (Fig. 14.2). The fetal bladder (Fig. 14.3) should always be seen by 16 weeks and if it is not the scan should be repeated. However, amniotic fluid volume, even in the absence of functioning kidneys, may well be within normal limits at this stage.

Abnormal prenatal appearances

Bilateral renal agenesis. This is potentially detectable as early as 16–18 weeks (Fig. 14.4) with absent renal images and failure to demonstrate

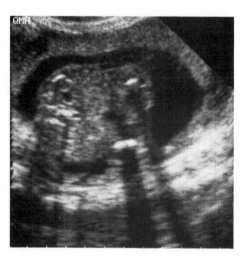

Fig. 14.2 Renal pelvis seen in a 20-week fetus — transverse section.

164

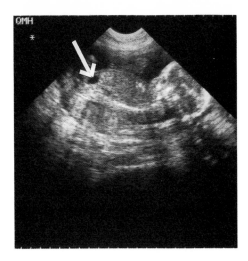

Fig. 14.3 Bladder seen in a 16-week fetus — longitudinal scan.

bladder filling on repeated examinations. Romero *et al.* (1985) made a positive diagnosis of renal agenesis by 24 weeks in all cases. This may seem late but the diagnosis of renal agenesis can be difficult because of the adverse effect of oligohydramnios on ultrasound imaging (see Management).

Cystic renal disease. The heterogeneity of cystic renal disease results in a variety of appearances prenatally and a range of gestational ages of detection. Figure 14.5 shows an affected fetus with infantile polycystic kidney disease. This condition carries a one in four recurrence risk and Romero *et al.* (1984) correctly diagnosed the condition in 9 out of 10 cases, amongst 19 at-risk pregnancies, by 22–23 weeks. A positive diagnosis had not been possible in 4 of the 10 affected cases when they were first scanned at 18 weeks.

Dysplastic kidneys. Cystic dysplastic kidneys (Fig. 14.6) may present early in pregnancy, although this will depend upon the underlying aetiology and whether or not the condition is bilateral. D'Alton *et al.* (1986) were able to establish a diagnosis in seven of nine cases by 24 weeks using the criteria of abnormal kidneys, absent bladder and oligohydramnios. There may be two main aetiologies. One results from absent or incomplete differentiation of mesoderm such that glomeruli may not be seen on histology. When unilateral, these kidneys will usually disappear leaving the individual with a single remaining normal kidney. The other aetiology arises from chronic outflow obstruction of an originally 'normal' kidney.

Pelviureteric junction (PUJ) obstruction. Pelviureteric junction obstruction (Fig. 14.7) may occur at any stage in pregnancy and is most likely to be

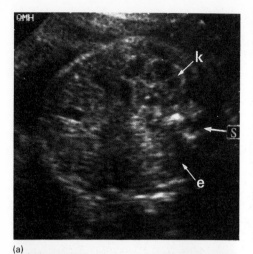

(a)

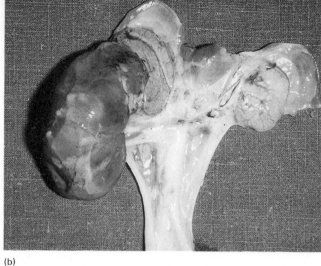

(b)

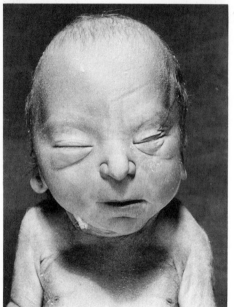

(c)

Fig. 14.4 Renal agenesis. (a) Ultrasound appearance in a 30-week
fetus with unilateral renal agenesis: k, kidney outline; s, spine;
e, empty renal fossa. (b) Pathological appearance in a fetus with
unilateral renal agenesis. (c) Potter facies in a neonate with
oligohydramnios due to bilateral renal agenesis.

discovered as a chance finding during an ultrasound investigation for some
other problem. Since the majority of these abnormalities are unilateral they
will not interfere with urine production in the fetus and so will not tend to
be obvious clinically, although polyhydramnios may be a feature (Kleiner
et al., 1987). Some cases of bilateral PUJ obstruction with minor hydronephrosis have been found to have poorer renal function as neonates than
had been anticipated. These changes can serve as a marker for karyotypic
abnormalities. Postnatal follow-up is currently recommended if the diameter
of the pelvis exceeds 0.5 cm as some of the children may subsequently be
shown to have reflux.

166

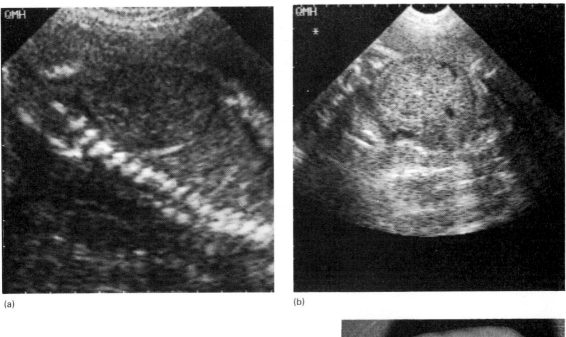

(a)

(b)

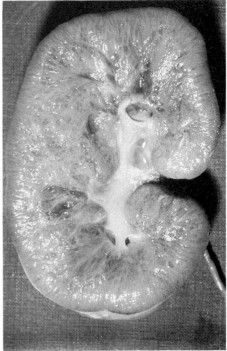

Fig. 14.5 Polycystic renal disease (infantile polycystic disease).
(a) Longitudinal section. (b) Transverse section. (c) Pathological
appearance in a fetus.

(c)

Urethral obstruction. Complete obstructive uropathy may only present late
in pregnancy usually as a small-for-dates uterus. Scanning reveals oligohydramnios but the appearances of the renal tract will depend on the level
of the obstruction and its duration. Thus, in urethral obstruction due to

167

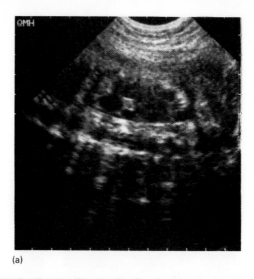

(a)

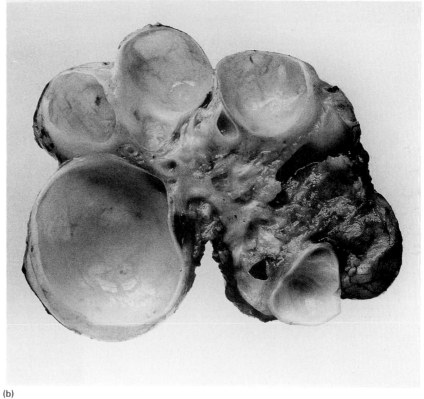

(b)

Fig. 14.6 Cystic dysplastic kidney. (a) Longitudinal section at 24 weeks. (b) Pathological appearance in a fetus.

posterior valves or atresia, the bladder will often be enormous and sometimes almost impossible to distinguish from the amniotic cavity, a source of confusion if an amniocentesis is attempted (Fig. 14.8). The ureters will

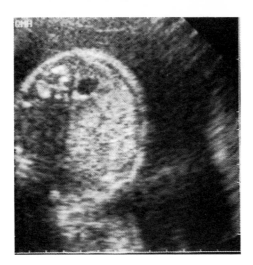

Fig. 14.7 Pelviureteric junction obstruction in a 22-week fetus — transverse section.

usually be dilated but occasionally they are small, indicating that renal failure has probably intervened. The renal pelves may show an extensive hydronephrosis with very little renal cortex remaining (Fig. 14.9). Conversely, the kidneys may show secondary cystic changes.

Most cases of obstructive uropathy present with cortex remaining (Fig. 14.9). Conversely, the kidneys may show secondary cystic changes. Although many cases with obstructive uropathy, usually due to urethral valves, present in early neonatal life, there is undoubtedly a potentially important role for second trimester ultrasound screening. Overall, about one-third of clinically important renal tract abnormalities might be missed in neonatal life without prenatal screening (Greig *et al.*, 1989).

Management

Fetal renal tract anomalies will usually be detected either as a result of an abnormal routine scan at 16 or 18 weeks or because clinical examination has suggested the presence of a small-for-dates uterus. Once the suspicion of a fetal renal anomaly has been raised it is important that the mother is counselled accordingly and then referred for a detailed anomaly scan both to confirm the renal tract malformation and to exclude other malformations. Since renal tract abnormalities may be secondary to chromosomal syndromes, fetal blood sampling for a rapid karyotype should also be considered in addition to an assessment of prognosis for the lesion.

The assessment of renal function is a difficult but important area of fetal evaluation. If it is clear that the fetus has bilateral renal agenesis then there is little else to be done.

169

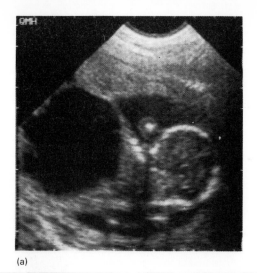

(a)

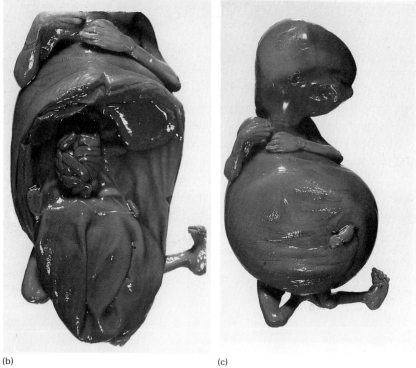

(b)   (c)

Fig. 14.8 (a) Enormous bladder in an 18-week fetus with urethral atresia. (b) and (c) Prune belly appearance in a fetus due to a greatly distended bladder.

When the fetal bladder is clearly seen, renal function can be determined by aspirating the urine under ultrasound control and testing it biochemically. The best parameters of renal function have yet to be established but crudely a sodium below 100 mmol/l and an osmolarity below 210 mosmol/l suggest adequate functioning renal tissue. However, it seems important to

170

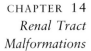

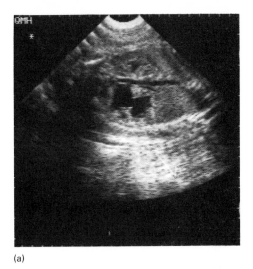

(a)

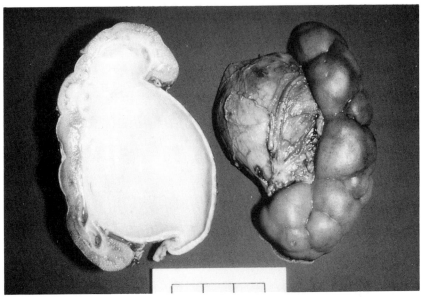

(b)

Fig. 14.9 Extensive hydronephrosis of one kidney. (a) Longitudinal section.
(b) Pathological appearance.

take into account the gestational age at the time of sampling so that
towards term a sodium of above 50 mmol/l may indicate impaired renal
function. A further test of renal function is to aspirate all the urine from
the bladder and then see how long it takes to refill.

The presence of oligohydramnios is likely to have profound effects on
the development of the fetal lungs. Indeed in many cases in which the renal
tract is abnormal, neonatal loss is due to the problems of lung hypoplasia
rather than renal failure. Unfortunately, there is currently no reliable

171

method of assessing the state of the fetal lungs although hypoplasia might be suspected when a narrow and funnel-shaped fetal chest wall is observed on ultrasound.

Once the prognosis has been established, a plan of management can be developed. Figure 14.10 illustrates a flow diagram for a management plan, based on the volume of amniotic fluid and the type of renal malformation. On this basis, three main prognostic groups can be identified: hopeless, good and doubtful.

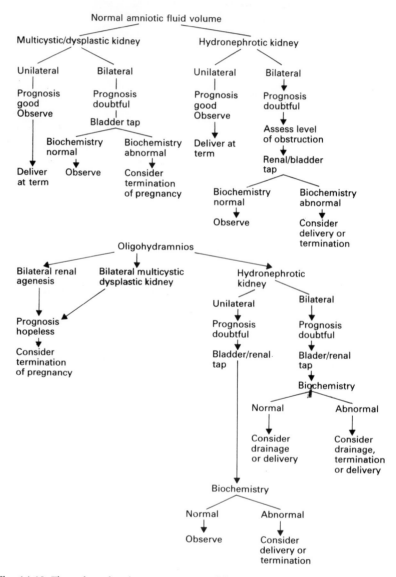

Fig. 14.10 Flow chart for the management of fetal renal problems. (Adapted from Harrison *et al.*, 1984.)

1. Hopeless prognosis

These are cases in which there is bilateral renal agenesis or in which renal tissue has been clearly damaged and tests have conclusively shown that it is non-functioning. Once it is clear that the prognosis is hopeless the couple should be told and, if appropriate, arrangements made to terminate the pregnancy. When the diagnosis is made in late pregnancy, it may be best to await the spontaneous onset of labour. Careful instructions should be placed in the patient's chart, however, so that an inappropriate caesarean section is not performed. It should be noted that fetal distress is a common feature during labour when the pregnancy is complicated by oligohydramnios.

2. Good prognosis

In these cases, the abnormality is usually unilateral and isolated. The management should be expectant but careful and repeated observation of the renal tract is necessary.

An indication from ultrasonography that the condition in the affected kidney is deteriorating or even more importantly that the contralateral kidney is beginning to show abnormal features are indications that delivery and/or treatment should be considered.

3. Doubtful prognosis

In practice many of the cases will fall into this category because the correct approach is to give most babies the benefit of the doubt. Two main categories exist — the cases with clearly multicystic disease but with reasonable amounts of amniotic fluid and the cases with obstructive uropathy.

It seems reasonable to continue observing the fetus with dysplastic kidneys so long as the amniotic fluid volume is stable and adequate, although the long-term prognosis for the neonate should be guarded. We believe that the mother should be made aware of this, although with future advances in transplant surgery it is always possible that a baby who has sufficient renal function to survive the first year or two may ultimately become a potential kidney recipient.

Obstructive uropathy gives the option of intrauterine drainage which has been attempted both by the insertion of pigtail catheters under ultrasound control and by direct exteriorization of the fetal bladder (see Chapter 17).

The major problem with most cases of obstructive uropathy is that they often present rather late in pregnancy when damage to kidneys and lungs has already occurred. Conversely, when the presentation is before 20–22 weeks, treatment is not an option because of the size of the fetus. In the collaborative review (Manning *et al.*, 1986) of 73 cases of obstructive uropathy, catheters were not inserted on average until about 24 weeks and the overall survival was 41%. Of the 29 neonatal deaths, however, 27 were the result of lung hypoplasia.

Although the current view of drainage procedures tends to be pessimistic, the early diagnosis of obstructive problems may improve their effectiveness.

The timing of delivery will depend on the state of the fetal kidneys and the underlying condition. Evidence that renal function is deteriorating suggests that delivery should be expedited if the pregnancy is beyond about 34 weeks at which time the baby is unlikely to develop severe respiratory problems related solely to immaturity. We believe that there is still an important case to consider testing amniotic fluid for the presence of adequate surfactant prior to elective delivery.

These babies should be delivered only in hospitals with adequately equipped and staffed neonatal units since the babies may have early and severe respiratory problems.

The route of delivery should be dictated on obstetric grounds alone.

Postnatal assessment

All couples who have had a baby with a renal tract malformation should be offered genetic counselling to discuss the condition's recurrence risk, range of prognosis and potential for future prenatal diagnosis.

REFERENCES

Bankier, A., Campo, M., Newell, R., Rogers, J.G. and Danks, D.M. (1985) A pedigree study of perinatally lethal disease. *Journal of Medical Genetics*, **22**, 104−11.

D'Alton, M., Romero, R., Grannum, P., DePalma, L., Jeanty, P. and Hobbins, J.C. (1986) Antenatal diagnosis of renal anomalies with ultrasound IV. Bilateral multicystic disease. *American Journal of Obstetrics and Gynecology*, **154**, 532−37.

Evans, B.B. (1981) Obstructive uropathy in the neonate, in *Perinatal Nephropathy, Clinics in Perinatology* (ed. J.E. Lewy), W.B. Saunders, London, pp. 273−86.

Fitzsimmons, P.J., Frost, R.A., Millward, S., Demaria, J. and Toi, A. (1986) Prenatal and immediate postnatal ultrasound diagnosis of ureterocele. *Journal of the Canadian Association of Radiology*, **37**, 189−91.

Greig, J.D., Raine, P.A.M., Young, D.G. *et al.* (1989) Value of antenatal diagnosis of abnormalities of the urinary tract. *British Medical Journal*, **298**, 1417−19.

Harrison, M.R., Golbus, M.S. and Filly, R.A. (eds.) (1984) Congenital hydronephrosis, in *The Unborn Patient*, pp. 277−348. Grune & Stratton, Florida.

Kleiner, B., Callen, P.W. and Filly, R.A. (1987) Sonographic analysis of the fetus with uretero-pelvic junction obstruction. *American Journal of Radiology*, **148**, 359−63.

Manning, F.A., Harrison, M.R. and Rodeck, C.H. (1986) Catheter shunts for fetal hydronephrosis and hydrocephalus. *New England Journal of Medicine*, **315**, 336−40.

Romero, R., Cullen, M., Jeanty, P. *et al.* (1984) Diagnosis of congenital renal anomalies with ultrasound. II. Infantile polycystic kidney disease. *American Journal of Obstetrics and Gynecology*, **150**, 259−62.

Romero, R., Cullen, M., Grannum, P. *et al.* (1985) Antenatal diagnosis of renal abnormalities with ultrasound. III. Bilateral renal agenesis. *American Journal of Obstetrics and Gynecology*, **151**, 38–43.

Roodhooft, A.M., Birnholz, J.C. and Holmes, L.B. (1984) Familial nature of congenital absence and severe dysgenesis of both kidneys. *New England Journal of Medicine*, **310**, 1341–45.

Wigglesworth, J.S. (1984) The kidneys and urinary tract, in *Perinatal Pathology*, W.B. Saunders, London, pp. 348–70.

Chapter 15
Skeletal Malformations and Dysplasias

J. McHUGO

Two main groups of skeletal abnormalities can be defined, namely those associated with malformations and those which are truly dysplasias. Skeletal malformations represent local problems due to failure of development or disruption of previously normal parts (e.g. amniotic bands). Major malformations are more common than dysplasias, and have a birth frequency of 1 in 500.

Skeletal dysplasias are characterized by generalized defective development of bone and cartilage. Dysplasias are rare but many distinct entities have been described and collectively they have a frequency of about 1 in 5000 births.

The fetal skeleton starts to ossify early in pregnancy (Table 15.1). Membranous ossification occurs in bones like the clavicle and mandible but most bones ossify from existing cartilage. The primary centre in long bones begins in the diaphysis (Fig. 15.1). The extent of ossification at 15–16 weeks is shown in Fig. 15.2 and although the majority of the diaphyses are ossified by term, most of the secondary centres in the epiphyses do not appear until after birth, the exceptions being the distal femur, proximal tibia and sometimes the proximal humerus (Fig. 15.3).

PRENATAL CLASSIFICATION

Skeletal malformations correlate reasonably well with the pathological classification but the dysplasias are much more difficult to categorize (Table 15.2). Broad groups include the extent of bone shortening, whether they are straight or bowed, abnormal ossification and the association of other anomalies particularly involving the spine and thorax.

Table 15.1 Fetal ossification

Structure	Gestation (weeks)
Clavicle	8
Mandible/palate	9
Vertebral bodies	9
Neural arches	9
Frontal bone	10–11
Long bones	11

176

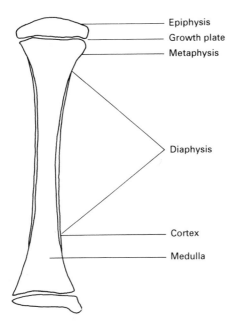

Fig. 15.1 Normal bone nomenclature.

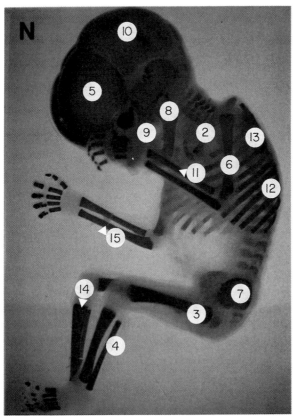

Fig. 15.2 Ossification at 15–16 weeks' gestation. 2, Clavicle; 3, femur; 4, fibula; 5, frontal bone; 6, humerus; 7, ilium; 8, mandible; 9, maxilla; 10, occipital bone; 11, radius; 12, ribs; 13, scapula; 14, tibia; 15, ulna. (From England, 1983.)

177

Table 15.2 Classification of skeletal malformations

Ultrasound diagnosis	Pathological diagnosis	Comments
Polydactyly	Same	May be isolated or a component of a syndrome (e.g. trisomy 13 or Meckel syndrome). Isolated polydactyly may be sporadic or inherited as an autosomal dominant trait. Short rib dysplasias
Syndactyly	Same	May be isolated or a component of a syndrome
Amelia	Same	Absence of a limb (amelia) or a seal-like extremity (phocomelia) are rare. Thalidomide is the classic environmental cause but this may occur sporadically or as a feature of the Holt−Oram syndrome (see Radial aplasia) or as a result of maternal diabetes mellitus
Ectrodactyly	Same	Split hands and or feet. May be isolated or a component of a syndrome (e.g. EEC syndrome — ectrodactyly, ectodermal dysplasia, and cleft lip)
Transverse limb defect	Same	Usually sporadic due to amniotic bands
Radial aplasia	Same	May be isolated or a component of a syndrome (e.g. trisomy 18, Fanconi syndrome, the autosomal recessive TAR syndrome — thrombocytopenia, absent radii but preserved thumbs, or the autosomal dominant Holt−Oram syndrome — variable limb defects and congenital heart disease)
Talipes	Same	Trisomy 18, 13, 4p−, 18q skeletal dysplasias Roberts syndrome Pena−Shokier Arthrogryposis

IDENTIFICATION OF AT-RISK PREGNANCIES

The majority of skeletal malformations are not inherited and thus the affected pregnancy occurs unexpectedly and will only be diagnosed by routine or indicated ultrasound examination. Several teratogens have been implicated in the causation of skeletal malformations (see Table 10.3).

In contrast, the majority of skeletal dysplasias are inherited (see Table 15.3). Thus a family history, especially an affected parent or a previously affected child, is an important clue to an at-risk pregnancy. In this respect accurate diagnosis is vital for prediction of the correct recurrence risk and this may be impossible if no post-mortem radiograph was taken. Poly-hydramnios occurs in about a third of lethal dysplasias and may provoke the need for a diagnostic ultrasound scan investigation.

Table 15.3 Classification of skeletal dysplasias

Ultrasound diagnosis	Pathological diagnosis	Comments
Short limbs		
Severe micromelia	Achondrogenesis type I, II, III	Hypomineralized. Rib fractures only type I. Autosomal recessive
Mild micromelia but marked bowing	Campomelic dysplasia	Scapulae hypoplastic/absent, scoliosis from vertebral anomalies. Often autosomal recessive
Marked rhizomelia hypertelorism	Rhizomelic chondrodysplasia punctata	Similar syndrome follows warfarin therapy. Autosomal recessive
Mild micromelia talipes, facial clefting. Hitch-hiker thumb	Diastrophic dysplasia	Autosomal recessive
Mild rhizomelia. Often normal at 20 weeks, apparent by 27/28 weeks. Distal long bones normal	Heterozygous achondroplasia	Autosomal dominant. 80% new mutations
Thoracic deformity		
Multiple vertebral/spinal rib abnormalities	Spondylothoracic dysostosis (Jarcho–Levin syndrome)	Autosomal recessive. Lethal
Thoracic/spinal deformity		
Profound micromelia Camptomelia of long bones Narrow thorax — short ribs Polyhydramnios	Thanatophoric dysplasia	Commonest lethal dysplasia 1 in 30 000. Sporadic but recurrences have been seen if associated with clover leaf skull.
Mild micromelia Marked thoracic hypoplasia. Polydactyly may be present	Asphyxiating thoracic dysplasia (Jeune's)	Often lethal but survivors exist. Autosomal recessive
As for Jeune's but with renal and cardiac anomalies	Chondroectodermal dysplasia (Ellis van Creveld)	Autosomal recessive
Short ribs, polydactyly. Narrow thorax. Cardiac and renal malformations. Short or absent tibias	Type I Saldino–Noonan Type II Majewski Type III Naumoff	All autosomal recessive and lethal

(Continued)

Table 15.3 (*Cont.*)

Ultrasound diagnosis	Pathological diagnosis	Comments
Mineralization defects Severe hypo-mineralization without fractures	Hypophosphatasia	Autosomal recessive. Absent or low alkaline phosphatase. Lethal
Hypomineralization. Severe micromelia due to multiple fractures. Bones appear broad. Rib fractures	Osteogenesis imperfecta IIa	Lethal. Recurrence risk non-consanguineous parents 3%. About 90% autosomal dominant new mutations, 10% autosomal recessive
As for osteogenesis imperfecta IIa. Less extensive fractures	Osteogenesis imperfecta III	Autosomal recessive. Non-lethal but progressive. Other types see Appendix

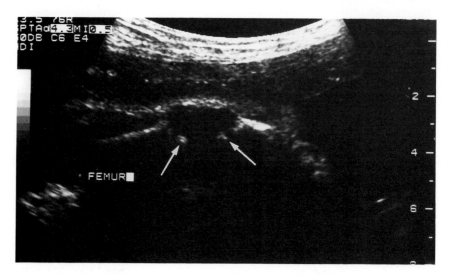

Fig. 15.3 Ossification at the knee at 34 weeks.

Prenatal diagnosis guidelines

Normal prenatal appearance

The skeleton is easily identified in the normal fetus, bone being a strong reflector of ultrasound. The optimal time for examination is between 18 and 20 weeks when biometry provides accurate information on gestational age. Reductions in bone length even at this stage will often be apparent and these allow the diagnosis of most lethal short limb dysplasias. Routine ultrasound measurements must include the femoral length (Fig. 15.4).

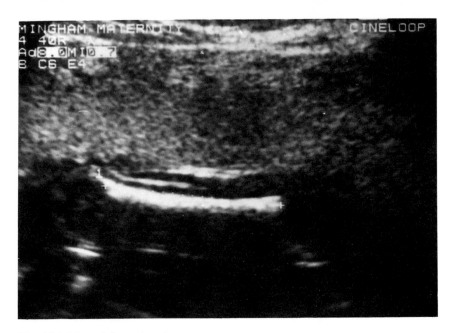

Fig. 15.4 Normal femur length.

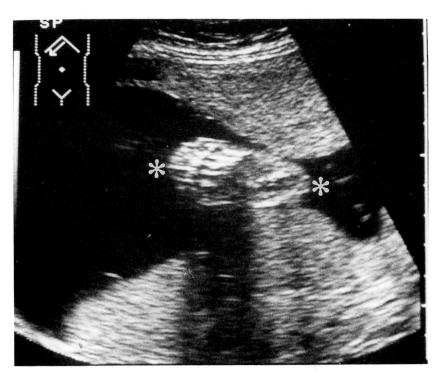

Fig. 15.5 Foot length.

Normograms are available for all the long bones (Table 15.4): the foot length (Fig. 15.5) should be equivalent to the femur length. Detailed skeletal assessment should include the items in Table 15.5.

181

Table 15.4 Normograms for long bones

(a) Normal values for the arm

Age (weeks)	Humerus (mm) Percentile			Ulna (mm) Percentile			Radius (mm) Percentile		
	5th	50th	95th	5th	50th	95th	5th	50th	95th
12	—	9	—	—	7	—	—	7	—
13	6	11	16	5	10	15	6	10	14
14	9	14	19	8	13	18	8	13	17
15	12	17	22	11	16	21	11	15	20
16	15	20	25	13	18	23	13	18	22
17	18	22	27	16	21	26	14	20	26
18	20	25	30	19	24	29	15	22	29
19	23	28	33	21	26	31	20	24	29
20	25	30	35	24	29	34	22	27	32
21	28	33	38	26	31	36	24	29	33
22	30	35	40	28	33	38	27	31	34
23	33	38	42	31	36	41	26	32	39
24	35	40	45	33	38	43	26	34	42
25	37	42	47	35	40	45	31	36	41
26	39	44	49	37	42	47	32	37	43
27	41	46	51	39	44	49	33	39	45
28	43	48	53	41	46	51	33	40	48
29	45	50	55	43	48	53	36	42	47
30	47	51	56	44	49	54	36	43	49
31	48	53	58	46	51	56	38	44	50
32	50	55	60	48	53	58	37	45	53
33	51	56	61	49	54	59	41	46	51
34	53	58	63	51	56	61	40	47	53
35	54	59	64	52	57	62	41	48	54
36	56	61	65	53	58	63	39	48	57
37	57	62	67	55	60	65	45	49	53
38	59	63	68	56	61	66	45	49	54
39	60	65	70	57	62	67	45	50	54
40	61	66	71	58	63	68	46	50	55

Reprinted with permission from Romero *et al.*, 1990.

(b) Normal values for the leg

Age (weeks)	Tibia (mm) Percentile			Fibula (mm) Percentile			Femur (mm) Percentile		
	5th	50th	95th	5th	50th	95th	5th	50th	95th
12	—	7	—	—	6	—	4	8	13
13	—	10	—	—	9	—	6	11	16
14	7	12	17	6	12	19	9	14	18
15	9	15	20	9	15	21	12	17	21
16	12	17	22	13	18	23	15	20	24
17	15	20	25	13	21	28	18	23	27
18	17	22	27	15	23	31	21	25	30
19	20	25	30	19	26	33	24	28	33

Table 15.4 (*Cont.*)

Age (weeks)	Humerus (mm) Percentile			Ulna (mm) Percentile			Radius (mm) Percentile		
	5th	50th	95th	5th	50th	95th	5th	50th	95th
20	22	27	33	21	28	36	26	31	36
21	25	30	35	24	31	37	29	34	38
22	27	32	38	27	33	39	32	36	41
23	30	35	40	28	35	42	35	39	44
24	32	37	42	29	37	45	37	42	46
25	34	40	45	34	40	45	40	44	49
26	37	42	47	36	42	47	42	47	51
27	39	44	49	37	44	50	45	49	54
28	41	46	51	38	45	53	47	52	56
29	43	48	53	41	47	54	50	54	59
30	45	50	55	43	49	56	52	56	61
31	47	52	57	42	51	59	54	59	63
32	48	54	59	42	52	63	56	61	65
33	50	55	60	46	54	62	58	63	67
34	52	57	62	46	55	65	60	65	69
35	53	58	64	51	57	62	62	67	71
36	55	60	65	54	58	63	64	68	73
37	56	61	67	54	59	65	65	70	74
38	58	63	68	56	61	65	67	71	76
39	59	64	69	56	62	67	68	73	77
40	61	66	71	59	63	67	70	74	79

Reprinted with permission from Romero *et al.*, 1990.

Table 15.5 Detailed assessment of the fetal skeleton

Image all long bones and measure	Length Width Structure Texture Fractures?
Cranium	Vault bones Facial profile
Ribs	Length Shape Fractures?
Spine Hands Feet	
Associated abnormalities	Cardiac Facial clefting Renal

Abnormal prenatal appearance

The lethal dysplasias should be identifiable in most cases by 20 weeks and long bones will show a persistent low growth profile. If a dysplasia is suspected gestational age is best assessed from fetal foot length; fetal head measurements can be unreliable because the skull may also be involved.

Non-lethal dysplasias (Table 15.6) may not be obvious until the time of birth. This may be of distress to parents who have previously had an affected child but it is important in counselling such couples that they are made aware that prenatal diagnosis may not be feasible. In some cases, such as heterozygous achondroplasia, an abnormal growth profile may be apparent by 22–24 weeks but absolute femoral shortening may not be noted until 26 or 27 weeks.

The complexity of the differential diagnosis of skeletal dysplasias demands a systematic approach as outlined below.

Short femur. This may arise because the gestational age is incorrect, the baby is dysmorphic, growth retarded, has a chromosome abnormality or, indeed, has a skeletal dysplasia. The morphology of the bone must be noted with particular reference to whether the bone is straight or bowed. The type of shortening, and whether it affects mainly the proximal or distal long bones, needs to be defined (Fig. 15.6).

Bone ossification. This can be difficult to assess but one guide is the extent of the calcification in the calvarium which is usually a strong reflector of ultrasound. When there are ossification problems, such as with osteogenesis imperfecta, the intracranial contents are seen with exceptional clarity and the falx will be a particularly strong reflector. The bone may also be

Table 15.6 Non-lethal short limbed dysplasias apparent at birth

Achondroplasia	AD
Chondroectodermal dysplasia (Ellis van Creveld)	AR
Mesomelic dysplasias (various types)	AD/AR
Rhizomelic dysplasias (various types)	AD/AR
Spondyloepiphyseal dysplasia	AD
Spondylometaphyseal dysplasia	AD/AR
Metatrophic dysplasia	AR?
Kniest syndrome	AD
Diastrophic dysplasia	AR
Parastremmatic dysplasia	AD?
Opsismodysplasia	AR?
Kyphomelic dysplasia	XL? AR?
Grebe chondrodysplasia	AR

AD, autosomal dominant; AR, autosomal recessive; XL, X-linked.

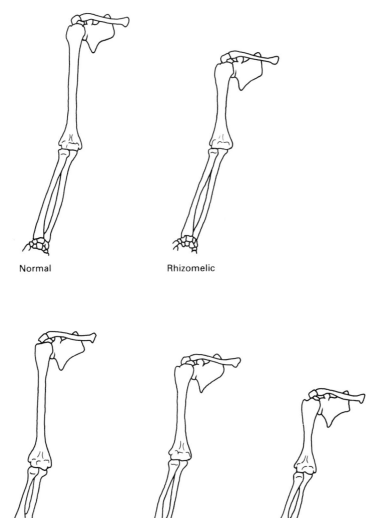

Normal   Rhizomelic

Mesomelia   Mild micromelia   Severe micromelia

Fig. 15.6 Types of limb shortening.

depressed by quite gentle pressure on the ultrasound probe. The presence
of fractures should be diligently sought, particularly in the long bones and
ribs. The ribs appear shortened and angulated (Fig. 15.7).

The appearance of the thorax is important. As mentioned above, there
may be rib fractures but in addition the ribs may be shortened, splayed or
bifid. The short-rib group of dysplasias are important to diagnose, being
autosomal recessive: they are often associated with other abnormalities
and most are lethal. A distorted thorax, which may be found in a variety
of other skeletal dysplasias, will lead to respiratory failure at birth, typically
seen in thanatophoric dwarfism.

185

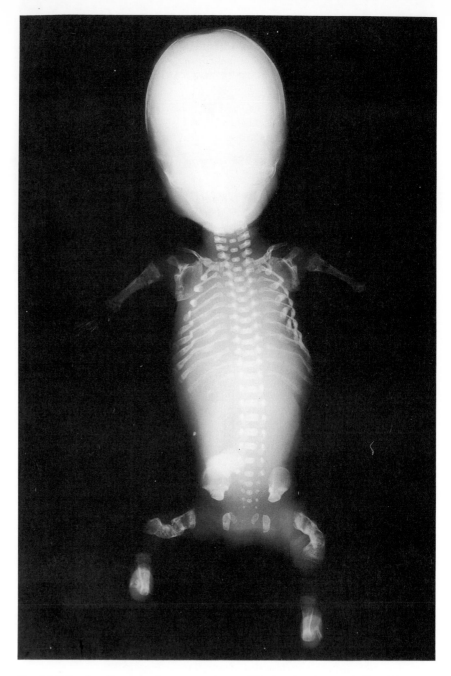

Fig. 15.7 Fetal radiograph of osteogenesis type IIA showing fractured ribs with angulation. Multiple long bone fractures with shortening.

Hands and feet must be examined for abnormal positioning of the fingers, polydactyly, rockerbottom feet or talipes.

Some abnormalities of the face, heart and kidneys are associated with skeletal dysplasias (Table 15.7).

Table 15.7 Commonly associated abnormalities seen with dysplasias

Polydactyly	Short-rib polydactyl syndrome
	Chondroectodermal dysplasia
	Asphyxiating thoracic dysplasia
Talipes	Campomelic dysplasia
	Diastrophic dysplasia
	Osteogenesis imperfecta
	Chondrodysplasia punctata
Small thorax	Achondrogenesis
	Hypochondrogenesis
	Thanatophoric dysplasia
	Short-rib polydactyl syndromes
	Chondroectodermal dysplasia
	Campomelic dysplasia
Cleft palate	Campomelic dysplasia
	Diastrophic dysplasia
Congenital heart disease	Chondrectodermal dysplasia ASD/Common atria
	Short-rib polydactyl type I transposition/double outflow right ventricle VSD
	Short rib-polydactyl type II transposition

VSD, ventricular septal defect; ASD, atrial septal defect.

Management

Skeletal dysplasias are rare (see Table 15.2) and it is unlikely that the average, busy unit will see more than a handful of cases each year. Once suspected it is advisable to refer the case to a tertiary centre so that an accurate diagnosis can be attempted. X-ray studies are of limited value in early pregnancy but may prove invaluable after about 24 weeks, at which time the classical radiological appearances of the various dysplasias may start to become apparent. Appropriate radiological assistance should then be sought.

A thorough ultrasound examination is mandatory to narrow the diagnosis but in contrast to other circumstances in which several abnormalities coexist, rapid fetal karyotyping may have little value. Pregnancy management is usually dictated by the ultrasound appearances alone and, if the condition is considered to be lethal, the matter of termination should be discussed.

Postnatal assessment

It cannot be over emphasized how important it is to have photographic and X-ray evidence in all skeletal dysplasias to enable a precise diagnosis to be made and to facilitate subsequent genetic counselling. The Appendix indicates which of the skeletal dysplasias have been successfully prenatally diagnosed. In general, the lethal chondrodysplasias can be recognized during the second trimester by serial ultrasound examinations but the non-lethal types will often present late or even postnatally.

REFERENCE

England, M.A. (1983) Normal fetal development. In *A Colour Atlas of Life Before Birth*, Wolfe Medical Publications, Netherlands.
Romero, R. (1990) Fetal skeletal anomalies. *Radiological Clinics of North America*, **28**(1), 75–99.

Chapter 16
Neck and Thorax Malformations

M. ROBSON and M. PEARCE

NECK SWELLINGS

The neck carries important structures between head and body so that masses and other abnormalities in this region are usually of serious consequence.

Prenatal classification

There are a number of important conditions presenting as neck swellings and these are shown in Table 16.1. The precise diagnosis of a neck mass in the fetus is vital because of the different implications.

Identification of at-risk pregnancies

Whilst there are some familial causes of recurrent neck lesions, e.g. Noonan syndrome, most affected pregnancies are not predictable but are diagnosed incidentally at routine ultrasound examination. Polyhydramnios may arise because a neck mass interferes with fetal swallowing and cystic hygromata may be associated with raised maternal α-fetoprotein levels.

Prenatal diagnostic guidelines

The differential diagnosis of neck lesions is shown in Table 16.2.

Abnormal prenatal appearances

Cystic hygromata

These may arise from a congenital malformation of the lymphatic system in which the sacs into which lymph drains do not communicate with the venous system as they should. Steady dilatation occurs although the hygromata may well regress eventually leaving the typical postnatal appearances seen in Turner's syndrome.

Diagnosis is usually easy with a cystic structure with multiple septi surrounding the neck (Fig. 16.1). Visualization may sometimes be difficult

Table 16.1 Important conditions presenting as neck swellings

Ultrasound diagnosis	Pathological diagnosis	Comments
Cystic hygroma	Lymphangiectasis. Mainly thin-walled cysts; occasionally more solid with cystic areas	Typical thin-walled cysts associated with 45,X in 50%; also seen with trisomy 21, 18 or 13, Noonan syndrome. AFP may be raised
Teratoma	Same	Generally anterior midline structures; can cause local bone erosions. Very rare; may affect swallowing and so is a cause of polyhydramnios
Haemangioma	Same	Vary in size/site; may show multiple septa. Some become organized
Goitre	Same	Bilobed mass anterior neck. TSH levels high in amniotic fluid
Branchial cleft	Same	Smooth cyst in anterior neck
Nuchal oedema	Same	Exclude trisomy 21
Klippel–Trenaunay–Weber syndrome	Same	Vascular and skeletal malformations. Sporadic

AFP, α-fetoprotein.

Table 16.2 Differential diagnosis of neck lesions

	Cystic hygroma	Encephalocele	Hydrops	Teratoma
Site	Posterior/ occasionally anterior	Posterior	Extensive	Anterior/lateral
Bilateral	85%	Midline	Extensive	Single
Wall	Thin	Thin	Oedema	Skin
Midline Septum	Present	Absent	Absent	Absent
Septation	Multiple	Unilocular	Variable	Variable
Content	Fluid	CSF/brain	Fluid	Semi-solid
Bony defect	None	Present	None	Erosion possible
Hydrops	Common	Rare	Present	Rare
Other anomalies	45,X; Trisomy 18, 13	See Chapter 11	See NIH	Rare

CSF, cerebrospinal fluid; NIH, non-immune hydrops.

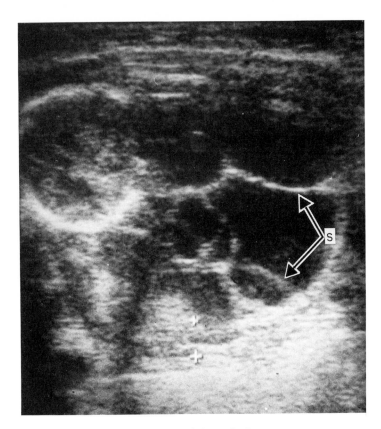

Fig. 16.1 Typical multicystic hygromata of the neck. S, septa.

if the lesion is pressed against the side of the placenta. There should be a midline septum (Fig. 16.2) and differentiation from encephalocele is important. Isolated cysts (Fig. 16.3) can cause difficulties.

Fetal goitre

This a rare condition occurring most often when the mother has taken iodides or other thyroid-blocking agents. An enlarged thyroid gland will appear as a solid bilobed anterior neck mass. It may be associated with polyhydramnios, presumably as a result of oesophageal compression.

Nuchal skin thickness

The pathogenesis of nuchal skin thickness is probably different to that of cystic hygromata and may reflect local oedema rather than anything to do with the lymphatic system. Changes have been described in both first and second trimesters. In the first trimester a nuchal thickness of 3 mm or more, measured in the saggital plane used for crown–rump length, has been associated with a tenfold increase in the individual risk of trisomy, its

191

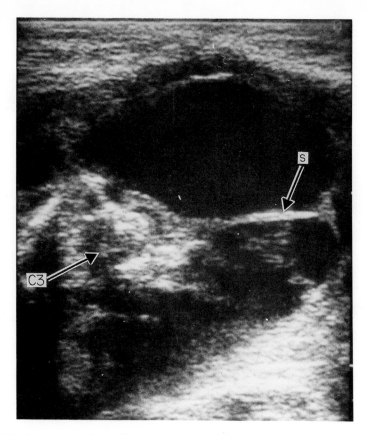

Fig. 16.2 Appearance of a midline septum in cystic hydroma. s, septum; c3, cerebellum — normal shape.

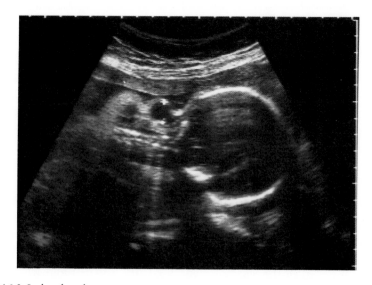

Fig. 16.3 Isolated neck cyst.

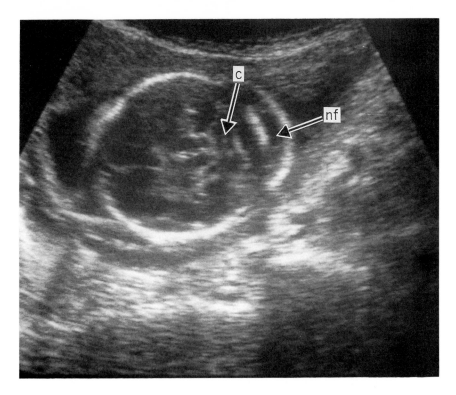

Fig. 16.4 Nuchal oedema. c, cerebellum; nf, nuchal fold.

absence a threefold reduction in risk. In the second trimester a nuchal fold of 6 mm or more, measured in the suboccipito-bregmatic plane (Fig. 16.4), is associated with an increased risk of fetal trisomy. Figure 16.5 shows a saggital view of the nuchal fold in a fetus with Down syndrome. Interestingly these changes are more likely to be associated with trisomies than Turner's syndrome.

Teratomata

Teratomata are composed of a variety of tissues foreign to the anatomical sites in which they find themselves. Although the majority of teratomata in the neck are benign, their situation in the neck can cause compressive problems *in utero* and difficulties with respiration and intubation following delivery.

Teratomata are most often located in the anterior and lateral regions of the neck and so are easily differentiated from cystic hygromata. Additionally they tend to comprise cystic and solid areas (Fig. 16.6) and may extend upwards to involve the maxilla (Fig. 16.7).

193

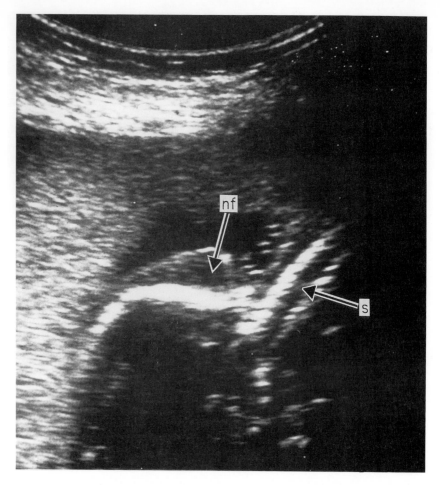

Fig. 16.5 Nuchal fold in saggital plane. s, spine; nf, nuchal fold.

Management

Detection of cystic hygromata must lead to a search for fetal skin oedema, ascites, pleural and pericardial effusions and for cardiac and renal anomalies. Because some hygromata are associated with mosaics, the fetal karyotype should be determined by amniocentesis or, preferably, from fetal blood obtained by cordocentesis; this is advised even if termination is contemplated since knowledge of the karyotype aids subsequent counselling.

In the case of goitre, fetal thyroid function can be established either from amniotic fluid or, preferably, from fetal blood. Hypothyroidism can be corrected indirectly by giving the mother 3,5 dimethyl-3-isopropyl thyronine and thyroxine or directly to the fetus via an injection into the amniotic fluid or cord vessels.

Teratomata can be managed by excision after delivery but the prognosis is usually particularly poor if the tumour has extended to the mandible.

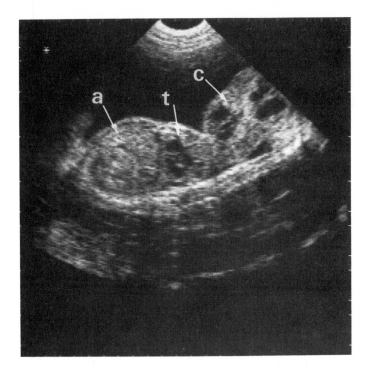

Fig. 16.6 Solid/cystic hygroma in longitudinal plane. c, solid/cystic hygroma; t, thorax; a, abdomen.

PULMONARY ANOMALIES

Prenatal classification

Pleural effusions are the commonest prenatally detected pulmonary anomalies and are most often associated with non-immune hydrops (NIH). Malformations and tumours are rare but careful differentiation is essential (Table 16.3).

Identification of at-risk pregnancies

Polyhydramnios is the most likely presenting feature and may be found in association with pleural effusions or tumours. This is presumably as a result either of increased intrathoracic pressure or compression by the mass itself, both having the potential to interfere with fetal swallowing.

Prenatal diagnosis guidelines

The normal appearances of the fetal chest are shown in Figs. 16.8 and 16.9. Diagnostically, it is important to establish whether or not the lesion is bilateral, if there is midline shift and if other structures, such as bowel, can be seen in the chest. As always, other anomalies should be looked for.

195

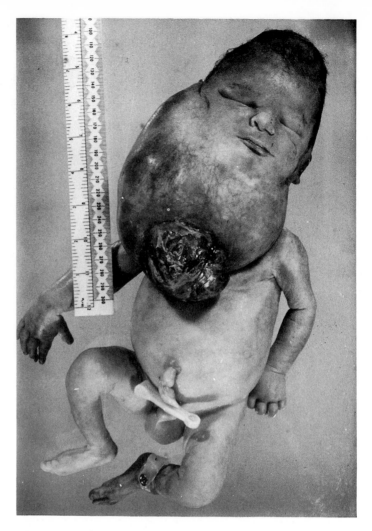

Fig. 16.7 Appearance of a teratoma.

Pleural effusion

These may be unilateral or bilateral and may often be associated with non-immune hydrops (NIH). Often the pleural effusion will be a feature of NIH and the underlying cause will be the same (see Table 16.3) but in some circumstances it would appear that the hydrops has occurred as a result of the pulmonary problem.

Thus 'chylothorax', cystic adenomatoid lung and diaphragmatic hernia, especially when situated on the right, may all be seen as a cause of hydropic change.

'Chylothorax' is a misnomer since chyle is not present until the baby takes oral feeds. Nevertheless, there is evidence that the observed pleural effusion may originate from lymphatic drainage; the chest fluid aspirated

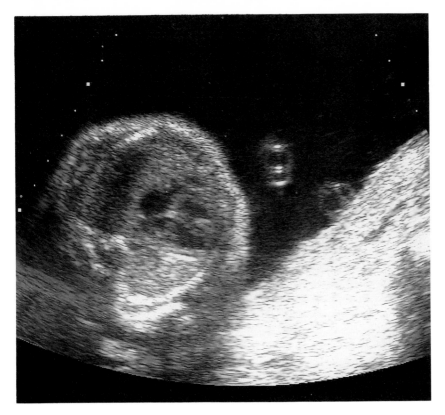

Fig. 16.8 Normal transverse section of fetal chest.

Table 16.3 Pulmonary anomalies

Ultrasound diagnosis	Pathological diagnosis	Comments
Pleural effusions	Chylothorax	May be unilateral or bilateral. *In utero* drainage possible but role unclear
	Pulmonary lymphangiectasia	Poor prognosis
	Non-immune hydrops (NIH)	Commonest cause of fetal pleural effusions. Poor prognosis
Cystic	Macrocysts >5 mm Microcysts about 50% association with other anomalies	Macrocysts prognosis good. Microcysts poor prognosis particularly with hydrops. Differential diagnosis is diaphragmatic hernia

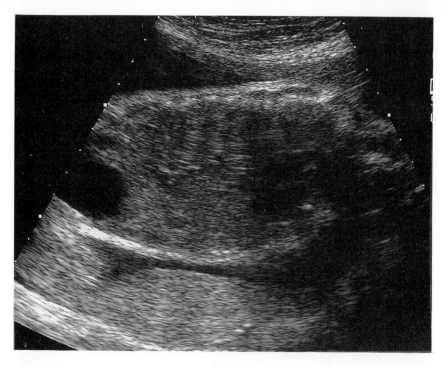

Fig. 16.9 Normal longitudinal section of fetal chest.

from the fetus has a relatively high lymphocyte count and is often under considerable pressure. There is often associated polyhydramnios.

Cystic adenomatoid malformation of the lung (CAM)

This is a rare abnormality with an incidence of about 1 in 4000 and is characterized by an overgrowth of the terminal bronchioles. The problem may be discrete but if more generalized, the expanding tissue may cause mediastinal shift and pulmonary, oesophageal and vena caval compression leading to polyhydramnios and hydrops. The lesions are usually unilateral and confined to a lobe but the whole lung may be involved. Associated problems include renal abnormalities, hydrocephalus and diaphragmatic hernia; the karyotype may be abnormal.

The original classification into three types has been replaced by organization into two groups: macrocystic (cysts > 5 mm diameter) (Fig. 16.10) and microcystic, which are highly echogenic on ultrasound (Fig. 16.11).

Pulmonary sequestration

There are two forms of this condition, extralobar and intralobar. In extralobar forms, the lobe is supplied by the systemic circulation and there are no tracheobronchial connections between normal and abnormal lung;

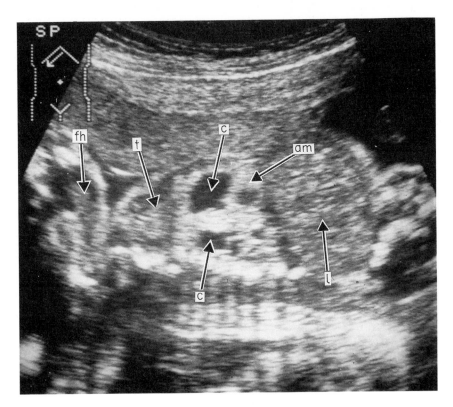

Fig. 16.10 CAM — macrocystic type. fh, fetal head; t, thorax; c, cyst; am, adenomatous malformation; l, liver.

venous drainage is not to the left atrium. The postero-medial segment of the left lung is most frequently involved.

In intralobar sequestration, the normal and abnormal lungs share the same pleura and venous drainage is normal. Fluid produced by the sequestered segment accumulates between the two pleural layers to form a large echogenic mass which displaces and compresses the heart and surrounding lung tissue. Non-immune hydrops may well develop.

Sequestration may be found with CAM; about 10% of cases with intralobar problems are associated with other anomalies including skeletal deformities, diaphragmatic hernia and heart, renal and intracranial malformations.

Pulmonary hypoplasia

Pulmonary hypoplasia may be a primary disorder or, most likely, may arise as a secondary effect. Conditions associated with abnormal lung growth include: diaphragmatic hernia, pleural effusion, CAM, oligohydramnios due to renal agenesis or membrane rupture prior to 20 weeks and rare neuromuscular disorders.

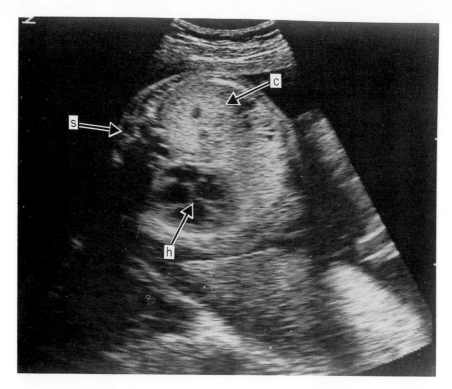

Fig. 16.11 CAM — microcystic type. s, spine; h, heart; c, CAM II/III.

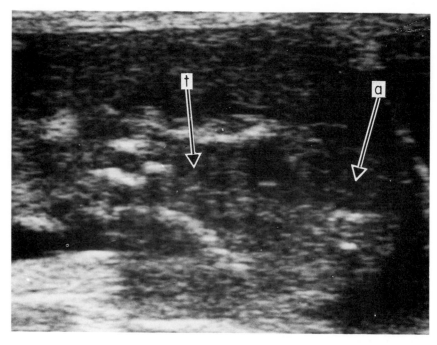

Fig. 16.12 Champagne cork appearance of osteochondrodysplasia. t, thorax; a, abdomen.

Unilateral hypoplasia will be recognized from the mediastinal shift with normal hypertrophied lung occupying the affected hemithorax. The assessment of lung size using ultrasound has been attempted but the technique seems to provide only a rough guide.

Thoracic hypoplasia

Malformations of the chest wall itself may arise in a number of conditions especially those involving the skeleton (see Chapter 15).

Osteochondrodysplasia will produce a deformed chest with the appearances of a champagne cork (Fig. 16.12). The heart seems to fill the thoracic cavity.

Table 16.4 Investigations for non-immune hydrops

Test for:	Amount	Bottle	Lab.
Maternal bloods			
Group	5 ml	BTS	Haematology
Antibodies screen	5 ml	BTS	Haematology
FBC and film	5 ml	EDTA	Haematology
Haemoglobinopathy	10 ml	5 ml (White clotted) 5 ml EDTA	Haematology
TORCH Parvovirus	5 ml × 2	5 ml clotted 5 ml clotted	Microbiology
Fetal bloods			
Karyotype	1 ml	Heparin	Cytogenetics
Gases	1 ml	Heparinized 1 ml syringe	Clinical chemistry
Liver enzymes	1 ml	Heparin	Clinical chemistry
TORCH and Parvovirus	1 ml 2 samples if possible	5 ml clotted white	Microbiology
Full Blood Count Film Group/Coombs'	0.5 ml	EDTA	Haematology
Amniocentesis Virology CMV and Parvovirus B19	10 ml	Plain bottle	Microbiology

BTS, Blood Transfusion Service.

Management

Unless the fetal condition is obviously fatal, detailed investigation of each case is advisable so that an accurate diagnosis can be made. This may include the aspiration of pleural fluid for biochemistry and cytology and fetal blood sampling for karyotype, liver enzymes and infection screen. In addition, fetal haematology and, if appropriate, blood grouping should be performed as for NIH (Table 16.4).

Once a firm diagnosis is established, treatment can be planned. In appropriately selected cases with pleural effusions, the insertion of pleuro-amniotic shunts may help, the aim being to decompress the thorax. Macrocystic CAM may also benefit from drainage of the largest cysts by the placement of shunts *in utero* although many do well with no treatment. Extrauterine surgery has also been attempted. Most of these cases will require surgery following delivery (see Chapter 17).

FURTHER READING

Benacerraf, B.R., Laboda, L.A. and Frigoletto, F.D. (1992) Thickened nuchal fold in fetuses not at risk for aneuploidy. *Radiology*, **184**, 239–42.

D'Alton, M., Mercer, B., Riddick, E. and Dudley, D. (1992) Serial thoracic versus abdominal circumference ratios for the prediction of pulmonary hypoplasia in premature rupture of the membrane remote from term. *American Journal of Obstetrics and Gynecology*, **166**, 658–63.

Deacon, C.S., Smart, P.J. and Rimmer, S. (1990) The antenatal diagnosis of congenital cystic adenomatoid malformation of the lung. *British Journal of Radiology*, **63**, 968–70.

Nicolaides, K.H., Azar, G., Byrne, D., Mansur, C. and Marks, K. (1992) Fetal nuchal translucency: ultrasound screening for chromosomal defects in first trimester of pregnancy. *British Medical Journal*, **304**, 867–69.

Neilson, I.R., Russo, P., Laberge, J.M. *et al.* (1991) Congenital adenomatoid malformation of the lung: current management and progress. *Journal of Pediatric Surgery*, **26**(8), 975–81.

Roberts, A.B. and Mitchell, J.M. (1990) Direct ultrasonic measurement of fetal lung length in normal pregnancies complicated by prolonged rupture of membranes. *American Journal of Obstetrics and Gynecology*, **163**, 1560–66.

Thorpe-Beeston, J.G., Nicolaides, K.H., Felton, C.V., Butter, J. and McGregor, A.M. (1991) Maturation of the secretion of thyroid hormone and thyroid stimulating hormone in the fetus. *New England Journal of Medicine*, **324**, 532–36.

Chapter 17
Specific Diagnostic Techniques and Fetal Therapy

L. J. ROBERTS and C. H. RODECK

INTRODUCTION

The indications for each form of invasive sampling are in a state of flux, governed by improvements both in ultrasound scanning and DNA probes. For example, amniocentesis to determine fetal sex when there is a risk of an X-linked recessive condition has been replaced by DNA probe analysis of chorionic villus samples or sex determination by ultrasound scanning. Similarly, fetal blood is no longer required to diagnose haemoglobinopathies, but it is frequently used to karyotype fetuses whose anomaly scan suggests aneuploidy. The current indications for the various forms of invasive testing are listed in Table 17.1.

SPECIFIC DIAGNOSTIC TECHNIQUES

Amniocentesis

Amniocentesis is the simplest technique for obtaining fetal cells, and is most commonly performed at 15–18 weeks' gestation when the uterus is clearly an intra-abdominal structure.

As for all sampling methods, when the uterus is instrumented at this gestation, blood for screening of serum α-fetoprotein should be taken before the procedure and the patient's blood group should be known so that Anti-D can be given if it is Rhesus (Rh) negative. Ultrasound scanning is performed to confirm fetal viability, gestational age, placental site and to identify suitable liquor pools and rarely, fetal abnormalities which could make the procedure unnecessary. Should there be no access to a suitable liquor pool without traversing the placenta, the procedure should be delayed for a week. The situation is usually different after this interval and enables avoidance of transplacental taps which are associated with an increased incidence of maternal cell overgrowth in cultures and with a higher pregnancy loss rate.

There is now little doubt that the insertion of the needle into the amniotic fluid should be ultrasound-guided. The development of curvilinear transducers allows one to visualize both the entry point of the needle and its entire length during the procedure and using this technique 'dry' or

Table 17.1 Investigations made feasible by invasive testing

CVS	Amniocentesis	Blood sampling
Cells Karyotype from direct (48 hrs) and cultured (1−2 weeks) preparations FISH	*Cells* Karyotype from cultured preparations (2−3 weeks) FISH	*Cells* Karyotype directly from WBC (24−48 hours), usually in cases of late presentation, fetal anomaly, failed culture or possible mosaicism FISH
Sexing	Sexing	
Enzyme analysis in metabolic disorders	Enzyme analysis in metabolic disorders	Enzyme analysis in metabolic disorders
DNA analysis for single gene defects, Rh and Hpa¹a typing and fetal infections (e.g. rubella and CMV)	DNA analysis for single gene defects	DNA analysis for single gene defects and fetal infections (e.g. *Toxoplasma gondii*)
		Group and haematocrit in the investigation and treatment of Rh haemolytic disease Platelets in the assessment and treatment of alloimmune thrombocytopenic purpura
	Supernatant AFP and acetylcholinesterase for neural tube defects	*Serum* Viral or protozoal antibodies in cases of suspected infection
	Bilirubin in the assessment of Rh haemolytic disease in the third trimester. Surface active phospholipids, to assess lung maturity	

FISH, fluorescent *in situ* hybridization

making repeated taps has become rare. Complicated needle guides attached to or forming an integral part of the transducer are not required, neither are 'on-screen' angle guides, although some operators prefer to use them.

The procedure should be aseptic but the use of surgeons' gowns, abdominal drapes and transducer bags is unnecessary; using washed, gloved hands and cleaning the transducer and abdomen with chlorhexidine are all the precautions that are required. The image of the needle's length should be observed continuously and the angle of approach changed if necessary. Local anaesthesia is not required if a 22 G needle is used; it causes pain and if injected into the uterine wall, can produce an intense contraction.

The needle stylet should not be removed until the tip is clearly seen in the amniotic fluid and the first few millilitres of fluid should be discarded to reduce the risk of maternal contamination. Twenty millilitres of fluid should be withdrawn for analysis and decanted to a sterile container (light-proof if for spectrophotometry for bilirubin). An initial dry tap can often be overcome by rotating the needle shaft through 360 degrees but if this is not successful the stylet should be replaced before the needle is manipulated further. Cultures from bloody taps are more likely to fail than those where clear fluid is obtained but the addition of 0.1 ml of Heparin (1 in 10 000) to the liquor sample improves the chances of a successful culture in this situation.

If two attempts to obtain fluid have failed (i.e. after two needle insertions) the procedure should be abandoned, although it may be repeated after an interval of a week without extra risk to the pregnancy.

Following the procedure, Anti-D should be prescribed for Rh negative women (250 iu if less than 20 weeks, 500 iu if more). Patients should be advised not to return to work until the following day and to avoid strenuous activity (including housework) until then.

The major risk to the pregnancy lies in the precipitation of spontaneous abortion. Although the earliest studies which attempted to quantify this risk were either unable to demonstrate a significantly increased risk (NICHD, 1976) or apparently demonstrated an excess spontaneous abortion rate above that which we would now accept (1–1.5%), the first randomized study with sufficient patients to satisfy statistical power calculations revealed an excess pregnancy loss rate of 1% (Tabor *et al.*, 1986). This figure remains the one most widely quoted to patients although local audits may reveal *total* pregnancy loss rates after amniocentesis which consistently fall below this level.

Direct evidence in animals (Symchych and Winchester, 1978) and the indirect evidence of the association between anhydramnios and pulmonary hypoplasia has led to concerns over a possible link between amniocentesis and pulmonary dysfunction. Tabor *et al.* (1986) reported a relative risk of 2.1 and 2.5 for respiratory distress syndrome and neonatal pneumonia respectively. It may be that this was caused by chronic amniotic fluid leakage, not noticed by the patient.

Any possible link between the temporary reduction in amniotic fluid volume and limb flexion anomalies of the kind usually associated with more prolonged and marked oligohydramnios has been investigated. Despite early reports of such an association these have not been confirmed. At present there is no evidence to suggest that amniocentesis is responsible for orthopaedic deformities.

As with any invasive procedure, infection is a potential hazard but it is extremely uncommon; meta-analysis suggests that 1 case of chorioamnionitis occurs with every 8000 amniocenteses. At least one maternal death, caused by infection and septicaemia, has been reported.

Chorionic villus sampling

Chorionic villus sampling (CVS) has provided further choice for expectant parents, allowing fast and accurate assessment in the first trimester of a pregnancy at a time when it is not obvious to the couple's friends and relatives. Termination is then technically safest and easiest, even though the decision may not be. Either a transabdominal or transcervical approach to the chorion frondosum may be made, depending on operator experience and ability and the location of the developing placenta.

Prior to any referral, a basic ultrasound scan should be performed to exclude the possibility of an anembryonic pregnancy and confirm the gestation. The relatively high maternal age of referred patients leads to as many as 10% of pregnancies being found to be anembryonic (Silverman and Wapner, 1992). The patient's Rh group should be known *before* the patient arrives for the test.

After further confirmation of gestational age and fetal viability, the placental site is located by ultrasound. The internal cervical os can often be identified and is a useful guide as to the feasibility of a transcervical approach. A fundal placenta and an anterior placenta in an acutely ante-verted uterus can be impossible to sample transcervically; a posterior placenta in a retroverted uterus cannot be sampled transabdominally without traversing the amniotic cavity. It is useful for referral centres to be able to offer both approaches.

Transcervical (TC)

The patient is made comfortable in the lithotomy position (ideally in a colposcopy chair) and after vulval cleaning, visualization of the cervix with a Cusco's speculum and cervical cleansing with an antiseptic, a curved biopsy forceps (Fig. 17.1) is passed through the cervical canal whilst the uterus is observed by ultrasound scanning (ideally, this is performed by the operator). A tenaculum may be used, but it is often not necessary. As the diameter of the forceps is small (2 mm), care should be taken to avoid creating a 'false passage'. It is often noticed that the cervical canal has a distinct curve and the forceps may need to be directed initially posteriorly, then anteriorly, or *vice versa*. The tip of the sampling forceps is not visible until it has passed the shadow of the anterior blade of the speculum but from then on it should be clearly seen and can be directed towards the placenta. Considerable angulation of the forceps may be required in order to do so. Sampling is achieved by opening the jaws, closing them whilst advancing the forceps further into the placenta and then withdrawing. An

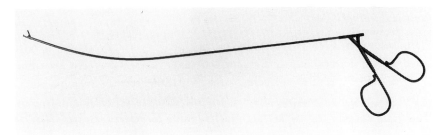

(a)

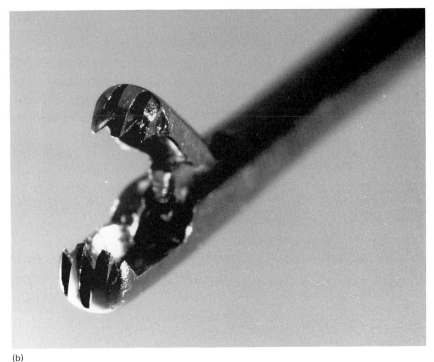

(b)

Fig. 17.1 (a) Transcervical CVS forceps; (b) The open tip in close-up.

adequate sample is obtained in a single passage in 95% of cases. The mass of tissue required will vary with the tests proposed: for karyotyping 5–10 mg may be enough but combinations such as karyotyping and diagnosis of complicated thalassaemia mutations will require up to 30 mg.

A major advantage of biopsy forceps is the clean, bloodless and decidua-free nature of the samples. This allows the operator to confirm that the appropriate amount of the correct tissue has been obtained and also makes handling the sample in the laboratory easier. The earliest techniques for TC CVS were developed using aspiration cannulae, either plastic or metal. The most widely used instrument is probably still the Portex cannula.

Transabdominal (TA)

Transabdominal CVS is a technique more easily learnt by those already familiar with amniocentesis. The aim is to achieve an instrument insertion along the long axis of the placenta, roughly parallel to the chorionic plate. Filling or partially emptying the bladder will often alter the orientation of the uterus enough to provide the most suitable angle of approach. Under ultrasound control an 18 G needle is passed through the skin to enter the placenta. 21 G forceps are advanced through the needle until visible on the scan within the placental substance. It is possible to repeat sampling several times through the same needle insertion. Each individual sample is small but clean, the latter being characteristic of biopsy forceps.

The first TA technique used a double needle system, where a 20 G sampling needle is passed through an 18 G outer needle. Suction is applied to the inner needle using a syringe containing culture medium whilst it is moved several times through the placenta (Smidt-Jensen and Hahnemann, 1984).

Recently, single needle aspiration using an 18 G or 20 G needle, has become widely used as it is attractively simple. However, if a 20 G needle is used, very vigorous movement of the needle tip within the placenta may be required to avulse sufficient villi. Furthermore, if the sample is inadequate, multiple transabdominal punctures may be required. Patients experience more pain and have more feto-maternal haemorrhage with this technique (Rodeck *et al.*, 1993). It has also been particularly associated with fetal limb reduction defects when performed before 9½ weeks and this may be related to placental trauma at a highly susceptible stage of development (Rodeck, 1993).

Risks and benefits of differing sampling techniques

CVS vs amniocentesis

The overwhelming advantages of the earliest possible diagnosis of fetal abnormality by CVS have already been alluded to but there are drawbacks associated with this technique. Firstly, reports of fetal limb defects following CVS before 10 weeks' gestation (Firth *et al.*, 1994) have led to the abandonment of the technique until after this time. Secondly, large multicentre trials confirm a higher pregnancy loss rate from CVS than from amniocentesis (Report of the Canadian Collaborative CVS–Amniocentesis Clinical Trial Group, 1989; MRC Working Party on the Evaluation of Chorion Villus Sampling, 1991) (Tables 17.2 and 17.3). Thirdly, the placenta is not necessarily genetically identical to the fetus, having been derived from the trophectoderm of the developing blastocyst, whilst the fetus develops from the inner cell mass. Discordance and mosaicism may

Table 17.2 Outcome following CVS. (From the Canadian Collaborative CVS–Amniocentesis Clinical Trial Group, 1989)

Outcome	CVS (%)	Amniocentesis (%)
Required re-testing (usually sampling failure)	6	2
Liveborn infant who survived	86	91
Abnormal diagnoses	5.6	3.9

Table 17.3 Outcome following CVS. (From MRC working party on the evaluation of chorion villus sampling, 1991)

Outcome	Disadvantage of CVS over amniocentesis (%)	95% CI	P
Decrease in percentage of a surviving liveborn infant	4.6	1.6–7.5%	<0.01
Increase in spontaneous fetal deaths <28 weeks	2.9	0.6–5.3%	
Increase in percentage of TOPs for chromosomal abnormalities	1.0	0.0–2.1%	
Increase in neonatal deaths	0.3	0.1–0.7%	

TOP, termination of pregnancy.

lead to a need for further sampling by amniocentesis, a procedure required after at least 6% of CVSs during the Canadian Collaborative CVS–Amniocentesis Trial.

Transcervical vs transabdominal CVS

The route to take in order to perform a CVS may be, as already mentioned, determined by the accessibility of the chorion frondosum. The learning curve for an operator already familiar with amniocentesis is likely to be quicker for the TA approach and the risk of infection is possibly greater via the TC route. However, neither large observational studies (Jahoda *et al.*, 1991) nor controlled trials (Jackson *et al.*, 1992) have shown any significant difference in pregnancy loss rates (Tables 17.4 and 17.5). CVS is not as easy as amniocentesis and will therefore not be as widely available. It should only be performed in tertiary referral centres by highly experienced individuals. The operator should ideally be equally good at TC and TA

Table 17.4 Outcome following TC and TA CVS. (From Jahoda *et al.*, 1991)

	Transcervical	Transabdominal
n	1780	1831
Gestational age (weeks)	9.3–11.6	9.3–20
Success at first attempt	86.5%	95%
Fetal loss rate (older women)	6.2%	5.8%*
Fetal loss rate (younger women)	2.8%	1.8%*

* Excludes procedures after 12 weeks' gestation.

Table 17.5 Outcome following TC and TA CVS. (From Jackson *et al.*, 1992)

	Transcervical	Transabdominal	Difference
n	1944	1929	
Sampling success in a single instrumentation (%)	90	94	
Spontaneous fetal loss <28/40* (%)	2.5	2.3	0.26 (95% CI −0.5 to 1.0%)

* Corrected for cytogenetic abnormalities.

CVS and will be able to select the most appropriate route for each patient. It should not be performed before 10 weeks, but this still enables a result to be obtained in the first trimester.

Early amniocentesis

In an effort to retain the advantage of early diagnosis made possible by CVS, but avoid some of the disadvantages of this test (see above), some obstetricians have explored the role of early amniocentesis. Fears that the establishment of suitable cell cultures from amniotic fluid at 12–14 weeks' gestation would fail have in the most part been proved groundless. The total number of cells and the viable fraction therein are comparable to those found after mid-second trimester amniocentesis. Before 12 weeks the culture failure rate increases as does the incidence of pseudomosaicism, possibly because of the relatively smaller proportion of viable cells that have arisen from the fetus (Kennerknecht *et al.*, 1992).

Technically, the procedure is little different from that in the mid-second trimester, but it is imperative that ultrasound control is used; success in obtaining a sample has been reported to be as low as 82% in one series where ultrasound was only used in two-thirds of cases. A vaginal approach both to scanning and needling is technically feasible and extremely accurate but there is a considerable problem with bacterial or fungal overgrowth in cultures, rendering up to 17% of samples unusable (Jorgansen *et al.*, 1992).

The volume of amniotic fluid at 10 weeks' gestation may be as little as 30 ml, and the proportion removed may therefore be as much as 30%. The effects of this on fetal development must still be established, with effects on lung and limb development being of most obvious concern. It is already known that amniocentesis in the second trimester can have an adverse effect on lung function (Milner *et al.*, 1992). Early amniocentesis also has an association with a reduced neonatal functional residual capacity, although this effect has also been described as a sequel to TA CVS (Thompson *et al.*, 1992).

The risks of pregnancy loss resulting from early amniocentesis are not yet fully established particularly in comparison to CVS or later amniocentesis. Hanson *et al.* (1992) reported a series of 936 procedures at less than 12.8 weeks in which 0.7% of pregnancies aborted within 2 weeks, 2.2% were lost before 28 weeks and there were four (0.4%) perinatal deaths. In a non-randomized trial Assel *et al.* (1992) were not able to demonstrate a higher spontaneous abortion rate after amniocentesis at 13–14 weeks compared to those performed at 16 weeks, although of those pregnancies lost, a higher proportion aborted within 4 weeks following early amniocentesis.

Because of the uncertainties surrounding the use of the procedure, the MRC Working Party on the evaluation of CVS (1991) expressed an opinion that early amniocentesis should only be offered as part of a randomized controlled trial, a view firmly endorsed by others (Neilson and Gosden, 1991). A multi-centre approach is required as it has been estimated that if the pregnancy loss rate after CVS is 4%, over 6000 patients are required to demonstrate or refute a difference of 1% in the loss rate between amniocentesis and CVS.

Fetal blood sampling

Although the fetal circulation was first punctured in 1963, when Freda and Adamsons (1964) exteriorized a fetus by hysterotomy, percutaneous access was not feasible until the development of a fine fetoscope. Pure fetal blood samples were first obtained by fetoscopic puncture of the umbilical cord (Rodeck and Campbell, 1978) but subsequently improved ultrasound scanning rendered the fetoscope obsolete. Under direct real time ultrasound guidance, fetal blood sampling is now feasible from the umbilical cord (Daffos *et al.*, 1983), the intrahepatic umbilical vein (Nicolini *et al.*, 1990) and the fetal heart (Bang, 1983), usually after 19 weeks' gestation. The exact site chosen will often prove to be that which is most accessible but the umbilical cord at the placental insertion can usually be easily identified and offers a fixed point for sampling. The umbilical vein is the vessel most commonly used, for although the umbilical artery offers the facility for admixture of transfused fluids with the placental circulation before return to the fetus, the risk of vascular spasm and cord tamponade leading to potentially fatal fetal bradycardia outweighs this theoretical benefit.

The intrahepatic portion of the umbilical vein is technically more difficult to sample but does offer some advantages over the cord insertion in specific situations. In the presence of allo-immune Rh haemolytic disease it can be disadvantageous to traverse the placenta with a needle; feto-maternal haemorrhage has been described in approximately 70% of cases where a cord insertion was sampled via an anterior placenta, and this may be responsible for rises in maternal Rh (D) antibody titres and an increased rate of fall in the fetal haematocrit. Cord tamponade is also impossible using this site and any fetal or transfused blood lost from the vessel after withdrawal of the needle may be reabsorbed from the peritoneal cavity (Nicolini *et al.*, 1990). On occasion the cord insertion can be quite inaccessible if the fetus is lying directly across it.

The positioning of the needle can be checked by the on-site determination of the fetal erythrocyte mean cell volume (which is much greater than in adult blood) and by the infusion of saline into the fetal vessel causing turbulent intravascular flow which is visible ultrasonically.

As the techniques of sampling have improved, the indications for its use have drastically changed mainly because of the rapid progress of genetic knowledge and technology. Linked DNA probes and direct gene analysis allow the diagnosis of many inherited disorders from chorionic villi and amniocytes where previously fetal blood was required to make a diagnosis. The haemoglobinopathies are the prime example. The direct analysis of fetal blood components is still required in cases of allo-immune haemolysis and thrombocytopenia (see below), in the confirmation of fetal infection, in cases of late presentation and in the investigation of fetuses discovered by ultrasound to have a fetal anomaly associated with aneuploidy.

The risks of fetal blood sampling to the fetus arise from the introduction of infection, from membrane rupture and also, significantly, from persistent bradycardia. Quantification of risk is complicated by the confounding variables involved such as the underlying fetal condition and its gestational age, the vessel chosen and the skill of the operator. In low-risk patients at 21 weeks' gestation the fetal loss rate following sampling of the cord insertion has been reported to be as low as 0.5%, although overall, 1.6% may be more realistic (Daffos, 1990). Sampling before 19 weeks has been reported to cause a fetal loss rate of 5% and bradycardia may follow 20%

of samples from the umbilical artery; these data suggest that sampling before 20 weeks and puncturing the artery should be avoided.

Fetal tissue biopsies

Skin

First performed fetoscopically for epidermolysis bullosa lethalis (Rodeck *et al.*, 1980), skin biopsies are now taken under ultrasound guidance from 15 weeks' gestation using 20 G forceps introduced through an 18 G cannula. Significant scarring did not follow any of 52 such cases (Nicolini and Rodeck, 1992). Congenital skin conditions requiring fetal skin biopsy for their diagnosis are shown in Table 17.6.

Liver

Initially a fetoscopic technique (Rodeck *et al.*, 1982), fetal liver biopsy is now done by an ultrasound-guided, double needle aspiration. It is indicated in conditions in which rare enzyme deficiencies cannot be diagnosed by DNA analysis (Table 17.7).

Muscle

Most families at risk of Duchenne muscular dystrophy (DMD) are informative for a variety of DNA probes, a few are not. Fetal muscle biopsy is

Table 17.6 Congenital skin conditions requiring fetal skin biopsy

Epidermolysis bullosa lethalis
Epidermolysis bullosa dystrophica
Harlequin ichthyosis
Oculocutaneous albinism
Epidermolytic hyperkeratosis
Sjögren–Larsson syndrome
Neuroaxonal degeneration

Table 17.7 Indications for fetal liver biopsy

Ornithine carbamyl transferase (OCT) deficiency, when DNA studies are not informative

Carbamyl phosphate synthetase (CPS) deficiency

Alanine glyoxalate aminotransferase (AGT) deficiency

Glucose-6-phosphatase (G6P) deficiency

213

then the only way of performing prenatal diagnosis. In several cases, DMD has been successfully excluded. Small fragments of muscle have been obtained with biopsy needles such as Tru-cut, which have then been stained for the presence of dystrophin (Evans *et al.*, 1991).

Other tissues

Fetal lung, kidney and tumours have been biopsied in a few cases for a variety of new indications, with varying degrees of success. In general, the risks of fetal tissue biopsy do not seem to be higher than for fetal blood sampling, but the numbers are far smaller so firm conclusions cannot be drawn.

Improving sonographic visualization

Despite the dramatic improvements in resolution achieved by contemporary ultrasound scanners, there remain situations in which the visualization of intrauterine structures is difficult, providing inadequate information for a reliable diagnosis or prognosis. One such condition is anhydramnios, where the acoustic window afforded by the amniotic fluid is unavailable. The differential diagnosis usually lies between premature preterm membrane rupture and renal agenesis, the prognoses being variable (dependent upon gestation) and fatal, respectively. The percutaneous instillation of warm normal saline into the amniotic cavity fulfils two functions: image definition may become sufficient to view the relevant structures (Quetel *et al.*, 1992) (in particular allowing differentiation between the kidney and adrenal gland) and leakage of fluid *per vaginam* infers a diagnosis of membrane rupture, unmasking rather than, as was previously thought, causing this condition.

Fluid instillation into the fetal body cavities can occasionally aid diagnoses; diaphragmatic hernias can be difficult to differentiate from cystic adenomatoid malformation of the lung or lung sequestration. Saline instilled into the fetal chest will remain there in the two latter conditions whereas the development of ascites indicates the presence of the former. Intraperitoneal instillation of saline may also help to confirm renal agenesis, a diagnosis that is frequently difficult to make (Haeusler *et al.*, 1993).

FETAL THERAPY

Allo-immune haemolytic anaemia

Despite the undoubted success of the prophylactic administration of anti-D to Rh negative women experiencing a potentially sensitizing event, some 600–700 UK women a year still develop anti-D antibodies, mainly because of sensitization in the first pregnancy, mismatched transfusions and the prescription of inadequate dosage of anti-D (Clarke *et al.*, 1985). Left untreated, 45–50% of fetuses would be mildly affected, 25–30% would develop hepatosplenomegaly, moderate anaemia and progressive jaundice and the remainder would develop hydrops and die *in utero* or in early neonatal life (Bowman and Pollock, 1965). Even as recently as 1983, 50 intrauterine and neonatal deaths were occurring annually as a result of rhesus alloimmune haemolysis. Anti-c and anti-Kell antibodies may also produce severe haemolytic disease in the Rh positive mother.

Prior to the feasibility of fetal blood sampling, management relied upon an indirect assessment of the degree of fetal haemolysis by the measurement of the optical density of amniotic fluid at 450 nm and hence its bilirubin content. Use of a Liley chart (Liley, 1961) allowed the obstetrician to plan the optimum time of delivery and occasionally to utilize intraperitoneal transfusion. Assessment by amniocentesis can still be useful in cases where antibodies develop in the third trimester but prior to this, Liley charts only have a 32% sensitivity for fetuses that are already severely affected and require treatment, a situation which becomes worse in those affected at less than 25 weeks' gestation (Nicolaides and Rodeck, 1985).

Attempts have been made to assess the fetal condition with non-invasive techniques, but results have been disappointing. Fetal hydrops can be detected with a high degree of accuracy with ultrasound and the early signs of increased visibility of the fetal gut and the development of a sonolucent crescent of fluid behind the liver may be easily recognized. Hydrops does not usually develop until the fetal haemoglobin falls below 4 g/dl in the second trimester and, on occasion, there is a time lag before hydrops develops, even at this degree of anaemia. The ultrasonic detection of hydrops can thus only detect a degree of haemolysis and does not exclude severe anaemia in all fetuses. Other ultrasonic markers, such as placental thickness, extra- and intrahepatic umbilical vein diameters, abdominal circumference (AC), head circumference (HC), AC : HC ratios and intraperitoneal volume, show little or no correlation with the degree of fetal anaemia (Nicolaides *et al.*, 1988). Measurement of fetal and umbilical blood flow by Doppler is similarly unhelpful; indices of impedance to flow in uterine, umbilical and fetal circulations are not altered significantly in the presence of fetal anaemia (Marsal *et al.*, 1992). Velocity measurements may, however, be more helpful (Oepkes *et al.*, in press).

The mainstay of the assessment and management of an affected pregnancy continues to be fetal blood sampling, measurement of the fetal haematocrit and transfusion where required. Timing of the first sample is governed by the father's genotype, the severity of the history and whether the antibodies are rising. If the father is heterozygous, an initial sample should be taken at 19–20 weeks in order to determine the fetal blood group although using polymerase chain reaction (PCR) technology fetal

Rh type can now be established from amniocytes taken by amniocentesis at 13/14 weeks (Fisk *et al.*, in press). If the Rh type is negative no further treatment is necessary. Sampling prior to this is technically more difficult and unnecessary as the fetal reticuloendothelial system is not sufficiently developed to mount a response to the immunoglobulin-coated erythrocytes. When the father is homozygous, ultrasound scanning should commence at 19 weeks and continue serially until 22−24 weeks when the first sample should be taken. Measurement of the degree of anaemia is undertaken on the same sample that confirms the presence of fetal, and not maternal, blood. If the history is severe, i.e. a previous second trimester fetal death, treatment may have to be earlier. In most exceptional circumstances, with a previous fetal death at 18−19 weeks, intraperitoneal transfusion may be performed at 14−15 weeks.

Whenever this initial sample is taken, screened O Rh negative blood, cross-matched against maternal serum and packed to a haematocrit (Hct) of 75−80%, should be instantly available for transfusion should the fetus be anaemic. Intravascular transfusion was initially performed fetoscopically (Rodeck *et al.*, 1981) but is now carried out with ultrasound guidance (Nicolaides and Rodeck, 1985). The volume of blood required can be calculated to within 10% from the formula:

$$\text{Donor volume} = \text{Fetoplacental volume} \times \frac{(\text{Target Hct} - \text{Fetal Hct})}{(\text{Donor Hct} - \text{Target Hct})}$$

the aim being a fetal haematocrit of 40−50%. The volume of the feto-placental circulation can be obtained from a normogram (Nicolaides and Rodeck, 1985). During transfusion the point of the needle and the fetal heart should be closely watched for signs of needle displacement, cord tamponade and bradycardia. The correct placement of the needle (in the umbilical or intrahepatic vein) is confirmed during transfusion by the observation of turbulence in the vessel. Excessive fetal movement can be controlled by the administration of pancuronium but this is usually un-necessary. At the end of the transfusion, the fetal haematocrit is rechecked to ensure that sufficient blood has been given. The second transfusion is usually performed 2 weeks after the first and subsequent transfusion intervals are based upon the rate of fall of the haematocrit over the 2 weeks. The trend is for a reduction in the rate of fall to about 1%/day as gestation advances and as fetal erythropoesis is suppressed: subsequent intervals are therefore usually 3 weeks. Performing transfusions by both intraperitoneal and intravascular routes simultaneously can extend the interval between transfusions (Nicolini *et al.*, 1989). The relatively increased longevity of adult red cells suppresses haemopoesis and paediatricians should be aware of the potential need for top-up transfusions postnatally.

This technique has been responsible for a remarkable improvement in the prognosis for affected pregnancies. Fetal survival rates following early fetoscopic transfusions were impressive, with 92% of non-hydropic and 71% of hydropic fetuses surviving. Utilizing ultrasound-guided transfusion, reports of more than 80% of hydropic fetuses surviving are commonplace.

Not all centres have had such uniform success, however, and alternative techniques have been suggested such as returning to the peritoneal cavity as the optimum site for transfusion following an assessment of the fetal condition by fetal blood sampling (MacKenzie et al., 1987). Case control studies do not, however, support any advantage to this method of treatment (Harman et al., 1990).

Allo-immune thrombocytopaenic purpura

The establishment of expertise in fetal blood sampling has allowed the development of therapies for other deficiencies of fetal blood components, most notably platelets. Fetal allo-immune thrombocytopenia is a rare condition, affecting 1 in 3000–5000 live births. Ninety-eight per cent of women express the platelet antigen Hpa[1]a, the 2% who do not may develop anti-Hpa[1]a if exposed to a sensitizing event, such as a transplacental haemorrhage in the index or previous pregnancy or a blood transfusion, particularly if she is HLA B8, DR3. Transplacental passage of the IgG antibody may occur from as early as 14 weeks' gestation (Svejgaard, 1969). The resultant fetal thrombocytopenia is associated with a perinatal mortality of 10–15% and severe neurological abnormalities in up to 25% of survivors, attributable to intracranial haemorrhage which may occur in the second trimester (Nicolini et al., 1990). Subsequent pregnancies are also invariably affected if the father is homozygous.

The extremely poor correlation between the fetal platelet count and the maternal serum antibody level (Svejgaard, 1969) necessitates that the assessment of the fetal condition depends on fetal blood sampling. Initial assessment is usually performed at 20–22 weeks and platelets should be immediately available for transfusion should the fetus be found to be thrombocytopenic; exsanguination may occur from the needle site if the platelet count is not corrected. Suitable platelets may be obtained from an Hpa[1]a negative donor or the mother (who is by definition Hpa[1]a negative) by centrifugal or plasmapheretic separation from other blood components, suspension in normal AB plasma to remove any circulating anti-Hpa[1]a antibody, and irradiation (Kaplan et al., 1988).

Platelet administration may be required at weekly intervals and the risks of repeated cord trauma and that of prematurity need to be carefully weighed in the third trimester. Administration of maternal high dose immunoglobulin or steroids is controversial and although possibly efficacious in mild to moderate cases, they cannot completely replace the need for transfusion in severe cases. Further therapeutic trials are required.

In such a rare condition it is difficult to report large series, but cases where the fetal platelet count has been corrected also show a reduction in the incidence of intracranial haemorrhage and perinatal mortality (Nicolini *et al.*, 1990; Kaplan *et al.*, 1988).

Fetal shunts

The antenatal drainage of pathological collections of fluid in the fetus is feasible both by direct needling and the placement of double pigtail-ended feto-amniotic shunts. In theory, drainage of abnormal fluid collections is possible from the fetal abdomen, brain, chest and renal tract, although it is only practised therapeutically in the latter two instances.

Pleural effusions

Pleural effusions can be of local or systemic origin. Drainage is of greatest benefit when the cause of the effusion is local as those of systemic origin (e.g. hydrops from fetal infection or anaemia) have their prognosis determined by the underlying cause. The finding of a fetal pleural effusion should lead to a detailed examination of the fetal anatomy (and karyotyping) with particular attention given to whether the effusion is uni- or bilateral and whether there is accompanying hydrops, which could be caused by the compression of the heart and inferior vena cava. Isolated effusions may resolve spontaneously and the insertion of a shunt should be limited to those without a systemic cause and which are causing hydrops fetalis (Fig. 17.2). After shunting, resolution of the effusion and associated hydrops is

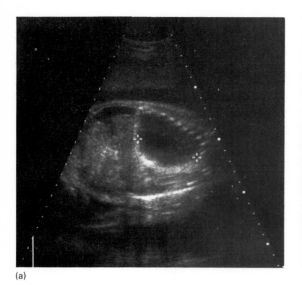
(a)

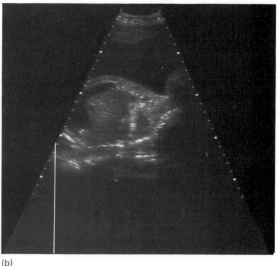
(b)

Fig. 17.2 (a) A sagittal section of a fetus with a unilateral pleural effusion and secondary ascites, (b) immediately after the insertion of a pleuro-amniotic shunt, the effusion has been completely drained.

a good prognostic indicator, as is the finding of large numbers of lymphocytes on microscopic examination of aspirated fluid. This indicates a
chylothorax which is due to a local cause (defective lymphatic drainage), a
form of effusion where fetal outcome is greatly improved by shunting
(Rodeck *et al.*, 1988).

Renal tract

Urinary tract dilatation is not always due to obstruction and may occur at
several anatomical levels, causing a variety of clinical appearances (Table
17.8). Uni- or bilateral hydronephrosis is usually due to uretero-pelvic
junction dysfunction and is normally benign. Urethral atresia carries a
hopeless prognosis whereas that of posterior urethral valves (Fig. 17.3) is
mixed.

The increased perinatal mortality rate associated with these cases arises
from three sources: (1) renal dysplasia; (2) pulmonary hypoplasia due to
chronic oligohydramnios; and (3) from associated congenital abnormalities.
Decompressing the dilated urinary tract should in theory relieve the first
two problems but in practice it must be done before renal and pulmonary
development are arrested. The selection of suitable cases for the continuance
of a pregnancy with a vesico-amniotic shunt *in situ* should therefore rely
upon the following criteria:
- no associated fetal abnormality
- normal karyotype
- urethral obstruction due to posterior urethral valves
- Oligohydramnios
- delivery not a viable alternative, (<32 weeks)
- normal or only moderately impaired renal function.
The full ultrasonic assessment of fetal anatomy will usually require amnio-
infusion and the determination of karyotype requires fetal blood sampling.

Table 17.8 The anatomical result of obstruction at varying levels in the fetal urinary
tract

Level of obstruction	Ultrasound appearance	
Pelviureteric junction	Renal pelvic dilatation	
Ureterovesical junction	Hydroureter Renal pelvic dilatation	+ Oligohydramnios if urine output and/or micturition sufficiently reduced
Urethra	Megacystis + Renal pelvic dilatation + Hydroureter +/− Prune belly	

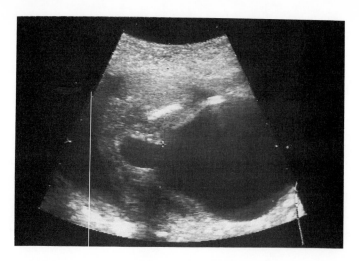

Fig. 17.3 A sagittal section of a grossly distended bladder in a male fetus. The distended posterior urethra suggests the presence of posterior urethral valves.

Fetal renal function is best assessed by biochemical analysis of aspirated urine. Fetal urine is kept relatively hypotonic by the kidneys and their ability to continue to do so up to the point of treatment is associated with an improved survival rate, (Table 17.9). Normal renal function and hence membership of a group with a good prognosis has been established (Cromblehome *et al.*, 1990) by the ability of the kidneys to maintain a urinary Na concentration of less than 100 mmol/l and a urinary Cl concentration of less than 90 mmol/l, measured on urine tapped at the time of shunt insertion. These criteria do not, however, take into account the normal fall in Na^+ osmolality in normal fetal urine. Publication of normal ranges for gestation (Nicolini *et al.*, 1992) has led to a refinement of these criteria and improved assessment of fetal renal function (Fig. 17.4).

Following insertion of the shunt, resolution of the urinary tract dilatation and a reaccumulation of the amniotic fluid point to a successful procedure with at least some surviving renal function. Failure of the oligohydramnios to resolve without redilatation of the urinary tract indicates renal failure

Table 17.9 Influence of prognostic group upon percentage fetal survival following decompressive treatment of urinary tract obstruction. (From Cromblehome *et al.*, 1990)

	Survivors		
	Treated	Untreated	Total
Good prognosis	8/9 (88.9%)	5/7 (71.4%)	13/16 (81.3%)
Poor prognosis	3/10 (30%)	0/14 (0%)	3/24 (12.5%)
Total	11/19 (57.9%)	5/21 (23.8%)	16/40 (40%)

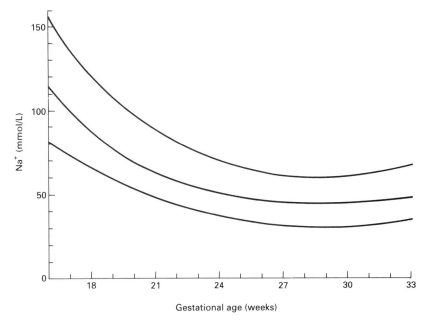

Fig. 17.4 Variation of fetal urinary Na$^+$ concentration with gestation. (After Nicolini *et al.*, 1992.)

rather than a shunt blockage in which case the outlook is invariably hopeless. Termination of pregnancy then has to be considered by the parents.

Relief of polyhydramnios

Excess amniotic fluid causes a rise in intramniotic pressure, increased myometrial tension, an increased incidence of premature labour and a reduction in the fetal Po_2 (Fisk *et al.*, 1990). Drainage of excess fluid should be beneficial in relieving these adverse conditions. Treatment is hampered, however, by the rapid reaccumulation of fluid, even when several litres are removed. The best that can usually be achieved is a temporary improvement in maternal discomfort.

Serial amniocentesis of huge amounts of liquor has been claimed to be beneficial in the 'stuck twin' syndrome (Fig. 17.5), the end stage of severe twin–twin transfusion. This condition, which occurs in monochorionic twin pregnancies with intraplacental vascular communications, can be recognized by the disparate growth between monochorionic twins and, in the advanced state of severe oligohydramnios of the donor twin, causing adherence of this twin to the uterine wall by its membranes. Fetal survival rates are poor without treatment (0–16%) but Mahoney *et al.* (1990) achieved an improvement to 69% (against historical controls of 20%) by serially removing enough fluid from the polyhydramniotic sac over 45–90

221

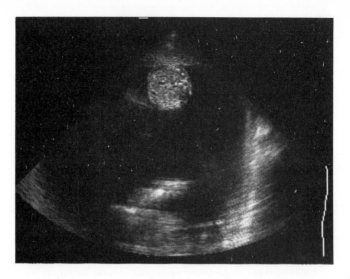

Fig. 17.5 The stuck twin phenomenon, the typical presentation of severe twin-twin transfusion syndrome. There is gross polyhydramnios, the donor fetus (abdominal circumference section) is fixed against the anterior wall of the uterus.

minutes with a 22 G needle to reduce the maximum column depth to about 7 cm.

Several alternative treatment options have been suggested and each continues to undergo evaluation:

1 Selective fetocide of the donor; this has been successfully performed but the presence of vascular communications places the recipient at high risk of porencephaly, probably due to the reversal of blood flow back to the original donor, as a result of its blood pressure being zero.

2 Removal of the donor twin; three cases of hysterotomy and removal of the stuck twin have been reported with a survival rate of one in three of the remaining twins (Kuller and Golbus, 1992).

3 Laser ablation of the communicating vessels via a fetoscope has been performed on three pregnancies and four out of the six infants survived (Delia *et al.*, 1990).

Therapeutic amnioinfusion

Oligohydramnios is associated with the occurrence of variable decelerations of the fetal heart rate during labour (most probably caused by transient umbilical cord or placental compression) and meconium aspiration syndrome. The instillation of normal saline in labour (via intrauterine pressure catheters) in attempts to reverse this situation has been reported in several small trials.

Miyasaki and Navarez (1985) relieved repetitive variable decelerations in 25 out of 49 cases treated by amnioinfusion, compared with 2 out of 47

222

randomized controls, $(P < 0.001)$ but only reduced the caesarean rate from 25.5% to 18.4% $(P < 0.547 \text{ NS})$. Their results were more impressive when primigravidae alone were considered. Variable decelerations were relieved in 18 out of 27 cases but in none of the 21 controls $(P = 0.001)$ and the caesarean section rate fell from 47.6% in the control to 14.8% in the treated groups. Strong *et al.* (1990) attempted this in fetuses at risk of developing, but not yet demonstrating, an abnormal CTG. Thirty women with oligohydramnios within the latent phase of labour underwent amnio-infusion. The fetal condition at birth was unaffected although the incidence of both fetal acidosis at delivery and caesarean section for fetal distress were significantly reduced.

In an attempt to reduce the incidence of meconium aspiration syndrome, Sadovsky *et al.* (1989) performed amnioinfusion on a randomly selected and controlled group of 40 women in labour with meconium stained liquor. Variable decelerations were commoner in the control group as was fetal acidosis and the presence of meconium seen below the vocal cords at delivery (Table 17.10).

Meconium aspiration syndrome is uncommon but has a high associated mortality. Amnioinfusion may go some way to prevent it but in order to demonstrate a significant reduction in its incidence, say from 3% to 1%, power calculations dictate the need for trials with in excess of 750 patients per arm. Clearly further work is required.

Open fetal surgery

Despite the undoubted advances in the field of fetal therapy, there remain some conditions which lie elusively beyond the ability of the most advanced centres to significantly influence their prognosis. Diaphragmatic hernias are a prime example; approximately 50% of affected infants who survive to undergo surgery die thereafter, despite optimal care, primarily from pulmonary insufficiency and hypertension secondary to chronic lung compression. Attempts have been made to improve on this situation by reversing

Table 17.10 Effects of amnioinfusion on women in labour with meconium stained liquor. (From Sadovsky *et al.*, 1989)

	Amnioinfusion (%)	Control (%)	P
Persistence of thick meconium	5	62	<0.0005
Cord arterial pH <7.2	16	38	<0.05
Meconium below vocal cords	0	29	<0.05
Need for PPV at birth	16	48	<0.05

PPV, positive pressure ventilation.

the trends in non-invasive treatment and reverting to partial exteriorization of the fetus (Harrison *et al.*, 1990), removing the abdominal contents from the chest and repairing the diaphragmatic defect with a plastic graft. Despite the technical expertise demonstrated during these procedures, success to date has been marred by a high incidence of fetal death, the not unexpected tendency of the uterus to enter premature labour and by pre-term, pre-labour membrane rupture.

Maternal outcome does not seem to be compromised but fetal outcome does not seem to be improved; operations performed on 15 high-risk cases show a 20% fetal survival and a 46% intraoperative fetal loss rate (Kuller and Golbus, 1992). This type of intervention has also been used by Harrison's group for some obstructive uropathies and congenital malformations of the lung, with variable success. With such a complicated and challenging technique, the learning curve is bound to be slow and the situation may improve as further experience is gathered. Clearly a great improvement is needed in outcome, however, if this management regime is to become accepted.

REFERENCES

Assel, B., Lewis, S., Dickerman, L., Park, V. and Jassani, M. (1992) Single operator comparison of early and mid-second-trimester amniocentesis. *Obstetrics and Gynecology*, **79**(6), 940–44.

Bang, J. (1983) Ultrasound guided fetal blood sampling, in *Progress in Perinatal Medicine* (eds. A. Albertini and Crosignani), Excerpta Medica, Amsterdam, pp. 223.

Bowman, J. and Pollock, J. (1978) Amniotic fluid, spectrophotometry and early delivery. *Paediatrics*, **35**, 815–35.

Canadian Collaborative CVS–Amniocentesis Clinical Trial Group (1989) Multicentre randomized clinical trial of chorion villus sampling and amniocentesis. First report. *Lancet*, **11**(1), 334–35.

Clarke, C., Mollison, P. and Whitfield, A. (1985) Deaths from Rhesus haemolytic disease in England and Wales in 1982 and 1983. *British Medical Journal*, **291**, 17–19.

Cromblehome, T., Harrison, M., Golbus, M. *et al.* (1990) Fetal intervention in obstructive uropathy: prognostic indicators and efficacy of intervention. *American Journal of Obstetrics and Gynecology*, **162**, 1239–44.

Daffos, F. (1990) Fetal blood sampling. In *The Unborn Patient* (eds. M.R. Harrison, M.S. Golbus and R.A. Filly), W.B. Saunders, Philadelphia, pp. 75–81.

Daffos, F., Capella-Pavlovsky, M. and Forestier, F. (1983) Fetal blood sampling via the umbilical cord using a needle guided by ultrasound. Report of 66 cases. *Prenatal Diagnosis*, **31**, 271–77.

Delia, J., Cruikshank, D. and Keye, W. (1990) Fetoscopic neodymium: YAG laser occlusion of placental vessels in severe twin–twin transfusion syndrome. *Obstetrics and Gynaecology*, **75**, 1046–53.

Evans, M., Greb, A., Kunkel, L.M. *et al.* (1991) *In utero* fetal muscle biopsy for the diagnosis of Duchenne muscular dystrophy. *American Journal of Obstetrics and Gynecology*, **165**, 728–32.

Firth, H., Boyd, P., Chamberlain, P., MacKenzie, I., Morriss-Kay, G.M. and Huson, S. (1994) Analysis of limb reduction defects in babies exposed to CVS. *Lancet*, **343**, 1069–71.

Fisk, N.M., Bennett, P., Warwick, R.M. *et al.* (1994) Clinical utility of fetal Rh typing in alloimmunized pregnancies using the polymerase chain reaction amniocytes or chorion villi. *American Journal of Obstetrics and Gynecology*, **171**, 50−54.

Fisk, N., Tannirandorn, Y., Nicolini, U., Talbert, D. and Rodeck, C.H. (1990) Amniotic pressure in disorders of amniotic fluid volume. *Obstetrics and Gynecology*, **76**, 210−14.

Freda, V. and Adamsons, K.J. (1964) Exchange transfusion *in utero*. *American Journal of Obstetrics and Gynecology*, **89**, 817.

Haeusler, M., Ryan, G., Robson, S., Lipitz, S. and Rodeck, C.H. (1993) The use of saline solution as a contrast medium in suspected diaphragmatic hernia and renal agenesis. *American Journal of Obstetrics and Gynecology*, **168**, 1486−92.

Hanson, F., Tennant, F., Hune, S. and Brookhyser, K. (1992) Early amniocentesis: outcome, risks, and technical problems at less than or equal to 12.8 weeks. *American Journal of Obstetrics and Gynecology*, **166**, 1707−11.

Harman, C.R., Bowman, J.M., Manning, F.A. and Menticoglou, S. (1990) Intrauterine transfusion — intraperitoneal versus intravascular approach. A case control comparison. *American Journal of Obstetrics and Gynaecology*, **162**(4), 1053−59.

Harrison, M., Adzick, N., Longaker, M. *et al.* (1990) Successful repair *in utero* of a fetal diaphragmatic hernia after removal of diaphragmatic viscera from the left thorax. *New England Journal of Medicine*, **322**, 1582−84.

Jackson, L., Zachary, J., Fowler, S. *et al.* (1992) A randomised comparison of transcervical and transabdominal chorionic-villus sampling. The US National Institute of Child Health and Human Development Chorionic-Villus Sampling and Amniocentesis Study Group. *New England Journal of Medicine*, **327**(9), 594−98.

Jahoda, M., Brandenburg, H., Reuss, A. *et al.* (1991) Transcervical (TC) and transabdominal (TA) CVS for prenatal diagnosis in Rotterdam: experience with 3611 cases. *Prenatal Diagnosis*, **11**(8), 559−61.

Jorgansen, F., Bang, J., Lind, A., Christensen, B., Lundsteen, C. and Philip, J. (1992) Genetic amniocentesis at 7−14 weeks of gestation. *Prenatal Diagnosis*, **12**(4), 277−83.

Kaplan, C., Daffos, F., Forester, F. *et al.* (1988) Management of alloimmune thrombocytopaenia. Antenatal diagnosis and *in utero* transfusion of maternal platelets. *Blood*, **72**, 340−43.

Kennerknecht, I., Baur-Aubele, S., Grab, D. and Terinde, R. (1992) First trimester amniocentesis between the seventh and thirteenth weeks: evaluation of the earliest possible genetic diagnosis. *Prenatal Diagnosis*, **12**(7), 595−601.

Kuller, J. and Golbus, M. (1992) Fetal therapy in Prenatal Diagnosis and Screening (eds. D. Brock, C.H. Rodeck and M. Ferguson-Smith), Churchill Livingstone, Edinburgh, pp. 703−717.

Liley, A.W. (1961) Liquor amnii analysis in the management of pregnancy complicated by rhesus sensitisation. *American Journal of Obstetrics and Gynecology*, **82**, 1359−70.

MacKenzie, I.Z., Bowell, P.J., Ferguson, J., Castle, B.M. and Entwhistle, C.C. (1987) *In utero* intravascular transfusion of the fetus for the management of severe rhesus isoimmunisation — a reappraisal. *British Journal of Obstetrics and Gynaecology*, **94**, 1068−73.

Mahoney, B., Petty, C., Nyberg, D., Luthy, D., Hictok, D. and Hirsch, J. (1990) The 'stuck-twin' phenomenom: ultrasonographic findings, pregnancy outcome and management with serial amniocentesis. *Obstetrics and Gynecology*, **77**, 537−40.

Marsal, K., Nicolaides, K.M., Kaminopetros, P. and Hackett, G. (1992) The clinical value of waveforms from the descending aorta, in *Doppler Ultrasound in Perinatal Medicine* (ed. J.M. Pearce), Oxford University Press, Oxford, pp. 257.

Milner, A., Hoskyns, E. and Hopkin, I. (1992) The effects of mid-trimester amniocentesis on lung function in the neonatal period. *European Journal of Pediatrics*, **161**(6), 458−60.

Milunsky, A. (1979) Prenatal diagnosis of neural tube defects, in *Genetic Disorders and the Fetus*, Plenum, New York, 379–430.

Miyasaki, F. and Navarez, F. (1985) Saline amnioinfusion for relief of repetitive variable decelerations: a prospective randomised study. *American Journal of Obstetrics and Gynecology*, **153**, 301–16.

MRC working party on the evaluation of chorion villus sampling (1991) Medical Research Council European trial of chorion villus sampling. *Lancet*, **337**, 1491–99.

Neilson, I. and Gosden, C. (1991) First trimester prenatal diagnosis: chorionic villus sampling or amniocentesis? *British Journal of Obstetrics and Gynaecology*, **98**, 849–52.

NICHD (1976) National Registry for Amniocentesis Study Group 1976. Midtrimester amniocentesis for prenatal diagnosis — safety and accuracy. *Journal of the American Medical Association*, **236**, 1471–76.

Nicolaides, K.H. and Rodeck, C.H. (1985) Rhesus disease: the model for fetal therapy. *British Journal of Hospital Medicine*, **34**, 141–8.

Nicolaides, K.H., Fontanarosa, M., Gabbe, S.G. and Rodeck, C.H. (1988) Failure of ultrasonographic parameters to predict the severity of fetal anaemia in rhesus iso-immunisation. *American Journal of Obstetrics and Gynecology*, **158**(4), 920–26.

Nicolini, U. and Rodeck, C.H. (1992) Fetal blood and tissue sampling, in *Prenatal Diagnosis and Screening* (eds. D. Brock, C.H. Rodeck and M. Ferguson-Smith), Churchill Livingstone, Edinburgh, pp. 47.

Nicolini, U., Kochenour, N.K., Greco, P., Letsky, F. and Rodeck, C.H. (1989) When to perform the next intrauterine transfusion in patients with Rhesus allo-immunisation: combined intravascular and intraperitoneal transfusion allows longer intervals. *Fetal Therapy*, **4**, 14–20.

Nicolini, U., Tannirandorn, Y., Gonzales, P. *et al.* (1990) Continuing controversy in alloimmune thrombocytopaenia. *American Journal of Obstetrics and Gynecology*, **163**, 1144–46.

Nicolini, U., Nicolaides, P., Fisk, N.M., Tannirandorn, Y. and Rodeck, C.H. (1990) Fetal blood sampling from the intrahepatic vein: analysis of safety and clinical experience with 214 procedures. *Obstetrics and Gynecology*, **76**, 47–53.

Nicolini, U., Fisk, N., Rodeck, C.H. and Beacham, J. (1992) Fetal urine biochemistry: an index of renal maturation and dysfunction. *British Journal of Obstetrics and Gynaecology*, **99**, 46–50.

Oepkes, D., Brand, R., Vandenbussche, F.P., Meerman, R.H. and Kanhai, H.H.H. (1994) The use of ultrasonography and Doppler in the prediction of fetal haemolytic anaemia: a multivariate analysis. *British Journal of Obstetrics and Gynaecology*, **101**, 680–84.

Quetel, T.A., Meijedes, A.A., Salman, F.A. and Torres Rodriguez, M.M. (1992) Amnio-infusion: an aid in the ultrasonographic evaluation of severe oligohydramnios in pregnancy. *American Journal of Obstetrics and Gynecology*, **167**(2), 333–36.

Rodeck, C.H. (1993) Prenatal diagnosis: fetal development after chorionic villus sampling. *Lancet*, **341**, 418–19.

Rodeck, C.H. and Campbell, S. (1978) Sampling pure fetal blood by fetoscopy in the second trimester of pregnancy. *British Medical Journal*, **ii**, 728–30.

Rodeck, C.H., Eady, R.A.J. and Gosden, C. (1980) Prenatal diagnosis of epidermolysis bullosa letalis. *Lancet*, **i**, 949–52.

Rodeck, C.H., Fisk, N.M., Fraser, D.I. and Nicolini, U. (1988) Long-term in-utero drainage of fetal hydrothorax. *New England Journal of Medicine*, **319**, 1135–38.

Rodeck, C.H., Kemp, J.R., Holman, C.A., Whitmore, D.N., Karnicki, J. and Austin, N.A. (1981) Direct intravascular fetal blood transfusion by fetoscopy in severe rhesus isoimmunization. *Lancet*, **i**, 625–27.

Rodeck, C.H., Patrick, A.D., Pembrey, M.E., Tzannatos, C. and Whitfield, A.E. (1982) Fetal liver biopsy for prenatal diagnosis of ornithine carbamyl transferase deficiency. *Lancet*, **ii**, 297–99.

Rodeck, C.H., Sheldrake, A., Beattie, B. and Whittle, M.J. (1993) Maternal serum alphafetoprotein after placental damage in chorionic villus sampling. *Lancet*, **341**, 500.

Sadovsky, Y., Amon, E., Bude, M. and Petrie, R. (1989) Prophylactic amnioinfusion during labour complicated by meconium: a preliminary report. *American Journal of Obstetrics and Gynecology*, **161**, 613–17.

Silverman, N. and Wapner, R. (1992) Chorionic villus sampling, in *Prenatal Diagnosis and Screening* (eds. D.J.H. Brock, C.H. Rodeck and M.A. Ferguson-Smith), Churchill Livingstone, Edinburgh, pp. 27.

Smidt-Jensen, S. and Hahnemann, N. (1984) Transabdominal fine-needle biopsy from chorionic villi in the first trimester. *Prenatal Diagnosis*, **4**, 163–69.

Smychych, P.S. and Winchester, P. (1978) Amniotic fluid deficiency and fetal lung growth in the rat. *American Journal of Pathology*, **90**, 779–82.

Strong, T., Hetzler, G., Sarno, A. and Paul, R. (1990) Prophylactic intrapartum amnio-infusion: a randomised clinical trial. *American Journal of Obstetrics and Gynecology*, **162**, 1370–74.

Svejgaard, A. (1969) Isoantigenic system of human blood platelets. A survey. *Series Haematologica*, **2**(3), 68.

Tabor, A., Philip, J., Madser, M., Bang, J., Obel, E.B. and Norgaard-Pederson, B. (1986) Randomised controlled trial of genetic amniocentesis in 4606 low risk women. *Lancet*, **i**, 1287–89.

Thompson, P., Greenhough, A. and Nicolaides K. (1992) Lung volume measured by functional residual capacity in infants following first trimester amniocentesis or chorion villus sampling. *British Journal of Obstetrics and Gynaecology*, **99**(6), 479–82.

Chapter 18
Paediatric Medical Management of Fetal Abnormality

I. MORGAN and G. DURBIN

Serious birth defects account for 20% of neonatal deaths, in addition to the toll of significant childhood illness. Caring for a child with major anatomical problems imposes great emotional and financial stresses on the parents and on elder or younger siblings.

Families who have already had one such child, whether surviving or not, can be enormously helped by the knowledge that prenatal diagnosis is available in a subsequent pregnancy.

It is likely that they will look upon this positively. They may have been directed to genetic counselling after the birth of the affected child, or later by their general practitioner. Even empirical recurrence risks, for instance 2% for congenital heart defects, allow some confidence in pregnancy planning and the organization of antenatal investigations. More commonly, with the advent of near-universal antenatal ultrasound screening, the suspicion of a fetal anomaly is, for the parents, a dreadful and unanticipated piece of news. Culturally they may be unable to accept the information they are given, particularly since the pregnancy may be progressing normally and there is no visible or external evidence of abnormality. A relationship of trust must be built up quickly between parents and the ultrasonologist if the information given, which may change with time, is to be accepted.

A team approach in planning appropriate counselling avoids delivery of inappropriate or conflicting information. The timing of information can also be planned ahead; for instance, details of surgical procedures necessary after delivery are best not approached until after 30 weeks' gestation.

LETHAL DEFECTS

Abnormalities likely to lead to the death of the fetus or neonate, and detected with confidence at around 20 weeks' gestation, for instance Potter's syndrome, seldom require planned antenatal paediatric involvement. A senior ultrasonologist, who will have seen the parents several times, can offer appropriate counselling. This will concentrate on accurate presentation of all the facts and options. If termination of pregnancy is decided on, the ultrasonologist will liaise with the obstetric team to organize this with speed and compassion.

If for cultural or religious reasons the parents decide to continue with the pregnancy, then ordinary obstetric supervision is appropriate. A clear plan for the management of the labour and the delivery must be agreed with the parents and prominently and clearly documented in case notes, so that the mother is protected from having an emergency caesarean section for a baby who has a lethal condition.

Regular interdepartmental meetings ensure that paediatricians are aware of such babies in advance. An experienced paediatrician will talk to the parents at 34–36 weeks if they so wish, and will attend the delivery.

A child with major, untreatable defects born alive can still be offered quality care. Active resuscitation will not be indicated. The baby needs to be examined thoroughly and the diagnosis confirmed to the parents. The baby can be kept warm and comfortable, either with his parents or in a cot on the neonatal unit until death supervenes. Request for a post-mortem examination to confirm antenatal findings is vital and must not be forgotten.

STILLBIRTHS

There is good evidence that parents can spend years regretting lost opportunities to see and hold their stillborn baby. This applies just as much if the baby is malformed; the defect in the parents' imagination may be worse than the reality. Peaceful time together, photographs, and mementoes may all be treasured. Consent for post-mortem is required and the parents need to be counselled by an experienced medical practitioner. If consent is refused, valuable genetic information can be obtained from clinical photographs and X-rays of the dead baby, as well as external examination by a geneticist if possible.

PRENATAL COUNSELLING

Serious defects suspected at 20 weeks' gestation may have unknown implications. Repeated imaging over time to clarify an anatomical lesion, for instance a congenital heart defect, may result in an eventual diagnosis with different implications from that initially suspected. Similarly, additional investigative tests may reveal a major chromosomal error which will transform the prognosis of an apparently minor anatomical abnormality. Caution must be exercised, therefore, in prognosticating in detail until a firm diagnosis is made.

Advice from surgical or neonatal colleagues may be indicated at 18–20 weeks when parents are attempting to decide whether to terminate the pregnancy. These interviews are often at parental request. Clinicians offering such counselling must be aware of the natural history of the presumed condition. Ideally, a small team who gain experience in this work can be used. Serious misinformation about likely benefits of surgery can result if surgeons base their counselling on their clinical postnatal experience; this usually represents a different population and has a higher proportion of less seriously affected babies. Counselling, as always, should be non-directive and needs to concentrate on accurate and comprehensible presentation of the facts and possible options.

Later in pregnancy, neonatal paediatricians and surgeons are very well placed to advise and inform the parents because of their experience in the management of babies with anomalies. Factual information as to what will happen to the baby at delivery, what the baby's external appearance is likely to be, and the likely timing and arrangements for surgery can be offered. Mothers may have questions about accommodation at the surgical centre, possibilities for breast-feeding etc. Useful information about the long-term outcome can be given, bearing in mind the possibility of undiagnosed additional defects or complications. The use of photographs, for instance of cleft lip and palate, or the chance to meet parents of similarly affected children can be very useful.

These interviews can be planned to coincide with antenatal clinic appointments but in any case should be booked in advance so that partners or extended family can attend. A private, quiet, unhurried approach is important, and a visit to the neonatal unit can add to the reassurance offered by such sessions.

IMMEDIATE POSTNATAL CARE

An equipped and experienced paediatric team needs to be available at the time of delivery. Indeed, this is one area that can be demonstrated to parents as an advantage of antenatal diagnosis. The major roles of the paediatrician will be to avoid treatable asphyxia and at the same time, rapidly to assess the external appearance and behaviour of the baby. Thus if the prognosis can be determined to be hopeless by an experienced paediatrician, vigorous and prolonged resuscitation can be avoided. The paediatric team should be informed in as much detail as possible prior to delivery so that they can anticipate problems. For instance, a baby with jejunal atresia may have an abdomen so distended as to split the diaphragm. Active resuscitation including gastric emptying with a large bore tube (8 FG) is important in any gut atresia to prevent inadvertent later tracheal aspiration of regurgitated gastric contents. A baby with a left sided diaphragmatic hernia may need to be intubated and needs to be laid head up and left side down, then rapidly transferred to the neonatal unit. A baby with exteriorized abdominal contents will require to have these wrapped immediately in an impermeable sac, (i.e. 'clingfilm' around the trunk and contents) to be kept adequately warm and to receive intravenous protein solution commenced shortly after delivery. A hydropic baby may require immediate aspiration of pleural and peritoneal effusions at the same time as intubation and positive pressure ventilation (this requires two operators).

Compatible blood can be organized in advance to treat a severely anaemic baby within half an hour of birth.

However ill the baby and however complicated the resuscitation, there is always the opportunity to allow the conscious mother, and the father, to see and touch, even if they cannot hold their baby before he/she is taken from the delivery suite. They must be kept informed of his/her condition and his/her physical location; a polaroid photograph can always be taken, particularly if he/she is to be transferred to another unit.

Once the baby's condition has been stabilized after delivery, subsequent management depends on the underlying condition. Medical problems will require confirmation of diagnosis. Surgical problems will require transfer to a specialized neonatal surgical unit if this is not on site.

While some conditions will require surgery the same day, others, notably diaphragmatic hernia, benefit from a period of stabilization in a neonatal intensive care unit so that lung function can be assessed and the appropriateness of surgery discussed.

MEDICAL CONDITIONS DIAGNOSED ANTENATALLY

The list of medical conditions (Table 18.1) is not exhaustive and details of management may vary; advance discussion with the neonatologist, the surgical team and the parents is vital to optimize care. A large number of single gene defects can now be detected antenatally, usually in families with a previous affected child. Specific tests of blood and/or urine will confirm the diagnosis postnatally in almost all cases. Management is of the underlying condition.

Table 18.1 Medical conditions and their management

Condition	Management	Comment
Inherited		
Cystic fibrosis	Confirm in first few days from immune-reactive trypsin using blood spot. Sweat test only of use later. Check for gene deletion	For meconium ileus see Table 19.1
Duchenne muscular dystrophy	Check dystrophin levels in muscle biopsy. Confirm creatine kinase levels after first week	
Congenital adrenal hyperplasia	Confirm 17-hydroxyprogesterone levels at about 3 days of age	Cortisone replacement plus aldosterone if necessary
Inborn errors of metabolism (IEM)	Confirm diagnosis and pending confirmation exclude fat and protein from diet and use only carbohydrate	Investigate blood gases, electrolytes, ammonia and amino acid profiles. Full blood count, urinalysis, urine amino and organic acid analysis
	If infant fails to respond and no diagnosis reached samples must be stored. This is particularly important if the child dies	Blood — separate and store plasma frozen. Urine — store frozen. Skin — keep in culture medium. Post-mortem aqueous humour — store frozen
		Liver biopsy — store frozen, some for electron microscopy. Muscle biopsy — frozen DNA extraction from anticoagulated blood or post-mortem spleen
Severe immune deficiencies	Infant should be delivered by caesarean section, wrapped in a sterile gown and nursed in a sterile, laminar flow tent until prenatal diagnosis confirmed	Feeds irradiated, all articles sterilized. Treatment by enzyme replacement or bone marrow transplantation
Non-genetic Hydrops fetalis (a) Immune	Adequate prenatal transfusion essential. Immediate resuscitation vital. Exchange transfusion if cord Hb <10 g/100 ml or bilirubin rising >12 µmol/hour	Investigations — cord Hb, bilirubin. Coombs' test and blood group Blood for transfusion should be fresh, CMV negative, concentrated and irradiated

Condition	Management	Comment
(b) Non-immune	Active resuscitation is vital with para- and thoracocentesis. Prognosis poor, usually <50%. Support until diagnosis clear	Investigations — FBC, blood for haemoglobinopathies, glucose 6-phosphate dehydrogenase (G6PD) deficiency, karyotype, viral studies; skeletal survey; echocardiography

Chapter 19
Paediatric Surgical Management of Fetal Anomaly

P. A. M. RAINE

Detection by prenatal diagnosis of a fetus with a structural anomaly immediately raises a series of questions and problems. It is an event of major importance for the parents and must be handled expertly, sympathetically and expeditiously to lessen the chances of serious distress and anxiety. A team approach is the surest way to achieve this; the perinatal team will usually include an obstetrician/ultrasonologist, neonatologist, neonatal surgeon and geneticist as well as other counsellors and specialists.

Accurate interpretation of ultrasound scan and biochemical analyses is essential in arriving at a precise diagnosis. However, the natural history and pathophysiology of *in utero* anomalies are only partly understood and not always predictable. The knowledge base is gradually expanding by careful collection and analysis of all data relating to *in utero* diagnosis i.e. ultrasound, biochemical, genetic, anatomical, pathological and histological.

Advice to the parents may of necessity be qualified and the prognosis for the fetus guarded. A series of interviews with reiteration of explanations may be needed. Photographs may help the parents to form a perception of their baby's anomaly and a chance to meet other couples with similarly affected children can be of great value.

Once the diagnosis is established, the principal objective is to determine which of a number of options is most appropriate in further management of the pregnancy. The options include:
- termination of the pregnancy
- *in utero* fetal surgery
- early (preterm) delivery and urgent surgery
- term delivery followed by surgery
- caesarean in preference to vaginal delivery
- delivery in a main centre close to neonatal intensive care and surgical facilities.

Termination of pregnancy

Termination of pregnancy on the grounds of anomaly may be considered when the prognosis for the fetus is unmistakably poor and when residual, severe disability is certain. The decision will be taken against a background of cultural, social, religious, ethical and moral considerations. The parents' previous experiences and the likely impact of a newborn with serious problems on the family are important factors. Extensive thoraco–lumbar myelomeningocele with hydrocephalus is such a problem. Full and careful counselling is imperative prior to the termination and the necessary certification and notification to authorities are both a statutory requirement and important for completion of accurate records and anomaly registers.

In utero fetal surgery

A knowledge of the natural history and pathophysiology of some structural anomalies shows that survival after birth will be impossible for severely affected fetuses. *In utero* fetal surgery is the only option if every effort to save the life of the fetus is to be made. Major moral and ethical dilemmas arise; paramount among these is the need to ensure that the risk to the mother is minimal. Extensive laboratory and animal experimental work (principally at the Fetal Treatment Centre, University of California, San Francisco) has led to development of strategies for safe hysterotomy, fetal exposure, closure of the uterus and control of preterm labour. Corrections of fetal anomalies *in utero* have been performed. The main areas of interest and potential progress are listed below.

- Congenital diaphragmatic hernia — early gestation fetal diagnosis and polyhydramnios are prognostic signs of poor outcome with perinatal death from pulmonary hypoplasia. *In utero* correction of the hernia may allow adequate lung growth.
- Bilateral urinary tract obstruction — hydronephrosis and renal dysplasia leading to oligohydramnios may cause irreversible pulmonary hypoplasia and renal failure. Decompression of kidneys or bladder by renal pelvis drainage or vesicostomy may preserve sufficient renal and pulmonary function.
- Hydrocephalus — progressive cerebrospinal fluid accumulation may cause more extensive cerebral atrophy and neuronal damage. Ventriculostomy may reduce this.
- Fetal intrathoracic masses (e.g. cystic adenomatoid malformation) — compression of normal lung tissue leads to pulmonary hypoplasia and hydrops. Excision of abnormal lung or drainage of cysts may encourage lung growth.
- Sacrococcygeal teratoma — these vascular lesions cause a 'steal' syndrome leading to high output cardiac failure with hydrops and placentomegaly. Tumour resection may protect against this.

Early (preterm) delivery

When early delivery and surgery are considered, a careful balance must be made between the putative advantages of organ preservation for the fetus and the increased risks associated with premature delivery and surgery. Progressive bowel obstruction and distention (e.g. gastroschisis complicated by atresia) or bilateral renal dilatation (e.g. posterior urethral valve obstruction) may provide indications for early delivery.

Term delivery followed by surgery

This is the usual choice for treatment of the majority of structural anomalies diagnosed *in utero*. Oesophageal and other intestinal atresias, intra-abdominal cystic lesions, neural tube defects and facial clefts are all best managed in a mature neonate after postnatal confirmation of the diagnosis, full assessment and identification of associated abnormalities.

Caesarean delivery

Caesarean delivery may be indicated either because of anticipated difficulty with vaginal delivery or to diminish the risks of fetal damage. Examples are:
- massive hydrocephalus and large sacrococcygeal teratoma may cause obstruction to vaginal delivery
- major exomphalos (extra-abdominal liver) may be ruptured during vaginal delivery and therefore require surgery when conservative treatment might have been the preferred option.

Delivery in a main centre adjacent to
neonatal intensive care and surgical units

When it is likely that the newborn will need immediate resuscitation and support, or when prompt assessment and preparation for surgery is necessary, there is obviously a clear advantage in delivery in a main centre. Additional advantages are that separation of the baby from the mother may be less abrupt and both parents will be able to be involved in discussions with the neonatal paediatrician and surgeon about the baby's management. Babies with diaphragmatic hernia and anterior abdominal wall defects (gastroschisis and exomphalos) should be delivered as close as possible to the neonatal surgical unit for these reasons. In other cases (e.g. duodenal atresia, unilateral renal dilatation) postnatal transfer of the baby may be appropriate.

AT DELIVERY

The majority of infants with anomalies are at substantial risk of birth asphyxia which can be minimized by ensuring that a fully equipped and prepared paediatric team is available at the time of delivery. An experienced paediatrician should head the team so that logical decisions can be made about the wisdom of aggressive resuscitation in circumstances in which the prognosis is clearly hopeless. However, it is also very important that those in attendance have a good understanding of the considerations underlying the immediate management so that the baby can be prepared appropriately and rapidly for surgery. This may make the difference between intact and damaged survival. Immediate passage of a nasogastric tube to deflate the stomach and endotracheal intubation for ventilation may avoid serious hypoxia in a case of diaphragmatic hernia. It is the objective that all babies undergoing surgery should leave the neonatal intensive care unit with stable blood gases, ventilation if necessary, normothermia, corrected acidosis, appropriate intravenous and intra-arterial lines in place, blood cross-matched and parental consent for surgery.

Brief details of the surgical management and outcome for various anomalies are shown in Table 19.1.

Table 19.1 Surgical conditions and their management

Condition	Management/Comment	Prognosis
Abdominal wall defects		
Exomphalos	Exclude chromosomal and other anomalies (e.g. cardiac) Occasional major epigastric and hypogastric associated defects Deliver at term — by caesarean section if major exomphalos (liver in sac) Protect sac membrane with warm sterile saline pack or 'cling-film' Surgery — primary closure or 'staged' closure using silastic silo Conservative — preserve sac membrane and encourage epithelialization	Prognosis good for minor exomphalos (<5 cm) and isolated lesions
Gastroschisis	Deliver at term, vaginally if possible Inspect for bowel atresia or stenosis Protect bowel with warm sterile saline pack and 'cling-film' Surgery — primary closure (possible in > 80%) — otherwise 'staged' closure using silastic silo	Prognosis good — up to 90% survival. May be slow (>30 days) to establish enteral feeding with delayed growth in first year

(Continued)

237

Table 19.1 (*Cont.*)

Condition	Management/Comment	Prognosis
Bowel atresia		
Oesophageal	Associated malformations in 50% — VACTERL syndrome Diagnosis by failure to pass nasogastric tube and plain X-ray of opaque catheter to confirm arrest in oesophagus Frequent suction of upper oesophagus to prevent aspiration pneumonia Surgery — primary end-to-end repair possible in 80% — otherwise 'staged' procedures, oesophagostomy/gastrostomy	Up to 80% survival May have early respiratory problems associated with tracheomalacia Gastro-oesophageal reflux may need treatment Good long term prognosis
Duodenal	Trisomy 21 in 30% Initial large bile-stained gastric aspirate common — aspirate not always bile-stained Surgery not urgent — full assessment for other anomalies important Naso-jejunal tube feeding necessary until pyloric/duodenal function recovers	Good prognosis if lesion isolated
Jejuno-ileal	Marked abdominal distension with visible bowel loops Atresias usually developmental or ischaemic — but possibility of meconium ileus must be considered Atresias single or multiple — sometimes with obvious short length of small bowel (suggests prenatal volvulus) Surgery — primary anastomosis preferable but proximal dilated bowel may require partial excision or tapering	Prognosis good even if only 20% of small bowel remains
Ano-rectal	Variety of perineal appearances — complete absence of anus or anterior stenotic anal fistula Passage of meconium *per urethram* or *per vaginam* may be noted Associated renal tract anomalies common Type of surgery depends on length of atretic segment (high, intermediate or low anomaly) Initial colostomy may be needed	Low malformations — outcome good High malformations — higher incidence of associated anomalies and long term problems with faecal continence

Condition	Management/Comment	Prognosis
Other gastrointestinal disorders		
Meconium ileus	Distal small bowel obstruction due to inspissated meconium pellets in terminal ileum Characteristic X-ray 'ground-glass' appearance Conservative treatment with series of gastrografin enemas Associated atresia, perforation or ischaemia will require surgery *In utero* perforation may lead to meconium cyst and peritonitis Ileostomy often necessary	Prognosis variable. Most cases due to cystic fibrosis with long term chest, liver, pancreatic complications
Hirschsprung's disease	Aganglionosis of distal bowel — commonly up to recto-sigmoid junction level Presents with failure to pass meconium in first 12–24 hours Diagnosis by rectal biopsy and barium enema preferably before rectal washouts Resection of aganglionic segment and pull-through either primarily or following initial proximal colostomy Risk of enterocolitis (10%)	Prognosis good
Intra-abdominal cysts		
Liver/spleen	Cysts may be very large but are often unilocular Excision usually possible	Prognosis good
Choledochal	Presents with jaundice Various types and degrees of biliary tract dilatation Excision of cyst if possible but drainage into Roux jejunal loop often necessary	Prognosis good though long term risks of ascending cholangitis, portal hypertension and malignancy in residual cyst wall
Ovarian	Usually follicular or luteal — very rarely malignant May tort or rupture — but can spontaneously regress Small cysts (<6 cm) can usually be managed conservatively	Prognosis good

(Continued)

Table 19.1 (*Cont.*)

Condition	Management/Comment	Prognosis
Urinary tract Multicystic kidney	Large, non-functioning, cystic mass replacing kidney — ureter usually atretic Contralateral kidney may be abnormal in up to 50% Risks of hypertension or malignancy in multicystic kidney probably minimal and excision now not usually advocated — mass may shrivel and disappear	Prognosis good provided contralateral kidney normal
Unilateral hydronephrosis (caused by reflux or PUJ obstruction)	Antibiotic prophylaxis from birth (trimethoprim). Investigate postnatally to exclude reflux and PUJ obstruction	Reflux often improves with time. Occasionally ureteric reimplantation needed PUJ obstruction can improve spontaneously or deteriorate postnatally. Early nephrostomy drainage if severe. Surgery (pyeloplasty)
Bilateral hydronephrosis/ hydroureter. (In a male may be due to posterior urethral valves, or bilateral reflux or PUJ obstruction)	In male, urgent MCUG to assess bladder outlet. Investigate as above. Monitor renal function and BP	Variable prognosis. Difficult to predict residual renal function until postnatal investigations complete. Early renal failure leading to death or dialysis may develop
Posterior urethral valves	Obstruction may be relieved by urethral catheter though secondary uretero-vesical obstruction may prevent renal decompression Upper renal tract drainage and reconstruction may be needed in addition to ablation of valves	Risk of progressive renal failure in up to 50% despite surgical decompression
Ectopia vesicae	Complex anatomical abnormality — upper renal tracts may also be abnormal Reconstructive surgery difficult but option of immediate repair should be considered	Prognosis good overall but prospects for urinary continence poor and permanent diversion may be needed

Condition	Management/Comment	Prognosis
Sacrococcygeal teratoma	Caesarean section may be needed in case of massive extrapelvic tumour. Secondary urinary tract obstruction should be investigated Early surgery indicated — complete excision may occasionally require both perineal and abdominal approach Risk of malignancy (10–15%) especially if residual tumour	Usually good — depends on type of tumour (intra/extrapelvic) Faecal continence may be affected
Neural tube defects Spina bifida	Detailed post-natal assessment of lower limb, bladder and anal function, kyphoscoliosis, hydrocephalus and size of back lesion is basis of policy of selection for early surgery Aim is to prevent further neurological damage Long term follow-up and support essential	Prognosis variable — may be poor due to lower limb paralysis, lack of sphincter control, renal failure and psychomotor retardation
Hydrocephalus	Post-natal assessment by serial measurements, ultrasound and computed tomography scan Progressive hydrocephalus requires lateral ventriculo-peritoneal or ventriculo-atrial valve drainage Occasionally direct surgery or drainage of posterior fossa (Dandy–Walker) cyst needed	Prognosis variable — depends on aetiology and extent of prenatal compression and dysplasia
Encephalocele	Anterior usually well covered, posterior (more common) may be enormous, thin-walled sacs Urgent surgery required	Prognosis usually poor especially if containing brain tissue — major disability due to severe psychomotor retardation, ataxia, and cortical blindness

(Continued)

Table 19.1 (*Cont.*)

Condition	Management/Comment	Prognosis
Thorax		
Diaphragmatic hernia	Immediate resuscitation essential — passage of nasogastric tube for aspiration and endotracheal tube for ventilation Maximum supportive therapy necessary to stabilize baby. Delayed surgery now preferable to immediate surgery to close defect. Vital to carefully assess lung function. May require pulmonary vasodilation Possibility of extra-corporeal membrane oxygenation if immediate lung function inadequate	Early *in utero* diagnosis and polyhydramnios prognostic signs of bad outcome. Prognosis for survival at time of prenatal diagnosis only 10–20% Survival approximately 50% if baby survives the first 48 hours of life. Long-term outlook good for survivors
Intrathoracic cysts	May have immediate respiratory problems requiring support Surgery not always urgent; precise diagnosis important — congenital cystic adenomatoid malformation, sequestration, congenital lobar emphysema Urgent surgery necessary for expanding lesion	Prognosis good
Hydrothorax	Chylothorax is a common cause but also found in hydrops, fetal infection and some chromosomal anomalies. Lung hypoplasia may be a problem	Prognosis for chylothorax good — may need repeated drainage. Feeding with medium chain triglycerides helps
Other		
Cystic hygroma	75% found in neck, some extend into thorax, lymphangiomata occasionally regress but usually require surgical removal — may be difficult and incomplete Recurrence in approximately 20%	Prognosis usually good
Cleft lip/palate	Common (incidence 1/600) Many associated syndromes — may be associated with extensive craniofacial anomalies Cleft lip closed at 3 months, palate at 6–9 months Treatment requires a team approach and long term follow-up	Prognosis good

FURTHER READING

Adzick, N.S. and Harrison, M.R. (1993) The fetus as a surgical patient. *Seminars in Pediatric Surgery*, **2**, 83–146.

Bagolan, P., Rivosecchi, C., Giorlandino, E. *et al.* (1992) Prenatal diagnosis and clinical outcome of ovarian cysts. *Journal of Pediatric Surgery*, **27**, 879–81.

Clayton-Smith, J., Farndon, P.A., McKeown, C. *et al.* (1990) Examination of fetuses after induced abortion for fetal abnormality. *British Medical Journal*, **300**, 295–97.

dell'Agnola, C.A., Tadini, B., Mosca, F. *et al.* (1992) Prenatal ultrasonography and early surgery for congenital cystic disease of the lung. *Journal of Pediatric Surgery*, **27**, 1414–17.

Elder, J.S., Duckett, J.W. and Snyder, H.M. (1987) Intervention for fetal obstructive uropathy; has it been effective? *Lancet*, **ii**, 1007–1010.

Goh, D.W. and Brereton, R.J. (1991) Success and failure with neonatal tracheo-oesophageal anomalies. *British Journal of Surgery*, **78**, 834–37.

Goh, D.W., Drake, D.P. Brereton, R.J. *et al.* (1992) Delayed surgery for congenital diaphragmatic hernia *British Journal of Surgery*, **79**, 644–46.

Grant, H.W., MacKinley, G.A., Chambers, S.E. *et al.* (1993) Prenatal ultrasound diagnosis: a review of fetal outcome. *Pediatric Surgery International*, **8**, 469–71.

Greig, J.D., Raine, P.A.M., Young, D.G. *et al.* (1989) Value of antenatal diagnosis of abnormalities of the urinary tract. *British Medical Journal*, **298**, 1417–19.

Harrison, M.R. (1988) The fetus with a diaphragmatic hernia. *Pediatric Surgery International*, **3**, 15–22.

Hutson, J.M., McNay, M.B., MacKenzie, J.R., Whittle, M.J., Young, D.J. & Raine, P.A.M. (1985) Antenatal diagnosis of surgical disorders by ultrasonography. *Lancet*, **i**, 621–23.

de Luca, F.G. (1987) The status of prenatal diagnosis and fetal surgery. *Pediatric Surgery*, **2**, 259–66.

Raine, P.A.M. (1991) Anterior abdominal wall defects. *Current Obstetrics and Gynaecology*, **1**, 147–53.

Revillon, Y., Jan, D., Plattner, V. *et al.* (1993) Congenital cystic adenomatoid malformation of the lung: prenatal management and prognosis. *Journal of Pediatric Surgery*, **28**, 1009–11.

Chapter 20
Termination of Pregnancy for Fetal Abnormality: A Practical Guide

R. B. BEATTIE

INTRODUCTION

Termination of pregnancy for a major fetal abnormality presents a problem not only for around 2000 parents and their families in the UK each year, but also for their attendants. The diagnosis of a major fetal abnormality is both distressing and shocking in itself but the decision to terminate causes a complex mixture of both acute grief and some relief.

PREPARING FOR TERMINATION

Although individual responses are varied, the factors associated with least mental trauma include termination in early pregnancy, termination for a lethal abnormality and good support from partners, families and friends (Black, 1989). It has been suggested that when counselling parents of fetuses with a major abnormality, the option to terminate is not assumed and other alternatives should be discussed, including continuing the pregnancy. Even couples who had previously stated that they would terminate based on an abnormal result may have some difficulty reaching a final decision when their fears become a reality. Various authors have stressed the need to respect parents' choices whether they choose to terminate or to continue the pregnancy in conditions incompatible with fetal survival (Whelton, 1990). The parents in this latter group carry both the burden of coping with a doomed pregnancy and the perceived need to defend their decision to health professionals. An interesting paradox, however, is that in the USA some disabled children, including those with Down syndrome, have been awarded damages for 'wrongful life' on the grounds that their parents did not choose the option of prenatal diagnosis and termination.

It is important that health care professionals are appropriately trained and discharge their duties both compassionately and efficiently at a time of strong and conflicting emotions if they are to best serve the immediate and long-term needs of the parents. It is thus highly desirable that a single individual in each centre is responsible for the co-ordination and audit of the prenatal testing and to supervise training for other involved staff. This chapter emphasizes some of the more important aspects of this difficult area, but proper training in counselling, the appointment of a specific

Bereavement Officer and the referral to established support groups are just as important as the clinical management.

Usually the decision to terminate a pregnancy will be based on diagnostic tests such as ultrasound followed by counselling by an experienced senior member of staff who may not be involved in the termination process itself. It is useful if the discussions about the results and subsequent counselling can be conducted in a quiet room away from the main clinical areas. For those wishing to terminate, there will be some who need time to come to terms with the termination of a wanted pregnancy and they may wish to make arrangements for the care of other children whilst others will want admission to hospital as soon as possible. Often it will be appropriate to refer patients to other specialists in paediatrics or clinical genetics, especially when rarer diagnoses are made or those in which the prognosis is difficult to define. It is also important to ensure that there is adequate time for parents to fully discuss and understand the significance of the diagnosis and its implications. This may mean allowing them time at home to consult with family members, friends, religious leaders and their own GPs. They should also have the proposed termination procedure fully explained to them and have a clear idea of where and when they should attend hospital, who to ask for and how long they will spend there. The staff in the clinical area to which they will be admitted should have full patient details, a clear indication for the termination and a designated, named practitioner who will be performing the termination.

Legal issues

Since October 1992, changes in the law allow a pregnancy to be terminated at any gestational age when there is a significant risk that the baby will have serious mental or physical disability. This has eased some of the difficulties surrounding late diagnosis of serious abnormalities but can create major management problems.

It is important that the doctor making the diagnosis leading to the parents' decision to terminate completes a blue form, 'Certificate A', and ideally arranges for the medical practitioner responsible for the termination to see the parents prior to admission to hospital after full discussion of the reasons for offering that option. They will then also countersign 'Certificate A' (HSA 1 1991) which gives the legal permission to terminate the pregnancy under Section 1(1) of the 1967 Abortion Act. Both practitioners must complete this certificate of opinion before any commencement of treatment and will usually do so under section E saying that they feel 'there is substantial risk that if the child were born it would suffer from such physical or mental abnormalities as to be seriously handicapped'. This certificate must then be kept for at least 3 years. When individuals feel that they cannot provide impartial advice and counselling because of their particular moral, religious or ethical beliefs, they should refer to a colleague who can manage the case on clinical grounds free from such restraints and the referral should be done in a non-judgmental way.

The clinician making the diagnosis should also state in their report the further investigations which are needed to confirm the diagnosis after termination. There should be specific details of which samples are required and to whom they should be sent. The value of post-mortem examination should also be stressed prior to the termination, as subsequent discussions are then more easily initiated and important specific tests are not omitted. The routine appointments for antenatal clinics, ultrasound examinations etc. should be cancelled and the patient's consultant, GP and midwife informed of the proposed termination to prevent causing further distress (see Checklists A and B — Appendices 20.4 and 20.3). In the presence of a lethal structural abnormality, antenatal karyotyping from amniotic fluid, fetal blood or placental tissue should be considered for future counselling since post-mortem karyotyping is much less successful.

In many units, 'Certificate A' is either incomplete or forgotten by junior staff or they may feel that they do not have the authority or knowledge to complete it. This is an important issue since the termination then becomes illegal and no medical or surgical procedure should be initiated at any stage unless the form is properly completed.

The clinician performing the termination must see and examine the patient prior to the completion of part 1 of the yellow form, the 'Form of Notification' (HSA4 1991). This is for the statutory registration of all terminations of pregnancy but does not itself permit the termination and can be completed afterwards provided it is sent within 7 days of the procedure to the Chief Medical Officer at the Department of Health, Richmond House, 79 Whitehall, London SWA1 2NS. Ideally, the relevant parts should be filled in at the time the couple decide on termination, when the treatment has been initiated and finally completed and checked immediately after the termination. Bereavement Officers often find incomplete registration forms which will in fact be returned to the unit if the information is inadequate.

TERMINATION OF THE PREGNANCY

Usually this will take place in a gynaecology or maternity ward. It is useful in medical terminations for partners to have facilities to stay overnight in an area away from patients with ongoing pregnancies, preferably in their own room. The parents should be allowed ample opportunity to discuss both the diagnosis and the termination procedure before any intervention is made and consent must be obtained prior to surgical termination before any premedication is given. Appropriate pre-delivery investigations, such as maternal blood samples not already taken, should be obtained and the benefits of a post-mortem and the parents' wishes for burial discussed, although no decision need be made prior to completion. Guidelines should be available for all health professionals and a relevant excerpt from those used in the Birmingham Maternity Hospital is detailed in Appendix 20.1.

METHODS OF TERMINATION

Surgical termination

Under 14 weeks' gestation, surgical termination of pregnancy is a relatively safe and reliable procedure and can be performed on a day case basis under general anaesthesia. Patients should be fasted, given appropriate antacid prophylaxis and of course consented prior to any premedication. A basic anaesthetic assessment is important including a haemoglobin estimation if indicated. The blood group must be known and an appropriate dose of prophylactic anti-D given to rhesus negative mothers afterwards. The choice of anaesthetic drugs should be based on their suitability for day case procedures and combinations such as intravenous Propofol in combination with 0.1 mg fentanyl have been shown to be appropriate.

Cervical preparation has been advocated by some clinicians and Gemeprost 1 mg pessary (Cervagem) is effective if given 2 hours before surgery. This is particularly important in the primigravida and reduces cervical trauma during dilatation. Alternatively, mechanical pre-dilatation with laminaria may be preferred. Since there will usually be no recognizable fetus at the end of the procedure, some parents may want an ultrasound photograph to remember their baby and this should have already been taken in anticipation of this eventuality. Although karyotyping is often successful on the products obtained, the major disadvantage is the lack of an intact fetus for post-mortem examination. Remember that not all abnormalities are detectable on ultrasound and accurate diagnosis is essential for counselling in future pregnancies. Occasionally, there may be excessive bleeding and intravenous access with a large bore cannula should be obtained at the outset. These procedures should only be carried out by experienced staff because of the risks of cervical trauma, uterine perforation, haemorrhage and incomplete evacuation of the uterus.

Medical termination

Beyond 14 weeks' gestation there is an increased risk of bleeding and usually a medical termination of pregnancy will be advisable. There are various regimes but the use of Gemeprost (Cervagem) is widespread and reasonably well tolerated by most patients (Table 20.1). The effects of this drug may be even further enhanced by the use of Mifepristone (RU486) which has been shown to reduce the induction to delivery interval. One

Table 20.1 Success rates and therapeutic regimes for termination of pregnancy

Study	n	Drugs	Route	Success (24 hour) (%)	Comment
Thong and Baird, 1992	100	Gemeprost Gemeprost and Dilapan Gemeprost and Mifepristone	PV PV and oral PV and oral	72 85 95	GIT side-effects reduced with Mifepristone
Allahbadia, 1992	200	Prostaglandin F2a	IM repeatedly	90	Iodine-saline is a cheap technique with high success rate
		20% Hypertonic saline Ethacridine lactate 5% Povidone iodine-saline	Intra-amniotic Extra-amniotic Extra-amniotic	96 98 100	
Ferguson (2d) et al., 1993	62	Prostaglandin F2a Urea Laminaria tent	Intra-amniotic Cervical	97	Immediate and delayed complications rare in either group
		Prostaglandin F2a Urea Laminaria tent Prostaglandin E2 pessary	Intra-amniotic Cervical PV	73	
Kanhai and Keirse, 1993 (II Trimester)	32	Sulprostone	IV 1 µg	100	All aborted in 52 hours, range 8–52, median 23 hours

GIT, gastrointestinal tract.

regime using 200 mg Mifepristone 36 hours before 4×1 mg Gemeprost vaginal pessaries inserted 6 hourly resulted in a 96% success rate in 24 hours. The rate was 99% within 48 hours if the dose interval was reduced to 3 hourly for a further 12 hours after the first 4 doses. However, 33% of these women required surgical evacuation of uterus and vomiting (31%) and diarrhoea (5%) also remain a problem needing appropriate treatment (Thong and Baird, 1992, 1993). One study has also suggested a further refinement using 4 hourly repeated doses of 10 mg intravenous Meto-clopramide which reduced the patient's analgesic requirements and reduced the induction—delivery interval. Even in late pregnancy following caesarean section there is a high success rate for vaginal delivery (87%) with a risk of uterine rupture under 5% (Boulot *et al.*, 1993).

Intra-amniotic injection of a single dose of prostaglandin F2a has been useful in middle and late second-trimester terminations of pregnancy and has the advantage that amniotic fluid can be obtained for karyotyping if this has not already been done.

Early medical termination is now possible using the antiprogestin Mifepristone RU486 (Zaytseva *et al.*, 1993). Various dosage regimes have been described but a recent report on 1182 women by the World Health Organisation Task Force on post-ovulatory methods of Fertility Regulation suggests that a low dose of 200 mg Mifepristone is as effective as doses of 400 mg and 600 mg when combined with a vaginal pessary of 1 mg Gemeprost (WHO, 1993). Complete abortion was achieved in about 95% cases, 3.7% were incomplete, 0.3% had a missed abortion and 0.4% failed completely and the pregnancy continued. Of those with incomplete abortion, over 50% required emergency surgical evacuation of uterus and therefore facilities for this and the management of severe haemorrhage must be available for these women.

Feticide and selective feticide

One of the first case reports of selective termination in America was a pair of twins discordant for trisomy 21 diagnosed by amniocentesis. Following counselling the parents elected for selective termination which was carried out by ultrasound directed cardiocentesis and exsanguination of the affected twin. When selective termination is required, this can be achieved by ultrasound-guided intracardiac injection of 'strong' potassium chloride (20 mmol/10 ml) with survival rates of the remaining twin of up to 75%. A similar technique may also prove useful prior to late pregnancy medical terminations to ensure that the fetus is stillborn, thus sparing the parents unnecessary distress at the time of delivery.

AFTER THE TERMINATION

Following delivery of a medically induced termination there will usually be a recognizable fetus. Some parents may wish to hold or name their baby and may wish to lay him/her out with a toy, a family photograph or a shawl. Some time should be set aside for parents to spend with the baby on their own should they wish. It is important that parents have as much time as they wish with their baby and they should be as undisturbed as possible by any necessary routine midwifery activities. If the baby is to be kept in another room for any length of time it is important to inform other staff to prevent unnecessary distress to domestics, ward clerks etc. who may enter that room.

The maximum use should be made of what parents can remember and they should be encouraged to touch, hold and dress their dead baby. Indeed this opportunity should be offered to parents on more than one occasion. When an overt abnormality exists it is important to point out the normal features such as hair and feet before cautiously undressing the baby with the parents. Most parents have perceptions of fetal abnormality which are much worse than they actually appear. A suggested 'Last office pack' is listed in Appendix 20.2.

Documentation

If a termination for abnormality is performed (any gestation) a blue 'Certificate A' and a yellow 'Form of Notification' should have already been completed by the medical staff. If there is no identifiable baby, attendant staff must also complete Checklist B (Appendix 20.3) and a Histology form. If there is an identifiable baby (any gestation), the staff should complete Checklist A (Appendix 20.4), the Post-mortem consent form and the Stillbirth Certificate or Notice of Death. The attendant at the delivery should also complete the two forms 'Statement by the Doctor or Midwife present at delivery for fetuses under 24 weeks' gestation certifying that the baby was born dead before the legal age of viability' (Appendix 20.5) and 'Check Sheet for Babies Born with External Abnormalities or Terminated for Fetal Abnormality' (Appendix 20.6). They will only be asked to complete a Stillbirth Certificate if the fetus is more than 24 weeks' gestation.

The Still-birth (Definition) Act received royal assent in 1992 and effectively reduced the minimal gestational age by which a stillbirth is defined from 28 to 24 weeks. As a consequence, Statutory Maternity Pay, Maternity Allowance and Social Fund Maternity Payments as defined in the Social Security Contributions and Benefits Act of 1992 will now be paid to qualifying mothers who give birth to a stillborn child after 24 weeks' gestation on or after 1 October 1992 and stillbirth certification is required for all babies born dead after 24 weeks' gestation (NHS, 1992).

For fetuses delivering after 24 weeks a Stillbirth Certificate must therefore be completed by the doctor or midwife who attended the delivery, issued to the parents and taken to the Registrar for Births and Deaths for the sub-district where the birth or death took place within 42 days (21 days after delivery in Scotland). The Registrar will then enter the baby's name on the Stillbirth Register, record the full names and dates of birth of the mother and father, the date and time of delivery and will issue a Certificate for Burial or Cremation (and a Stillbirth Certificate if the parents wish). If the baby's father is not married to the mother then both must attend the registration if they wish the father's name to be entered on the register. If, however, the father is married to the mother then he may register the death on his own.

Before 24 weeks' gestation there is no requirement to register the death though a letter or certificate is required by funeral directors (see Appendix 20.5) before they will bury or cremate the baby to certify that the fetus 'was born before the age of viability and showed no signs of life.'

Viewing the baby

Parents should be able to see their baby at any reasonable time after the termination before the funeral. A contact number should be given to them and ideally he or she should be viewed fully dressed in a moses basket in the chapel or a suitable quite place. This is a particularly important time for both parents and relatives and a suitably trained member of staff should accompany the family and remain with them. Babies should not be taken for viewing back to the ward or delivery suite once they have been taken to the mortuary because of the risk of cross infection and for the same reason parents should not pick up the baby following post-mortem examination.

The funeral

Funerals are often arranged in a hurry by a grieving father who wishes to spare his partner further distress but it was been repeatedly found that the mother usually regrets not having the opportunity to share in the arrangements for her baby. It is often an important time for parents and their families to acknowledge the death of the baby and though painful and distressing, most parents are glad they went through it. Funerals can be arranged by either the hospital or a funeral director regardless of gestation. Although hospital burials are free of charge and may include a memorial service conducted by the couple's religious leaders or the hospital chaplain, the burial may be in unconsecrated ground some weeks after the death, and often in a common grave without specific memorial. Alternatively, parents may prefer to have a private funeral according to their own particular religious and cultural beliefs. The latter may be simple or elaborate, religious or non-religious and for those on low incomes (e.g. on Income Support or Family Credit) the Social Fund (Social Security) may be able to help with the expenses.

Regardless of the funeral arrangements, the parents can decide whether they wish their baby to be cremated or buried. Remember that cremation cannot occur until the cause of death is known and therefore a post-mortem may delay the proceedings. The cremation certificate must be signed by two doctors and other forms available from the funeral director must be signed by the next of kin and a medical referee at the crematorium.

The post-mortem

In 1989 the Royal College of Physicians (RCP, 1989) suggested that the main requirements for genetic counselling were as follows:

1 accurate diagnosis in the propositus
2 estimation of the genetic risk
3 communication of the genetic risks and options for avoiding them
4 assistance to the consultant to assimilate the information and reach an appropriate decision
5 accessibility for long term contact with genetic services when appropriate.
In order to properly answer the demands of both the first and second requirement following the diagnosis of a fetal abnormality, and to ensure the quality of the diagnostic services, an accurate diagnosis is essential. A 5 year audit examined the prenatal and postnatal diagnoses amongst fetuses who had a termination of pregnancy for either fetal structural abnormality on ultrasound ($N = 133$) or chromosomal abnormality on amniocentesis ($N = 115$). The diagnosis was modified or changed in 34% (53) of those with an abnormal scan and 2.6% (3) with an abnormal karyotype. Furthermore, the revised diagnosis in those with suspected structural abnormalities led to a significant change in the recurrence risk in over 90% of the revised cases which would have affected their post-termination counselling (Clayton-Smith *et al.*, 1990).

Even when a full post-mortem is not possible, consideration should be given to a partial post-mortem including needle biopsy of major organs, skin biopsy, X-rays and ultrasound, blood and urine examination. It is equally important to have close collaboration between the paediatric pathologists, cytogeneticists and clinical geneticists in such cases to maximize the accuracy of the diagnosis. The results of all the postnatal investigations should then be discussed with the parents in order to allay any fears about wrongful diagnosis and to help them make decisions about future pregnancies.

COUNSELLING AND LONG TERM SUPPORT

The proven harmful psychological sequelae after termination of pregnancy for fetal abnormality has prompted authorities in the field of prenatal diagnosis to recommend that a properly co-ordinated system of follow up is required, preferably by the primary care team. They suggest that as a minimum there should be a visit within 2 weeks and again 2–3 months later, though in our own unit there is also permanent access to a named nurse specialist who is known to the patient and familiar with their case and the Bereavement Officer. Certainly up to 30% of women with a perinatal death may have overt psychiatric problems up to 2 years afterwards and it is not unusual for some patients to telephone on a regular basis over a year later for psychological and moral support, even when all their questions have been answered to their satisfaction.

It is at this stage that voluntary support groups have an important role to play and indeed the work of groups such as SANDS, SATFA and others (Table 20.2) have done much to modify and enhance the training of the health professionals involved in this aspect of prenatal diagnosis. Local groups provide support long after contact with health professionals, and

Table 20.2 Voluntary support group addresses

A.S.B.H. (1994) Association for Spinal Bifida and Hydrocephalus. A.S.B.H. House, 42 Park Road, Peterborough PE1 2UQ. Tel. 01733-555 988

CARE (1994) Scottish Association for Care and Support after Diagnosis of Fetal Abnormality. Duncan Guthrie Institute of Medical Genetics, Yorkhill, Glasgow G3 8SJ. Tel. 0141-201 0365

SANDS (1994) Stillbirth and Neonatal Death Society. 28 Portland Place, London W1N 4DE. Tel. 0171-436 7940 or 5881

SATFA (1994) Support after termination for fetal abnormality. 29/30 Soho Square, London W1V 6JB. Tel. 0171-439 6124

SOFT (1994) Support Organization for Trisomy 13/18. Trisomy 13: Tudor Lodge, Redwood, Ross-on-Wye, Herefordshire HR9 5UD: Tel. 01989-567 480. Trisomy 18: 48 Froggats Ride, Walmley, Sutton Coldfield, West Midlands B76 8TQ. Tel. 0121-351 3122

DSA (1994) Down Syndrome Association. 155 Mitcham Road, London SW17 9PG. Tel. 0181-682 4001

Miscarriage Association (1994) Miscarriage Association c/o Playton Hospital, Northgate, Wakefield, West Yorkshire WF1 3JS. Tel. 01924 200799

---

their literature for parents has been carefully prepared by others in similar circumstances. They include useful lists of suggested keepsakes which are important during the grieving period such as the Stillbirth Certificate, a lock of hair, a footprint, a record of the baby's weight and measurements and an ultrasound or postnatal photograph. The latter two photographs should always be taken without necessarily consulting the patients as many will want such keepsakes at a later stage.

Caring for the carers

Just as parents and families need support following termination for fetal abnormality so too do their health care professionals. To this end many hospitals have a 'Staff Support Department' to provide a confidential, formal and structured staff support system in addition to the informal support gained from friendships and relationships with professional colleagues.

ROLE OF THE BEREAVEMENT OFFICER

The main role of the Bereavement Officer is to provide a constant contact point for staff, parents and other agencies. They give support, advice and information to bereaved parents and help with obtaining Death or Stillbirth Certificates from the doctor and explain to the parents when and where to register the death. They can discuss the advantagess and disadvantages of hospital versus private funerals and help with the arrangements. Other key roles include providing information about the 'Book of Remembrance' and long-term support for bereaved parents, families and the staff caring for them. They liaise with support groups, funeral directors, the Registrar's office, hospital chaplain, Histology Department and medical and midwifery staff. It is therefore incumbent upon them to ensure that they are well informed about various cultural and religious attitudes towards death and termination and to ensure that regularly updated guidelines are available to keep other health care professionals informed.

Birmingham Maternity Hospital guidelines

Termination of viable pregnancy <28 weeks

A single dose of Cervagem (Gemeprost) 1 mg per vaginam may be considered prior to surgical termination which may be carried out before 14 weeks' gestation. Beyond this either extra-amniotic prostaglandin E2 (EAPG) or Cervagem can be used to terminate the pregnancy. The method of inducing labour will depend on the state of the cervix and both are effective in early pregnancy.

Epidural analgesia may be offered if the patient wishes and is highly effective and appropriate. Ensure consent is obtained if for a surgical procedure and if this is a termination of a viable pregnancy (even if abnormal) a blue 'Certificate A' form must be completed by the consultant and/or Senior Registrar who has counselled the patient and agreed to termination *before any treatment is given*. Two signatures are required. Yellow 'notification forms' must be filled in by the doctor inserting the first pessary and completed by the doctor discharging the patient.

All staff must be familiar with the Checklists 'A' and 'B' available in the labour ward.

Cervagem

Cervagem (Gemeprost) is a prostaglandin preparation and should be used with care in patients with medical conditions in which it is contra-indicated such as asthma and cardiac disease or with a previous uterine scar. These must be stored at $-10°C$ and taken out of fridge 30 minutes before use. Medical staff should insert Cervagem pessaries (1 mg) at 3 hourly intervals up to a maximum of five pessaries. Patients should remain in bed for 30 minutes after each pessary is inserted. A pyrexia is not an unusual side effect with this preparation and some patients will also experience diarrhoea which may require treatment with 'Lomitol'. When the membranes are bulging, an amniotomy will often rapidly expedite labour though Syntocinon may occasionally be required to augment labour. The Syntocinon regime is the same as for induction of labour namely 6 units of Syntocinon in 44 ml 5% dextrose commenced at 1 ml/hour and increased at 15 minute intervals until contracting regularly or a maximum infusion rate of 10 ml/hour. Partograms are not usually completed as the interval to delivery may be quite prolonged though they are useful in documenting blood pressure recordings and top-ups when epidurals are sited.

EAPG E2

Use a special pack with 5 mg Prostin E2/50 ml diluent. Insert Foley catheter into cervix, and commence at 1 ml/hour increasing to a maximum rate of 2 ml/hour after 30 min. Once catheter falls out (cervix has dilated 2–3 cm) commence intravenous Syntocinon via infusion pump as for the Cervagem regimen.

APPENDIX 20.2

Last office pack — these should be readily available on the labour ward

---

Contents of pack

1 Large plastic bag
1 Baby shroud
1 Stillbirth sheet made from calico shrouding
6 Safety pins
1 Set of duplicate labels

Procedure

Wash infant as necessary
Weight and length recorded as necessary
Cord ligatured as necessary
Name bands on wrist and ankle
Shroud put on infant
Top copy of duplicate label stitched to shroud
Infant then wrapped in stillbirth sheet which is pinned (not sewn)
Second copy of duplicate label stitched on to this sheet
Contact mortuary porter for transfer of infant to mortuary
Complete notice of death forms and send to appropriate department

---

Checklist 'B' following a pregnancy loss
This checklist is to be used following an **abortion where there is no identifiable fetus.**

Mother's name ....   Partner's name ....

Unit No. ....   Telephone No. ....

E.D.D. ....   Gestation ....

	Tick	Signature	Date
Mother and partner seen by obstetrician			
Necessary bloods taken			
Bereavement Officer informed			
Histology form completed and sent with specimen			
Community midwife informed by telephone			

GP informed
   By telephone
   Discharge letter			

Discharged by obstetrician			
Discharged by anaesthetist			
Anti-D given YES/NO			
Rubella vaccination given YES/NO			
TTO DRUGS GIVEN YES/NO			
Antenatal appointment cancelled (if appropriate)			

(Continued)

APPENDIX 20.3 (*Cont.*)

Parentcraft/relaxation classes cancelled			

Contact groups
    SATFA
   Miscarriage Association			

Follow-up appointment arranged (Please ensure Medical Records staff are aware pregnancy loss has occurred)			
Genetic counselling appointment (if appropriate)			

(*Please tick, sign and date*)

Checklist 'A' following a pregnancy loss
This checklist is to be issued by delivery suite/ward staff following delivery of an identifiable fetus, stillbirth or neonatal death.

Mother's name .... Partner's name ....

Unit No. .... Telephone No. ....

Baby's Name .... Gestation ....

Unit No. .... E.D.D. ....

Checklist 'A' following a pregnancy loss — part 1

	Tick	Signature	Date
Both parents informed of stillbirth/death by			
Consultant obstetrician informed			
Parents given opportunity to see/handle baby			

Mementoes offered to parents
 	
Photographs
   Taken
   Accepted by parents
   Kept in notes
Lock of hair
Cot card
Name band
Foot/hand print			

Religious advisor notified (if desired by parents) Baptism or other religious ceremony offered			
Consent for post-mortem requested Consent given YES/REFUSED			

(Continued)

APPENDIX 20.4 (*Cont.*)

Post-mortem form completed by medical staff		
If baby under 24 weeks, statement by the doctor or midwife present at delivery certifying that the baby was born dead before the legal age of viability **completed, signed and witnessed.**	*See Appendix 20.5*	

(Please tick, sign and date)

Checklist 'A' following a pregnancy loss — part 2			
	Tick	Signature	Date
Bereavement Officer or Deputy informed			

GP informed
  By telephone
  Discharge letter			

Notice of Death form completed			
Health visitor informed			

Community midwife informed on day of discharge
  By telephone
  Discharge letter			

For South Birmingham residents Community computer 24 hour answerphone Tel. 0121-446-5346			
Anti-D given YES/NO			
Rubella vaccination given YES/NO			
Necessary bloods for investigations YES/NO			
Mother given information regarding suppression of lactation YES/NO			

Contact groups
   SANDS
   SATFA
   Miscarriage Association			

Parentcraft/relaxation classes cancelled			
Discharged by Obstetrician TTO DRUGS GIVEN YES/NO Postnatal appointment arranged (Please ensure Medical Records staff are aware pregnancy loss has occurred)			
Genetic counselling (if appropriate)			

(Please tick, sign and date)

(Continued)

APPENDIX 20.4 (*Cont.*)

	Tick	Signature	Date
Checklist 'A' following a pregnancy loss — part 3 (Bereavement Officer to complete)			
Death or stillbirth certificate completed, explained and given to parents			
Information on when/where to register stillbirth, birth and death			
Information on funeral arrangements given and discussed			
Parents' decision: HOSPITAL Burial/cremation/informal service PRIVATE Burial/cremation			
Gravecard requested YES/NO			
Chapel service requested YES/NO			
Parents given information about 'The Book of Remembrance'			

(*Please tick, sign and date*)

When completed, please retain this checklist in mother's notes

Statement by the doctor or midwife present at delivery for fetuses under 24 weeks' gestation certifying that the baby was born dead before the legal age of viability to be given to funeral directors.

Hospital name and address

I, Doctor/Midwife ....

was present at the birth of the Male/Female fetus of .... weeks'

gestation, born to

Mrs/Miss ....

of ....

....

....

at .... hours on ....

I certify that the fetus was not born alive and showed no signs of life.

Signature ....

Date ....

Signature witnessed by ....

APPENDIX 20.6

Check sheet for babies born with external abnormalities or terminated for fetal abnormality

Please complete for abortuses, stillbirths or babies dying in delivery suite/ postnatal wards.

Tick or describe briefly all abnormalities noted

SKIN			NECK		
Macerated	{	}	Webbing	{	}
Intact	{	}	Masses or lumps	{	}
Blistered	{	}	Describe		
Rash present	{	}			
Meconium staining	{	}	....		
Other	{	}	BODY		
Describe			Body wall defect	{	}
			Abdominal distension	{	}
....			Abnormal umb. cord	{	}
HEAD			Hernias	{	}
Large head	{	}	Abdominal massess	{	}
Small head	{	}	Describe		
Encephalocoele	{	}			
Other	{	}	....		
Describe			BACK		
			Spina bifida	{	}
....			Symmetrical	{	}
EYES			Patent anus	{	}
Lids fused	{	}	Describe		
Lids open	{	}			
Size abnormal	{	}	....		
Other	{	}	GENITALIA		
Describe			Normal male	{	}
			Normal female	{	}
....			Other	{	}
NOSE			Describe		
Nostrils patent	{	}			
Nostrils not patent	{	}	....		
Other	{	}	LIMBS		
Describe			Absent limbs	{	}
			Hypertrophied limbs	{	}
....			Curving limbs	{	}
EARS			Fractures	{	}
Normal	{	}	Contractures	{	}
Abnormal	{	}	Abnormal digit shape	{	}
Describe			Describe		
....			....		

MOUTH			OTHER FEATURES
Cleft lip	{	}	
Cleft palate	{	}	
Size abnormal	{	}	
Tongue abnormal	{	}	
Small chin	{	}	
Other	{	}	
Describe			

REFERENCES

Allahbadia, G. (1992) Comparative study of midtrimester termination of pregnancy using hypertonic saline, ethacridine lactate, prostaglandin analogue and iodine-saline. *Journal of the Indian Medical Association*, **90**(9), 237−39.

Black, R.B. (1989) A 1 month and 6 month follow-up of prenatal diagnosis patients who lost pregnancies. *Prenatal Diagnosis*, **9**, 798−804.

Boulot, P., Hoffet, M., Bachelard, B. *et al.* (1993) Late vaginal induced abortion after a previous cesarean birth: potential for uterine rupture. *Gynecological and Obstetrical Investigation*, **36**(2), 87−90.

Clayton-Smith, J., Farndon, P.A., Mckeown, C. *et al.* (1990) Examination of fetuses after induced abortion for fetal abnormality. *British Medical Journal*, **300**, 295−97.

Ferguson (2d), J.E., Burkett, B.J., Pinkerton, J.V. *et al.* (1993) Intra-amniotic 15(s)-15 methyl-prostaglandin F2a and termination of middle and late second-trimester pregnancy for genetic indications: a contemporary approach. *American Journal of Obstetrics and Gynaecology*, **169**(2(1)), 332−39.

Kanhai, H.H. and Keirse, M.J. (1993) Low-dose sulprostone for pregnancy termination in cases of fetal abnormality. *Prenatal Diagnosis*, **13**(2), 117−121.

NHS (1992) The Still-birth (Definition) Act. NHS Management Executive.

RCP (1989) A report of the Royal College of Physicians. *Prenatal diagnosis and genetic screening. Community and Service implications.* College of Physicians, London.

Thong, K.J. and Baird, D.T. (1992) A study of gemeprost alone, dilapan or mifepristone in combination with gemeprost for the termination of second trimester pregnancy. *Contraception*, **46**(1), 11−17.

Thong, K.J. and Baird, D.T. (1993) Induction of second trimester abortion with mifepristone and gemeprost. *British Journal of Obstetrics and Gynaecology*, **100**(8), 758−61.

Whelton, J.M. (1990) Sharing the dilemmas: midwives role in prenatal diagnosis and medicine. *Professional Nurse*, July, 514−18.

WHO (1993) Termination of pregnancy with reduced doses of Mifepristone. World Health Authority Task Force on Post-ovulatory Methods of Fertility Regulation. *British Medical Journal*, **307**, 532−37.

Zaytseva, T.S., Gonchorava, V.N., Morozova, M.S. *et al.* (1993) The effect of RU486 on progesterone and oestrogen receptors in human decidua on early pregnancy. *Human Reproduction (England)*, **8**(8), 1288−92.

Chapter 21
Fetal Pathology

W. J. A. PATRICK

The aim of this chapter is to provide a brief outline of perinatal pathology in the context of clinical practice. It is not intended to offer a detailed description of embryology, fetal pathology or post-mortem technique all of which can be found in standard textbooks. The relative frequency of abnormalities in fetuses following termination of pregnancy in recent years is shown in Table 21.1.

REQUEST FOR POST-MORTEM EXAMINATION

A brief summary of the clinical history should accompany the post-mortem request and history based on the headings listed in Table 21.2 usually covers the relevant points. Accurate categorization of fetal death is essential because of the important differences between late abortions and stillbirths with regard to consent for examination, certification and disposal of the body. The indication for a termination of pregnancy must be stated and a

Table 21.1 Pathology in 501 cases of termination of pregnancy (TOP) for fetal abnormality, 1983–1987

Neural tube defects		
Anencephaly	156	
Spina bifida	161	347
Encephalocele and other	30	
Chromosomal disorders		
Trisomy 21	31	
Trisomy 18	10	
Trisomy 13	4	82
Turner 45,X	15	
Klinefelter 47,XXY	10	
Other	12	
Other malformations		
Anterior abdominal wall defect	29	
Urethral obstruction	11	
Skeletal deformity	7	72
Renal malformation	3	
Miscellaneous	22	

Relevant history	Points of interest
Present obstetric history	
Category	Spontaneous abortion, therapeutic abortion (and indication), stillbirth
Gestational age	Assessment by dates and by ultrasound, maternal serum α-fetoprotein value
Abnormal clinical features	Spontaneous preterm rupture of membranes, premature labour, bleeding, prolonged rupture of membranes
Abnormal ultrasound scan features	Fetus, liquor or placenta
Invasive procedures and dates	Chorionic villus sampling, amniocentesis, fetoscopy, intrauterine transfusion, fetal blood sampling, coil, cervical suture
Mode of induction and delivery	Extra-amniotic prostaglandins, artificial rupture of membranes, Syntocinon
Previous obstetric history	
Parity	Conventional para x + y notation
Outcome	Specify cause of any stillbirth, neonatal death or abortion
Maternal history	
Pregnancy	Infectious disease contacts, drugs, alcohol abuse, toxaemia
Medical	Diabetes, hypertension, etc.
Family history	Genetic disorders, malformations

note of any invasive procedure and the date performed is helpful. The purpose of a clinical summary is to forewarn the pathologist of any special points of interest in addition to the core data of the case.

TRANSFER OF THE FETUS TO PATHOLOGY

The fetus (and placenta) should be transferred to the Pathology Department, preferably in a Regional Centre with a special interest in perinatal pathology, as soon as practicable. The fetus should be sent fresh, *not in fixative*, to allow the option of cytogenetic, microbiological or biochemical investigation if appropriate. In the interval between delivery and transfer the fetus should be kept in a refrigerator (4°C). Under these conditions a delay in transport is not disastrous since post-mortem autolysis occurs slowly in the fetus in the absence of bacterial colonization and fibroblast culture for karyotyping is still possible after 3 or 4 days. On no account should a fetus be stored in a deep freeze (−20°C) before transfer.

CATEGORIZATION

An accurate categorization of fetal and perinatally related wastage is necessary for epidemiological purposes. By convention, an abortion or stillbirth is termed a fetus and a livebirth an infant. The term 'therapeutic abortion' is entirely specific and should be used in preference to termination of a pregnancy for fetal abnormality. The latter can have a wider, less specific meaning, for example, if there is active intervention to terminate the pregnancy for a missed abortion.

The reduction of the age of viability from 28 weeks to 24 weeks' gestation in the UK and Northern Ireland came into law in October 1992. The change has reduced the time available for the exclusion of fetal anomalies but the Act provides for the termination of pregnancies with abnormalities of such severity that the fetus would inevitably be stillborn or die early in the neonatal period.

The gestational age established clinically by dates or ultrasound examination is the determining factor for categorizing abortions or stillbirths but there will always be debate about the category of a missed abortion (defined as the death of a fetus *in utero* more than 2 weeks before delivery) which is delivered after 24 weeks' gestation in a single or multiple pregnancy (fetus papyraceous).

Fetuses of pregnancies terminated using intra-amniotic urea (not now in the UK) or following prior potassium chloride injection show a greater degree of autolysis than those terminated by Cervagem or prostaglandins (see Chapter 20). The tissues are usually soft and difficult to handle, changes which may compromise histological interpretation, chromosome analysis and the establishment of a cell line to exclude metabolic disorders.

Studies of perinatal mortality now need to include all second trimester abortions, stillbirths and neonatal deaths up to the end of the fourth week of life rather than, as previously, restricting perinatal mortality to stillbirths and first week deaths. It is now necessary to think of an extended perinatal period to take account of total perinatally related wastage.

Unfortunately, many of the definitions used in childhood mortality are not standard. For example, in the UK, stillbirth rates are expressed per 1000 total births, but in other countries the rate is expressed per 1000 live births. This, together with changes in the law which are not, of course, universally applied, makes comparisons of mortality rates impossible.

POST-MORTEM EXAMINATION

External appearances (Table 21.3)

The description of external appearances includes measurements of weight, crown-heel and crown-rump lengths, the occipito-frontal circumference

Table 21.3 Categories of fetal abnormality evident on external inspection

Nil
Normal

General
Maceration
Growth retardation
Oedema

Local
Neural tube defect
Signs of chromosomal disorder: dysmorphism, cystic hygroma
Anterior abdominal wall defect
Abdominal distension: urethral obstruction
Short-limbed dwarfism

and foot length. Certain anatomical planes are useful for excluding dysmorphic features. The corner of the mouth normally lies on the saggital plane passing through the junction of the inner and middle one-third of the palpebral fissure and the tragus of the auricle should lie on the diagonal plane between the point of the chin and the posterior fontanelle. Any deviations from this may indicate small palpebral fissures, broad based nose, small mouth or low set ears. Choanal atresia is excluded by passage of a probe into the nasopharynx and anal atresia by a probe into the rectum. The position and relative proportions of the limbs are noted and the fingers and toes individually examined so that minor degrees of syndactyly are not overlooked. A common error is in mistaking a female for a male because of the relative clitoral enlargement found in the second trimester.

Internal appearances

Examination of the organs is by body cavity unlike the systematic approach used in adult pathology. All fetuses should have a routine radiological skeletal survey (see below) and photographs should be taken of any dysmorphic features. This can be a considerable aid to genetic counselling.

Organ weights are routinely recorded and tables exist in standard textbooks. The weights are of greater significance if there are gross discrepancies and ratios of organ to body weight are being more widely used.

Histology

The minimum histology includes thymus, lung, kidney, gonad, pancreas, amnion and umbilical cord. The aim of lung histology is to assess maturity from the presence of hyaline membrane disease in preterm infants and to

269

exclude intrauterine pneumonia in the fetus. Histology of the pancreas will help to identify cystic fibrosis. The relative width of the subcapsular nephrogenic zone in the kidney is also a useful measure of maturity. The histology of the gonad obviously allows sexing and also excludes gonadal dysgenesis.

With regard to the placenta, a separate block of amnion from the fetal surface is taken to look for evidence of amnionitis (see below). This is almost invariably present in cases with prolonged rupture of the membranes.

GENERAL FETAL ABNORMALITIES

Maceration

Stillbirths may show varying degrees of maceration which is defined as the natural aseptic process of autolysis that a fetus undergoes following death *in utero* from whatever cause. A manifestation of fetal distress *in utero* is the passage of meconium which results in meconium contamination of the liquor and meconium staining of the fetal skin. At post-mortem there is a relative reduction of the amount of meconium in the large bowel and histological evidence of fetal squames in the periphery of the lungs. This is sometimes referred to as meconium aspiration but bile-stained material can rarely be identified.

The earliest sign of maceration in a fetus dying *in utero* some 12−24 hours before delivery is generalized dusky discolouration and some separation of the epidermis with gentle abrasion of the skin. With death *in utero* 24−48 hours before delivery, there is generalized dark haemic discolouration of the fetus due to blood leaking out and haemolysing in tissue spaces, with separation of the epidermis, laxity of the joints, collapse of skull bones and large volumes of haemolysed bloodstained fluid in body cavities. Over the subsequent few weeks the blood pigments break down and the fetus becomes increasingly pale and papyraceous as the body fluids are absorbed, resulting in the typical appearance of a missed abortion. Exceptions to this sequence of events are cases of feto-maternal haemorrhage and congenital human parvovirus infection (see below) in which the fetus is unusually pale and hydropic. Diffuse soft-tissue calcification due to the deposition of calcium in the autolysed tissues may be seen in the skeletal survey. The timing of the changes is arbitrary but usually corresponds fairly closely to the interval in which there was loss of fetal movements and delivery.

Infections

Essentially, intrauterine infections are of two types: ascending, usually bacterial, and giving rise to acute amnionitis, and haematogenous, which are mostly viral and transmitted from mother to fetus via the placenta.

Acute amnionitis (often incorrectly termed 'chorioamnionitis') usually results from prolonged rupture of the membranes but may also follow invasive procedures, the presence of an intrauterine contraceptive device or cervical suture. The membranes are thickened and show yellowish green discolouration. Histology shows an acute inflammatory cell infiltrate in the amnion and frequently a reactive migration of inflammatory cells from the vessels in the umbilical cord which should not be regarded as inflammation as such (funitis). Intrauterine pneumonia is also a feature of amnionitis.

A particularly severe form of amnionitis can result from infection by *Candida albicans*. The yeast and hyphial forms can be readily demonstrated using special stains and the infection can cause destruction of alveolar ducts and fungal abscesses in other organs.

Cytomegalovirus (CMV) is endemic in the community and involves the fetus by haematogenous spread. The fetus may develop splenomegaly but in severely affected fetuses there may be microcephaly with dystrophic calcification around the lateral ventricle in necrotic tissue. Similar findings occur in congenital toxoplasmosis.

Human parvovirus is now a well-recognized cause of fetal hydrops. The fetus is usually pale as a result of profound anaemia and nuclear inclusion bodies can be identified in circulating cells. *In situ* hybridization techniques have assisted the diagnosis of this condition. Treatment by intrauterine transfusion has been successful in some cases.

Listeriosis is blood-borne and seems to have become more prevalent in recent years. It causes pin-point necrosis or microabscesses and is often fatal.

Growth retardation

Routinely the pathologist attempts to assess if fetal growth is appropriate to the clinical estimate of gestational age or is impaired. Signs of intrauterine growth retardation (IUGR) are seldom evident until the second half of pregnancy. Two main patterns are recognized depending on the time of onset of growth inhibition. When occurring early in pregnancy the effect is more uniform and the infant is generally small but normally proportioned — the symmetrical form of IUGR. However, later in pregnancy the effect is to produce relative sparing of the growth of the brain at the expense of the skeletal frame, soft tissues and internal organs, particularly the liver — the asymmetrical form of IUGR. The symmetrical form is associated with intrauterine infections such as rubella and CMV and malformation syndromes, particularly chromosomal. The asymmetrical form is essentially a problem of fetal malnutrition and is commonly seen with maternal pre-eclampsia.

Maturation of organs is not impaired in IUGR and the state of gyral development in the brain and nephrogenesis in the kidney provide useful gestational milestones. The ratio of brain weight to liver weight is increased in late-onset growth retardation.

Oedema

A mild degree of oedema is often present in the preterm fetus and is of no importance. Severe generalized oedema (hydrops fetalis) is always pathological and has many different causes (Table 21.4). A significant proportion remain unexplained after the most detailed investigation.

External inspection may give a clue to the underlying cause when there is associated local pathology in the form of cystic hygroma of the neck which supports a chromosomal disorder, most commonly Turner syndrome.

LOCAL FETAL ABNORMALITY

Neural tube defects (NTDs)

Failure of the neural tube and its related structures to close during the fourth week of development is the basic cause of NTDs. In the occult lesion there is a limited defect in the spinal arches extending over 2–3 vertebrae with in some cases an overlying skin lesion such as a sacral pit, pigmented patch, tuft of hair or a lipomatous mass. The defect in the

Table 21.4 Mechanisms and causes of fetal hydrops

Chronic intrauterine anaemia
  α-thalassaemia
  Rhesus isoimmunization
  Intrauterine infection

Intrauterine fetal cardiac failure
  Cardiac malformations
  Endocardial fibroelastosis
  Conduction defects

Hypoproteinaemia
  Congenital nephrotic syndrome

Obstruction of fetal circulation
  Premature closure of ductus arteriosus or foramen ovale
  Thoracic malformations and tumours
  Abdominal neuroblastoma

Miscellaneous
  Chromosomal disorders
  Skeletal dysplasias
  Metabolic storage disorders

Idiopathic

spinal arches is of greater extent in the more severe cystic forms of spina bifida and associated with protrusion of the meninges through the defect. There is no spinal cord involvement or neurological deficit in a simple meningocele, but in a myelomeningocele the spinal cord also protrudes through the defect in the spinal arches and is splayed out immediately below the surface where it is covered by a thin transparent membrane which is readily traumatized during delivery. A neurological deficit distal to a myelomeningocele is inevitable and an early indication of this is the varus deformity of the feet that is almost invariably present in these cases.

Meningoceles and myelomeningoceles occur most frequently in the lumbo-sacral region but other sites may be involved and skip lesions can occur. Occasionally in the extreme form the whole spine may be involved. Absent, fused or hemivertebrae, and short, absent or fused ribs are some of the other associated skeletal abnormalities that can occur; occasionally a spur of bone may project backwards from a vertebral body above the main defect causing a worsening or late onset of a neurological deficit due to splitting of the spinal cord with growth (diastematomyelia). A neurological deficit may also be a late complication of a meningocele if there is some tethering of the cauda equina.

At the level of a myelomeningocele there is usually a sharp angular kyphosis which may restrict both the thoracic and abdominal cavities. Myelomeningoceles are almost invariably (95%) associated with an Arnold–Chiari malformation. In these severe forms of spina bifida, the posterior cranial fossa is small and funnel-shaped and in order to allow for normal development there is downward protrusion of the cerebellum (Arnold) and medulla (Chiari) into the cervical spinal canal. This causes cerebrospinal fluid outflow, tract obstruction in the roof of the fourth ventricle and secondary hydrocephalus which may be present as early as 20–24 weeks' gestation. Hyperextension and a short neck (iniencephaly) is due to a defective closure of the neural tube in the cervical region which, in association with a low hairline and fused or hemivertebrae, is characteristic of a Klippel–Feil anomaly. Neural tube defects may also form part of other syndromes such as trisomy 18 (Fig. 21.1).

Anencephalus is the most severe form of NTD and is due to the failure of the neural tube to close at the cranial end of the embryo towards the end of the fourth week of development. The cranial vault in these cases is absent and the brain is represented by a soft haemorrhage mass of amorphous tissue overlying the base of the skull. The base of the skull is foreshortened making the eyes unduly prominent. The neck is not usually restricted in defects confined to the head (anencephalus acrania) but in cases in which the defect extends downwards to involve the spine (anencephalus cranio-rachischisis) the restriction of the neck can be severe. If the spinal involvement is extensive there is likely to be deformity and some restriction of the thoracic and abdominal cavities with an exomphalus. Internally the adrenal

273

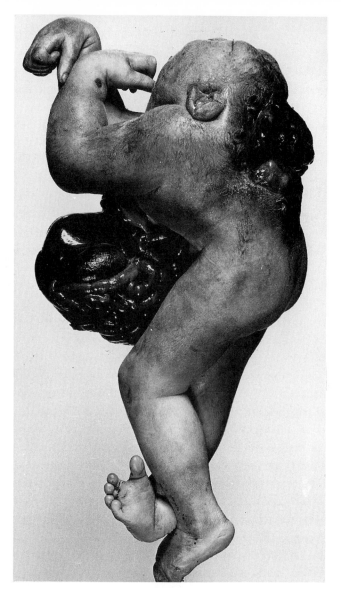

Fig. 21.1 Multiple congenital abnormalities — exomphalos, spina bifida and iniencephaly. Fascia lata should be taken for chromosomal analysis.

glands are unusually small, probably as a result of the lack of trophic factors of the hypothalamic/pituitary axis as the pituitary gland is rarely identified. The only other anomaly frequently encountered in these cases is a horse-shoe kidney in which there is fusion of the lower poles of the kidneys across the midline. Sometimes anencephaly can result from an amniotic band (Fig. 21.2).

Faulty ossification of skull bones can result in an encephalocoele. This occurs most frequently in the squamous part of the occipital bone and

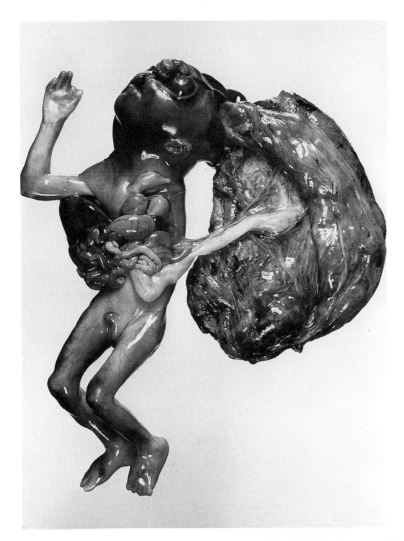

Fig. 21.2 Amputation of one arm and several digits and facial clefting due to amniotic bands in a fetus.

often involves the foramen magnum. An occipital encephalocele almost always contains cerebellum. Occasionally, an encephalocele presents through defects in the base of the skull anteriorly where it may be mistaken for a teratoma. The combination of an encephalocele, polydactyly, large polycystic kidneys and hepatic fibrosis (Meckel–Gruber syndrome) is a severe disorder with an autosomal recessive inheritance (Fig. 21.3).

Abnormalities at the aqueduct of Sylvius are the usual cause of hydrocephalus in which, characteristically, there is dilation of the lateral ventricles, thinning of the cerebral cortex and, in the mature fetus or neonate, polygyria. Hydrocephalus can also be caused by a subarachnoid cyst in the roof of the fourth ventricle (Dandy–Walker anomaly). Care should be taken,

275

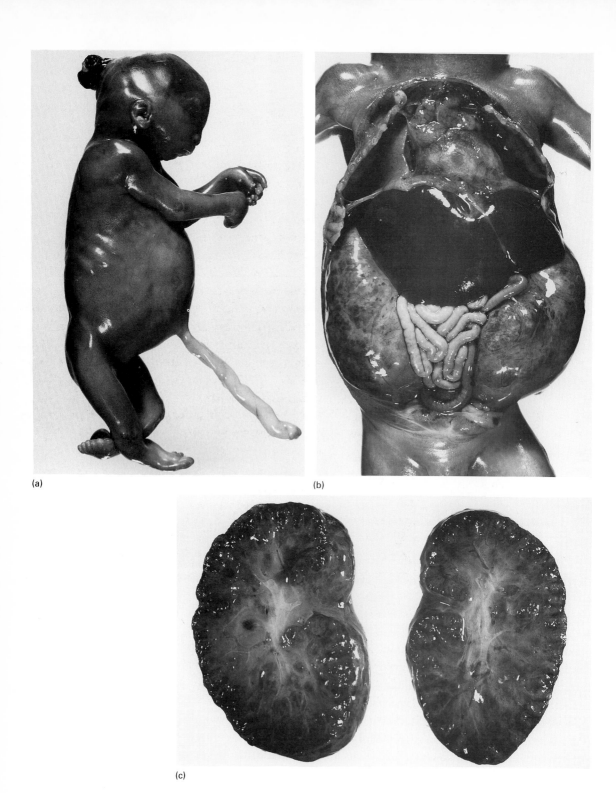

(a)

(b)

(c)

Fig. 21.3 (a) Meckel syndrome showing occipital encephalocele, abdominal distension due to polycystic kidneys, and polydactyly. (b) Enormous polycystic kidneys in Meckel syndrome. (c) Pathological appearance of polycystic kidneys in Meckel syndrome.

276

however, not to mistake the normal relatively large lateral ventricles in
second trimester fetuses for hydrocephalus in the absence of other anomalies.

Cardiac anomalies

A basic knowledge of embryology is helpful in understanding most cardiac
anomalies. Briefly, during the fifth week of development septae form
within the now folding simple tubular heart of the embryo, to transform it
into the definitive four chamber mammalian structure. Essential to this
process is the proliferation of anterior and posterior endocardial cushions
which grow towards each other fusing in the midline to divide the atrioventricular canal into right and left sides and create the tricuspid and
mitral valve orifices. At the same time, the atrial septum primum grows
downwards and fuses with the endocardial cushions. After fusion it separates from the roof of the atrium and is followed by similar downward
growth of the septum secundum, the lower free border of which overlaps
the septum primum and forms the valve-like orifice of foramen ovale
allowing oxygenated blood preferentially to pass *in utero* from the right to
the left atrium. Meanwhile the muscular part of the interventricular septum is
formed by anterior and posterior arms passing upwards to fuse also with
the endocardial cushions; the final membranous part of the interventricular
septum being closed by the spiral growth downwards of the trunco-conal
septum which separates the right and left ventricular outflow tracts as well
as the main pulmonary and aortic trunks.

Failure of endocardial cushion development therefore results in a persistent atrioventricular canal, a fundamental cardiac anomaly in which
there is a central defect with low atrial and high ventricular septal components. The tricuspid and mitral valves are abnormal in that split septal
leaflets of the valves fuse with their counterparts across the midline to
form common anterior and posterior leaflets passing through the defect
from one side to the other. Asymmetrical fusion of the endocardial cushions
causes tricuspid or mitral stenosis which may or may not be associated
with a ventricular septal defect. It is of particular interest that the persistent
atrioventricular canal, the most primitive of all cardiac anomalies, is the
one most frequently associated with Down syndrome.

An understanding of the pivotal role played by the endocardial cushions
in the development of the four chamber heart helps to explain most other
cardiac anomalies. Anomalies of the atrial septum include low atrial septum
primum and high septum secundum defects, patent foramen ovale or, as in
cor triloculare, complete failure of the septum to develop. Occasionally,
the foramen ovale closes prematurely resulting in severe dilatation and
hypertrophy of the right atrium.

The most frequent ventricular septal defect is the high membranous
type which is best visualized from the left ventricle. This is due to failure of

277

the trunco-conal septum to close the final part of the interventricular septum, as described above. Less frequently, defects in the form of multiple fenestrations occur in the muscular part of the septum.

Trunco-conal (aorto-pulmonary) septal anomalies include persistent truncus arteriosus in which the septum fails to form as a whole or in part resulting in a single arterial trunk overriding a ventricular septal defect. Transposition of the great vessels is caused by the septum as if it were growing straight downwards instead of developing in a spiral fashion, and asymmetry in the formation of the septum results in aortic or pulmonary stenosis.

Abnormal development of the trunco-conal septum is also the basic cause of Fallot's tetralogy. This is a relatively common anomaly, in which there is narrowing of the right ventricular outflow tract, a defect in the membranous part of the interventricular septum, a large aortic trunk overriding the septal defect and subsequently, right ventricular hypertrophy. It may also be associated with bicuspid or other abnormalities of the pulmonary valve.

Asymmetry of trunco-conal septal development may result in aortic stenosis. If the aortic valve is completely atresic there is usually an associated mitral stenosis and under-development of the left ventricle comprising the hypoplastic left heart syndrome. In these circumstances, blood passes directly to the systemic circulation through a wide patent ductus arteriosus. The hypoplastic ventricle may only be a small slit-like opening and because of the outlet obstruction there is usually severe subendocardial fibroelastosis.

Dextrocardia with complete reversal of the heart is the most frequent positional abnormality resulting from failure of normal symmetry. In Kartagener's syndrome, for example, there is the interesting combination of situs inversus and asplenia in patients with recurrent respiratory infections and infertility due to ciliary dyskinesia. Abnormalities of the great arteries such as co-arctation of the aorta, double aortic arch, interrupted aortic arch, right-sided aortic arch and dorsal aorta arch are the result of persistent or abnormal obliteration of branchial arch arteries during development of the definitive vascular pattern. In cases of right aortic arch, the left arch artery and left dorsal aorta are both obliterated. In the fetus, the preductal part of the aorta is relatively narrow and this should not be mistaken for a co-arctation of the aorta.

In practice, a persistent left superior vena cava is the only significant anomaly of the venous system. The innominate or brachiocephalic vein is absent and blood from the left side of the head and neck region drains directly into the greatly enlarged coronary sinus at the left side of the heart. As an isolated anomaly, a persistent left superior vena cava is of little clinical significance.

Anomalous pulmonary venous drainage occurs when the pulmonary veins fail to enter the left atrium. In the incomplete or partial form, the right pulmonary veins drain into the right atrium, but in totally anomalous pulmonary venous drainage, large anastomotic channels may pass below the diaphragm to join the systemic venous circulation through the inferior vena cana.

Anterior abdominal wall defects

Defects of the anterior abdominal wall are the commonest fetal abnormality diagnosed prenatally after NTDs and chromosomal disorders. It is important to distinguish different types of defect in relation to their natural history and potential surgical repair. Characteristic features of each type are listed in Table 21.5.

Urethral obstruction

Complete outlet obstruction due to urethral atresia is a rare congenital malformation but because of the ease of prenatal detection and the increased risk of spontaneous intrauterine death it is not infrequent in second trimester fetal pathology. Massive abdominal distension, usually in a male fetus, is the external clue. Severe dilatation of the bladder and posterior urethra is present; the upper urinary tract may be relatively normal or show hydronephrosis and renal dysplasia.

Table 21.5 Anterior abdominal wall defects: types and pathological features

Gastroschisis	Small defect, close to normal cord, smooth margin
	Protruding loops of bowel, no covering sac
	Associated pathology (10%) includes areas of atretic intestine and congenital heart disease
	Normal karyotype
Exomphalos	Defect always involves umbilical cord, varies in size
	Minor: herniation into base of cord only
	Major: defect consists of large protruding sac containing bowel and part of liver
	Semitranslucent sac wall with amnion/peritoneum surface, incorporating umbilical vessels
	Associated malformations in 50%, especially NTD and congenital heart disease
	Abnormal karyotype common (30%)
Body stalk defect	Large irregular defect, filmy sac
	Almost whole of liver and bowel extruding
	Short umbilical cord
	Associated pathology almost invariable: major spinal and pelvic deformity, hypoplastic or absent lower limbs, closed NTD, etc.
	Normal karyotype

Incomplete forms of obstruction such as posterior urethral valves do not usually present until the third trimester.

Cystic kidneys

Congenital cysts of the kidney form a complex group of disorders, important because of their relative frequency and widely varying risk of recurrence. The main varieties of bilateral cystic kidney which occur in the fetus are summarized in Table 21.6.

External inspection may indicate grossly enlarged kidneys but features such as Potter facies and amnion nodosum (Fig. 21.4) typical of severe oligohydramnios at term are not seen in early pregnancy.

Skeletal deformity

Generalized skeletal deformity is seen in two main groups of disorder in the fetus, osteochondrodysplasias or short-limbed dwarfism and defects of bone formation such as osteogenesis imperfecta. There are many different forms which are lethal in the perinatal period. External inspection with a photographic record and radiographic examination of the whole skeleton are *obligatory*, even if consent for post-morten is withheld. Histopathology contributes additional information in only a proportion of the conditions

Table 21.6 Varieties of bilateral cystic kidney seen in fetuses

Cystic dysplasia	Generalized corticomedullary disorganization, typical histology
	Enlarged and grossly cystic ('multicystic') or small semisolid nodule with tiny cysts ('aplastic')
	Absent pelvicalyceal differentiation
	Hypoplastic and commonly atretic ureters
	Normal liver histology
Infantile polycystic disease	Massive renal enlargement, shape and lobulation preserved
	Uniform sponge-like structure, radially-aligned fusiform cysts, typical histology
	Small normal pelvicalyceal system and ureters
	Congenital hepatic fibrosis invariable
Adult polycystic disease	Modest renal enlargement
	Rounded cysts, ill-defined histology
	Small normal pelvicalyceal system and ureters
	Congenital hepatic fibrosis and liver cysts not described
Cysts associated with multiple malformation syndromes	Degree of involvement highly variable, non-specific changes

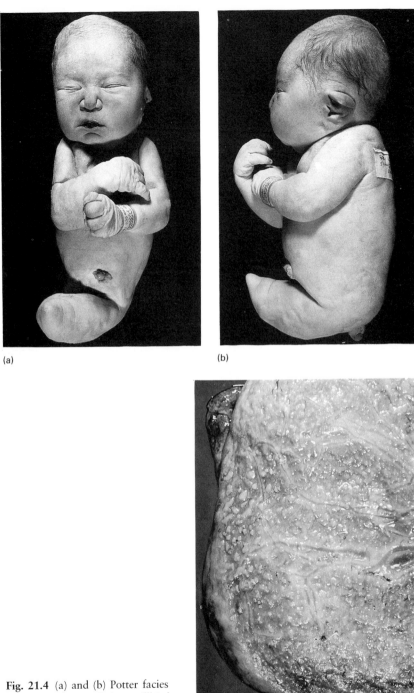

(a)

(b)

(c)

Fig. 21.4 (a) and (b) Potter facies due to renal agenesis in a stillbirth with sirenomelia. (c) Amnion nodosum due to oligohydramnios.

and it is essential to sample tracheal cartilage as well as a long bone, vertebrae and rib for examination of the growth plate.

Chromosomal anomalies (Table 21.7)

An abnormal external appearance of a fetus is usually an indication of an underlying chromosomal abnormality. In trisomy 21 (Down syndrome) (Fig. 21.5), for example, there may be generalized oedema or nuchal thickening as well as the usual features although these may be difficult to recognize early in the second trimester or in macerated stillbirths. Down syndrome is frequently associated with cardiac anomalies (see above), duodenal atresia, Meckel's diverticulum and Hirschsprung disease.

An enlarged head, small mouth and chin and marked incurving of the index and fifth fingers are typical of trisomy 18 (Edwards' syndrome) (Fig. 21.6). Internal anomalies are relatively minor with ventricular septal defects the most frequent abnormal finding. Despite the relatively minor nature of

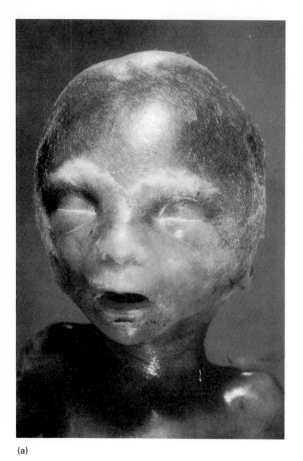
(a)

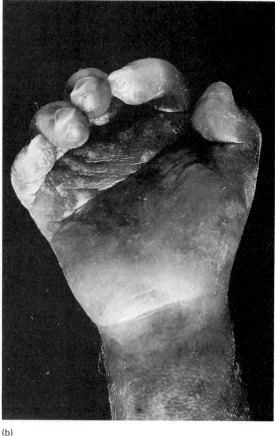
(b)

Fig. 21.5 Trisomy 21. (a) A 19-week fetus. The facial features are not characteristic at this gestation. (b) A fetus showing a single transverse palmar crease.

Table 21.7 Common chromosomal disorders seen after termination of pregnancy

Chromosomal disorder	Eponym	Karyotype	Major features	Associated anomalies	Outlook
Trisomy 21	Down syndrome	47,XX or XY,+21	Round brachycephalic head Flat facies Slightly protuberant tongue Upwards slanting eyes Prominent epicanthic folds Small ears Abnormal (single transverse) palmar creases Broad spatulate hands	Cardiac anomalies (persistent atrioventricular canal) Duodenal atresia Hirschsprung disease	Varying degrees of mental retardation
Trisomy 18	Edwards' syndrome	47,XX or XY,+18	Small chin and prominent occiput. Clenched hands with overlapping of index and fifth fingers Excess of digital arches Growth retardation Low set ears, short sternum, single palmar creases, rockerbottom feet	Ventricular septal defect Incompletely lobated lungs Meckel diverticulum Bicornuate uterus Single hypogastric (umbilical) artery Exomphalos	5% may survive first year
Trisomy 13	Patau syndrome	47,XX or XY,+13	Facial clefts Flat sloping forehead	Microcephaly Holoprosencephaly Arhinencephaly Microphthalmia	Usually fatal in first year
Triploidy	—	69,XXY,XXX or XYY	Relatively large head Syndactyly 3rd and 4th fingers (Vesicular) Hydatidiform change in the placenta	Hypospadias and cryptorchidism in males	Spontaneous second trimester abortion usual
Turner syndrome	Turner syndrome	45,X	Webbed neck Apparently broad chest with widely spaced nipples Generalized oedema	Dysplastic ovaries	Short stature and primary infertility usual if liveborn

283

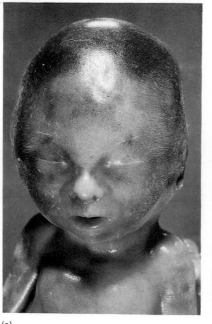

(a)

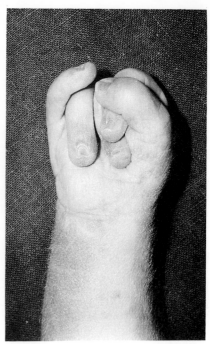

(b)

Fig. 21.6 Trisomy 18. (a) Facies in a fetus. (b) Characteristic overlapping fingers.

the anomalies, few infants survive beyond the first few months of life and any longer term survivors are severely retarded.

Facial clefts with holoprosencephaly cardial defects, bicornuate uterus and a single hypogastric (umbilical) artery are the anomalies usually associated with trisomy 13 (Patau's syndrome) (Fig. 21.7). This condition also has a high mortality in the first year of life and any survivors have severe mental retardation. In practice, any fetus or infant with facial clefts should be karyotyped.

Turner syndrome (Fig. 21.8) with an 45,X karyotype, or the Turner-like Noonan's syndrome in a male fetus, typically has soft tissue swelling and webbing of the neck. The condition is due to fertilization of the ovum lacking a sex chromosome following non-disjunction of the chromosomes during reduction division as opposed to the fertilization of the ovum with the extra sex chromosome in 47,XXY Klinefelter's syndrome.

Triploidy (Fig. 21.9) in which a fetus gains a complete extra set of chromosomes derived from the father is thought to occur in about 2% of conceptions (Smith, 1982). It is accompanied by hydatidiform change in the placenta and the fetus usually shows partial or complete syndactyly of the third and fourth fingers. All cases not diagnosed antenatally are stillborn or die early in the neonatal period.

Other chromosomal abnormalities are relatively rare. All cases which are diagnosed by chorionic villus sampling should have the result confirmed

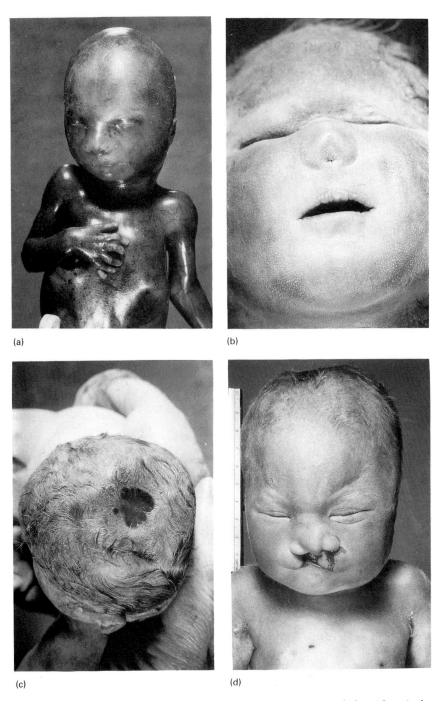

Fig. 21.7 Trisomy 13. (a) Polydactyly in a fetus. (b) Holoprosencephaly with a single nostril and microphthalmia in a fetus. (c) Scalp defect in trisomy 13 which led to raised MSAFP. (d) Bilateral cleft lip in a trisomy 13 neonate.

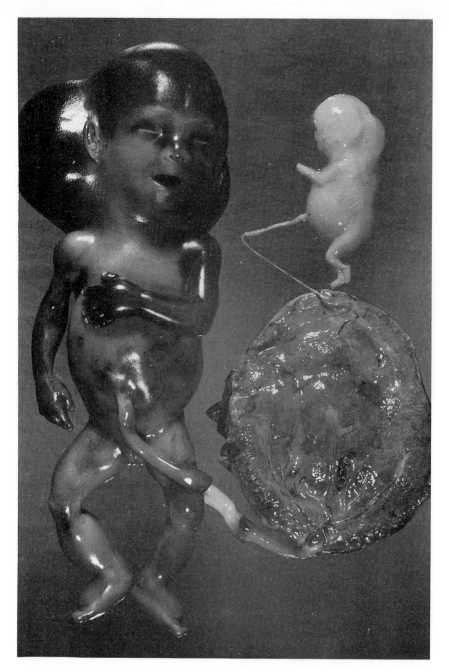

Fig. 21.8 Turner syndrome (45,X) in a fetus with generalized oedema and marked nuchal swelling. The twin died some weeks earlier and might also have been affected.

with tissue samples (fascia lata, amnion) taken from the fetus or placenta. In cases of parental consanguinity, suspected metabolic disorders or potential teratogenic agents (i.e. maternal medication) a cell line should be established and tissue (usually liver) stored in liquid nitrogen for subsequent DNA analysis.

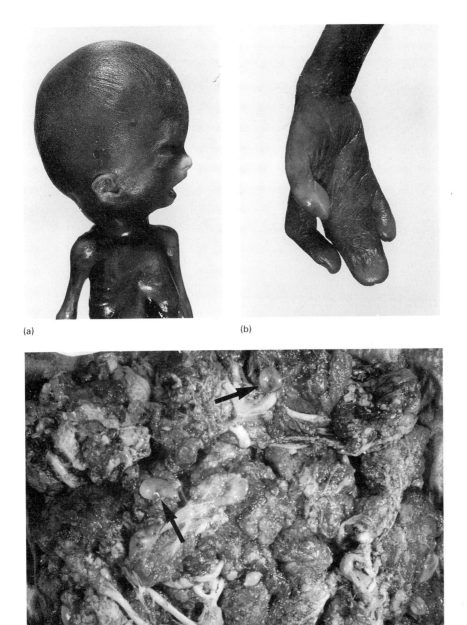

(a)

(b)

(c)

Fig. 21.9 Triploidy in a fetus showing: (a) large head in relation to trunk size; (b) syndactyly; (c) hydatidiform change in the placenta (as arrowed).

SPECIAL INVESTIGATIONS (Table 21.8)

Chromosome analysis

Fascia lata for karyotyping or fibroblast culture for enzyme analysis is

287

Table 21.8 Special post-mortem investigations

Special investigation	Indications	Specimen(s)	Urgent	Precautions	Alternatives
Chromosome analysis	Dysmorphic features Multiple anomalies Older women (>35 years) Translocation carriers Other siblings with chromosomal abnormalities	Heart blood and fascia lata	Yes	Culture medium	Amnion
DNA analysis	Known or suspected single gene disorder	Spleen or liver	Yes	Fresh or snap-frozen	Cultured amnion or fascia lata
Bacteriology	Acute amnionitis Intrauterine pneumonia Microabscesses	Heart blood and lung fluid	No	Aerobic and anaerobic culture Blood agar plate and Robertson medium	None
Virology	Haematogenous infections Hydrops fetalis (polyserositis) Hepatosplenomegaly Miliary necrotic foci	Brain, lung, liver, spleen, kidney, placenta	No	Fresh or in transport medium	None
Enzyme studies	Known or suspected inborn errors of metabolism	Liver	Yes	Liquid nitrogen	None
		Fascia lata	Yes	Culture medium	None
		Urine, aqueous humour, plasma	Yes	Frozen	None
Radiology	Skeletal dysplasia (dwarfism) Fetal maturity Intrauterine infections Chromosomal abnormalities Drugs and drug abuse Skeletal anomalies (e.g. neural tube defects)	Anteroposterior and lateral projections	No	Correct Positioning	None

obtained from the lateral aspect of the thigh of the fetus through a vertical incision taking reasonable precautions to minimize contamination of the specimen. The fascia is recognized as a tough membrane enclosing the muscles of the thigh which may lie close to the undersurface of the skin in second trimester abortions due to the lack of subcutaneous fat. In older fetuses it should be obtained free of fat so that it does not float on the surface of the culture medium.

Fascia remains viable for several days after delivery but should the viability be in doubt, as for example in the macerated fetus, amnion or a thin segment of umbilical cord close to its attachment to the placenta is taken as an alternative. Amnion is a thin semitransparent membrane that can be picked up with forceps from the fetal surface, ensuring that in so doing underlying chorion is not included, in order to minimize the risk of maternal contamination. In the presence of chorio-amnionitis, recognized as thickening and opacity of the membranes, or a history of prolonged rupture of the membranes, amnion should not be used in preference to fascia lata as this can give rise to contaminated cell culture lines and potentially spurious results despite the precaution of adding antibiotics to the culture medium.

Pericardium and gonad are also good sources of cells for fibroblast culture and can be readily obtained in the early stages of dissection in post-mortem examination of a fetus. A less labour intensive source of cells for chromosome analysis in a fresh non-macerated fetus is heart blood (heparinized) but the number of cells capable of further division may be limited and a back-up specimen of fascia lata should always be taken.

Bacteriology

Specimens for bacterial culture are taken routinely in potentially infected cases, for example a fetus with an unpleasant smell, the presence of chorio-amnionitis, or the knowledge of pathogenic organisms in high vaginal swabs taken at the antenatal clinic. The specimens should include heart blood for aerobic and anaerobic culture, lung fluid aspirate from the right lower lobe (intrauterine pneumonia) sprayed directly onto a blood agar plate or into Robertson meat medium, and a specimen or swab of amnion with due precautions, as for chromosome analysis, to avoid contaminants.

Virology

In cases of suspected congenital transplacental haematogenous infections, for example CMV and human parvovirus, fresh specimens of fetal brain, lung, liver, spleen, kidney and placenta are submitted for viral culture. Viral cultures are feasible in tissue obtained several days after delivery but should further delays be anticipated specimens should be placed in specially provided transport (as opposed to culture) medium. Fresh specimens have the advantage that they can be used for DNA hybridization techniques although immunohistochemical methods are becoming available for standard fixed paraffin embedded material.

Radiology

A skeletal survey of an aborted fetus or stillbirth is used to assess maturity, to define major skeletal abnormalities and to disclose any changes which would not otherwise be detected, for example fetal rickets in the immigrant population and congenital syphilis. It is essential in any case of suspected skeletal dysplasia but is also a useful non-invasive investigation should consent for a full post-mortem examination be withheld.

Anteroposterior and lateral projections are used and both projections can be included on a single X-ray plate in most cases. For the anteroposterior projection the fetus is placed in the standard anatomical position with the palm of the hand and dorsal aspect of the feet facing upward and held in position by surgical tape. For the lateral projection care should be taken to avoid overlapping of the limbs wherever possible.

Fetal maturity can be determined by centres of ossification, measurement of thoracic or lumbar vertebral height, biparietal diameter, or femoral length. In the lower extremity, the centres of ossification initially appear in the calcaneum at 22–24 weeks' gestation, lower femoral epiphysis at 36 weeks' gestation and in the upper tibial epiphysis at 40 weeks' gestation. This, however, is only a rough guide as a number of conditions such as a light-for-dates fetus, intrauterine infection, Down syndrome and skeletal dysplasia may delay their appearance. The femoral length measurement is the most practical method of assessing fetal maturity and this is carried out on either the anteroposterior or lateral projections selecting the femur with the least metaphyseal distortion. Standard charts for femoral length by gestational age are available in paediatric radiology textbooks.

Enzyme analysis

In suspected cases of inborn errors of metabolism, fresh fetal liver should be removed as soon after delivery as possible, snap-frozen in liquid nitrogen and stored for subsequent enzyme analysis in a deep freeze at $-20°C$. Deep-frozen samples of urine, vitreous humour and plasma may also be of value.

Fibroblast cultures (fascia lata) should also be established and cryo-preserved cell lines stored in liquid nitrogen for future analysis. Similar storage of material should always be considered for any condition in which the underlying aetiology is not understood or in which a fundamental biochemical defect may be defined in the future.

DNA analysis

DNA may be extracted from any source of nucleated cells. Fresh fetal spleen or liver should be removed as soon after delivery as possible and transported directly in a dry sterile tube to the genetics laboratory or if this is not possible, snap-frozen in liquid nitrogen and stored at −20°C pending transport on dry ice.

FURTHER READING

Keeling, J.W. (1993) *Fetal and Neonatal Pathology* 2nd edn, Springer-Verlag, London.
Larroche, J.C. (1977) *Developmental Pathology of the Neonate*, Excerpta Medica, Amsterdam.
Smith, D.W. (1982) *Recognizable Patterns of Human Malformation* 3rd edn, W.B. Saunders, Philadelphia.
Wigglesworth, J.S. (1984) *Perinatal Pathology*, W.B. Saunders, Philadelphia.

Appendix
Compendium of Prenatally
Diagnosable Diseases

J. M. CONNOR

This compendium aims to provide, in tabular form, details of conditions which have been prenatally diagnosed. If conditions are included in McKusick's *Mendelian inheritance in man* (McKusick, 1994) then the appropriate MIM number is given. This has advantages in providing consistency of nosology, and in allowing direct access to a summary and bibliography, but does have the potentially confusing limitation that inclusion does not mean that the condition is always or even usually inherited as a single gene disorder. Hence the Compendium should be used as a guide to the prenatal diagnostic situation for the condition and other data will be required to determine appropriate risks for genetic counselling. Furthermore, inclusion of a condition in the Compendium does not mean that prenatal diagnosis is necessarily indicated or desirable in each affected family.

The Compendium contains 622 entries, and approaches to prenatal diagnosis are divided into 'Imaging', 'Biochemistry', 'DNA' and 'Other'. Imaging is further subdivided into ultrasound and other (which includes fetoscopy, radiography, magnetic resonance imaging, and fetal echocardiography). Biochemistry is subdivided into amniotic fluid cells (AFC), amniotic fluid supernatant (AFS), chorionic villus samples (CVS) and other. (Mucolipidosis IV and neuronal ceroid lipofuscinosis are also included in the biochemical section even though electron microscopy of cultured cells is employed for prenatal diagnosis rather than biochemical analysis.) DNA is subdivided into gene tracking using linked probes, which may be either intragenic (ILP) or extragenic (ELP), and direct detection of molecular pathology (MP). The 'Other' category is subdivided into fetal blood sampling (FBS), fetal liver biopsy (FLB), fetal skin biopsy (FSKB) and chromosomal analysis (CHR). These approaches and the general pitfalls in relation to prenatal diagnosis are discussed elsewhere in this volume.

The current status of prenatal diagnosis is indicated under each subheading using +, (+), or (−). The symbol + indicates that successful prenatal diagnosis has been widely reported with a high degree of reliability in the second trimester or earlier. The symbol (+) indicates that prenatal diagnosis has been reported but with a limitation: (+)E, limited world experience (under 5−10 cases); (+)R, known reduced sensitivity or specificity or suspected limited reliability (see references); and (+)L, diagnosis may not be possible until the third trimester. The symbol (−) indicates that

293

prenatal diagnosis should be possible but as yet has not been reported and the symbol − indicates that prenatal diagnosis using that particular approach is impossible. For some conditions (for example hypophosphatasia and osteogenesis imperfecta) alternative approaches to prenatal diagnosis are available and these are indicated in the references for these entries.

For each entry one to five references are cited. These aim to be recent, easily accessible and to give good coverage of relevant previously published work. Currently, there are over 1500 publications each year in the field of prenatal diagnosis and hence selection of a limited number of key references is bound to generate some controversy. I look to the generosity of users to accept this limitation and also to help identify misconceptions and omissions.

ACKNOWLEDGEMENTS

I wish to thank Dr Guy Besley, Dr Margaret McNay and Professor Martin Whittle for their invaluable help in compiling and updating this database of prenatally diagnosable conditions.

REFERENCES

McKusick, V.A. (1994) *Mendelian inheritance in man. Catalogs of autosomal dominant, autosomal recessive and X-linked traits* 11th edn, Johns Hopkins University Press, Baltimore.

continued on p. 296

Disease	MIM	Imaging	Biochemistry	DNA	Other	References
Abruption, placental	—	US (+)R	—	—	—	Gottesfeld (1978)
Absent cerebellum	—	US +	—	—	—	Campbell and Pearce (1983) (see also Joubert syndrome)
Absent pulmonary valve	121000	US (+)E	—	—	—	Kleinman et al. (1982)
Acardius	—	US +	—	—	—	Wexler et al. (1985), Zanke (1986)
Acatalasia (Takahara disease)	115500	—	AFC (−), AFS —	ILP (−)	MP (−)	Quan et al. (1986)
Acetylgalactosaminidase deficiency (Schindler disease)	104170	—	AFC (−), CVS (−)	—	—	Schindler et al. (1989)
Achondrogenesis type IA (Parenti–Fraccaro syndrome)	200600	US (+)E	—	—	—	Benacerraf et al. (1984), Mahoney et al. (1984a), Glenn and Teng (1985)
Achondrogenesis type IB (Langer–Saldino syndrome)	200610	US (+)E	—	—	—	Wenstrom et al. (1989)
Achondroplasia	100800	US (+)L	AFC +, AFS −	ELP (−)	MP (−)	Kurtz et al. (1986)
Acid phosphatase deficiency	200950	—	AFC +, AFS −	—	—	Nadler and Egan (1970)
Acrorenal syndrome	102520	US (+)E	—	—	—	Meizner et al. (1986a)
Acute intermittent porphyria	176000	—	—	—	—	See Porphyria, acute intermittent
Acyl-CoA oxidase deficiency (pseudoneonatal adrenoleucodystrophy)	264470	—	AFC (+)E, CVS (+)E	—	—	Wanders et al. (1990)
Adenosine deaminase deficiency	102700	—	AFC (+)E, AFS (+)E, CVS (+)E	ILP (−)	FBS (+)E, MP (−)	Linch et al. (1984), Berkvens et al. (1987), Dooley et al. (1987)
Adrenal cysts	—	US (+)E	—	—	—	Patti et al. (1993)
Adrenal haemorrhage	—	US (+)E	—	—	—	Gotoh et al. (1989), Marino et al. (1990), Lee et al. (1992)
Adrenogenital syndrome (11-β-hydroxylase deficiency)	202010	—	AFC −, CVS −	—	—	Rosler et al. (1979), Schumert et al. (1980)
Adrenogenital syndrome (congenital adrenal hyperplasia, 21-hydroxylase deficiency)	201910	—	AFS +, AFC −, CVS −	ILP +	FBS (+)E, MP (+)P	Hughes et al. (1987), Speiser et al. (1990), Keller et al. (1991), Owerbach et al. (1992), Speiser et al. (1994)
Adrenoleucodystrophy (Schilder disease)	300100	—	AFS (+)R, AFC +, AFS —, CVS +	ELP +, ELP (+)E	—	Boue et al. (1985), Schutgens et al. (1989)

Disease	MIM	Imaging	Biochemistry	DNA	Other	References
Adrenoleucodystrophy, autosomal neonatal form	202370	–	AFC +, CVS (+)E	–	–	Schutgens et al. (1989)
Adrenoleucodystrophy, pseudoneonatal form	–	–	–	–	–	See Acyl-CoA oxidase deficiency
Adult polycystic kidney disease	173900	US (+)E	–	ELP (+)E, MP (–)	–	Ceccherini et al. (1989), Journel et al. (1989), Novelli et al. (1989), Turco et al. (1992)
Agammaglobulinaemia, X-linked	300300	–	–	ELP (+)P	FBS +	Lau et al. (1988), Journel et al. (1992)
Agenesis of corpus callosum	217990	–	–	–	–	See Corpus callosum, agenesis
Agnathia–holoprosencephaly syndrome	202650	US (+)E	–	–	–	Persutte et al. (1990), Rolland et al. (1991)
Agnathia–microstomia–synotia syndrome	–	US (+)E	–	–	–	Cayea et al. (1985)
Albinism, oculocutaneous (tyrosinase negative)	203100	–	AFC –, CVS –	MP (–)	FSKB (+)E	Hayes and Robertson (1981), Eady et al. (1983), Spritz et al. (1990), Shimizu et al. (1992)
Allantoic cyst	–	US (+)E	AFS –	–	–	Fink and Filly (1983)
Alpha-1-antitrypsin deficiency	107400	–	–	ILP +, MP (+)P	FBS +	Corney et al. (1987), Hejtmancik et al. (1989)
Alpha-thalassaemia mental retardation syndrome (X-linked)	301040	–	–	ELP (–)	–	Gibbons et al. (1992)
Alport syndrome	301050	–	–	ELP (–), MP (–)	–	Barker et al. (1990)
Ambiguous genitalia	–	US (+)E	–	–	–	Cooper et al. (1985)
Amelia	104400	US +	–	–	–	Campbell and Pearce (1983)
Amniotic bands	104400	US +	–	–	–	Mahony et al. (1985), Hill et al. (1988), Nishi and Nakano (1994)
Amyloidosis I (Portuguese type of familial amyloid neuropathy)	176300	–	AFS (+)R	MP +	–	Nichols et al. (1989), Morris et al. (1991), Almeida et al. (1990)
Amyloidosis II (Indiana/Swiss type, familial amyloidotic polyneuropathy type II)	176300	–	–	MP (+)E	–	Nichols et al. (1989), Nichols and Benson (1990)
Anal atresia (imperforate anus)	207500	US (+)R	–	–	–	Shalev (1983)
Anderson disease	232500	–	–	–	–	See Glycogen storage disease IV
Androgen insensitivity syndrome (testicular feminization)	313700	US (+)E	–	ILP (+)E, MP (–)	–	Stephens (1984), Wieacker et al. (1987), Brown et al. (1988), Lobaccaro et al. (1992)
	–	–	–	ELP (–)	–	

Disorder	MIM No.	US	AFC	AFS	CVS	ILP	ELP	MP	FBS	FSKB	Reference(s)
Anencephaly	182940	US +	–	–	–	–	–	–	–	–	Goldstein et al. (1989)
Aneurysm, left ventricular	–	US (+)E	–	–	–	–	–	–	–	–	Gembruch et al. (1990c)
Aneurysm, vein of Galen	–	US (+)E	–	–	–	–	–	–	–	–	Jeanty et al. (1990a), Ordorica et al. (1990)
Angiokeratoma corporis diffusum (Fabry disease)	301500	–	AFC +	–	CVS +	ILP (–)	–	MP (–)	–	–	Kleijer et al. (1987), MacDermot et al. (1987), Eng and Desnick (1994)
Angioneurotic oedema											See Hereditary angioedema
Anhidrotic (hypohidrotic) ectodermal dysplasia (Christ–Siemens–Touraine syndrome)	106100, 305100	–	–	AFS –	–	–	ELP (–)	–	–	FSKB (+)E	Arnold et al. (1984), Zonana et al. (1990)
Annular pancreas	–	US (+)E	–	–	–	–	–	–	–	–	Boomsa et al. (1982)
Anophthalmia	206900	US (+)E	–	–	–	–	–	–	–	–	Pilu et al. (1986a)
Antithrombin III deficiency	107300	–	–	–	–	ILP (–)	ELP (–)	MP (–)	–	–	Bock and Prochownik (1987)
Antley–Bixler syndrome	207410	US (+)E	–	–	–	–	ELP (+)E	–	–	–	Savodelli and Schinzel (1983), Schinzel et al. (1983), Jacobson et al. (1992)
Aortic atresia	121000	US (+)E	–	–	–	–	–	–	–	–	Silverman et al. (1984), Allan et al. (1985), Gembruch et al. (1990b)
Aortic stenosis	121000	US (+)E	–	–	–	–	–	–	–	–	Allan et al. (1985)
Apert syndrome (acrocephalosyndactyly type I)	101200	US (+)E	–	–	–	–	–	–	–	–	Hill et al. (1987), Narayan and Scott (1991)
Aplasia cutis congenita	107600	Other (+)E	–	–	–	–	–	–	–	–	Bick et al. (1987)
Arachnoid cyst	–	US (+)E	–	–	–	–	–	–	–	–	Chervenak et al. (1983)
Argininaemia	207800	–	AFC –	AFS –	CVS –	–	–	MP (–)	FBS (–)	–	Spector et al. (1980)
Argininosuccinicaciduria	207900	–	AFC +	AFS +	CVS +	–	–	–	–	–	Fleisher et al. (1979), Vimal et al. (1984), Chadefaux et al. (1990)
Arnold–Chiari malformation	207950	US +	–	–	–	–	–	–	–	–	Johnson et al. (1980)
Arterial calcification, idiopathic infantile	208000	US (+)E	–	–	–	–	–	–	–	–	Juul et al. (1990), Spear et al. (1990)
Arteriovenous fistula (brain)	–	US (+)E	–	–	–	–	–	–	–	–	Mao and Adams (1983)
Arteriovenous fistula (lung)	–	US (+)E	–	–	–	–	–	–	–	–	Kalugdan et al. (1989)
Arteriovenous malformation of the vein of Galen	–	US (+)E	–	–	–	–	–	–	–	–	Reiter et al. (1986)

continued on p. 298

Disease	MIM	Imaging	Biochemistry	DNA	Other		References
Arthrogryposis	108110	US (+)E	–	–	–	–	Baty et al. (1988), Gorczyca et al. (1989), Bui et al. (1992)
Aspartylglucosaminuria	208400	–	AFC +, CVS +, AFS +	ILP (–)	MP (–)	–	Aula et al. (1989), Voznyi et al. (1993)
Asphyxiating thoracic dysplasia (Jeune syndrome)	208500	US (+)E	–	–	–	–	Elejalde et al. (1985), Schinzel et al. (1985)
Asplenia syndrome	208530	–	–	–	–	–	See Ivemark syndrome
Asymmetric septal hypertrophy (hypertrophic obstructive cardiomyopathy)	192600	US (+)E	–	–	–	–	Allan et al. (1985), Stewart et al. (1986)
Ataxia telangiectasia	208900	–	–	ELP (–), ELP (+)E	–	CHR +	Schwartz et al. (1985), Gatti et al. (1988), Jaspers et al. (1990), Gatti et al. (1993)
Atelencephalic microcephaly	–	US (+)E	–	–	–	–	Siebert et al. (1986)
Atelosteogenesis	108720	US (+)E	–	–	–	–	Chervenak et al. (1986)
Atrial bigeminal rhythm	–	US (+)E	–	–	–	–	Steinfeld et al. (1986)
Atrial flutter	–	US (+)E	–	–	–	–	Kleinman et al. (1983)
Atrial haemangioma	–	US (+)E	–	–	–	–	Leitheser et al. (1986)
Atrial septal defect	108800	US (+)E	–	–	–	–	Allan et al. (1985)
Atrioventricular canal defect	–	US (+)E	–	–	–	–	Kleinman et al. (1983), Gembruch et al. (1990a)
Bare lymphocyte syndrome	209920	–	–	–	FBS (+)E	–	Durandy et al. (1982b), Schuurman et al. (1985), Durandy et al. (1987)
Bartter syndrome	241200	US (+)E	–	–	–	–	Sieck and Ohlsson (1984)
Becker muscular dystrophy	310200	–	–	ILP +	MP (+)P	–	Wood et al. (1987) (see also Allelic Duchenne muscular dystrophy)
Beckwith–Wiedmann syndrome (EMG syndrome)	130650	US (+)E	–	ELP +	–	–	Cobellis et al. (1988), Shah and Metlay (1990), Dahl et al. (1993)
Bernard–Soulier syndrome (giant platelet syndrome)	231200	–	–	–	FBS (+)E	–	Gruel et al. (1986)
Beta mannosidosis	248510	–	–	–	–	–	See Mannosidosis, beta
Beta-glucosidase deficiency (Gaucher disease, types I, II and III)	230800, 230900	–	AFC +, CVS +, AFS –	ILP +	MP (+)P	–	Besley et al. (1988), Dahl et al. (1992)
Beta-methylcrotonyl glycinuria I (3-methylcrotonyl-CoA-carboxylase deficiency)	210200	–	AFC (–), CVS (–), AFS (–)	–	–	–	Benson and Fensom (1985)

continued on p. 300

Syndrome	OMIM									Reference
Blackfan–Diamond syndrome	205900	US (+)E	—	—	—	—	—	—	—	Visser et al. (1988), Barth et al. (1990), Jaffe et al. (1990)
Bladder exstrophy	—	US (+)E	—	—	—	—	—	—	—	Blagowidow et al. (1986)
Blagowidow syndrome	—	US (+)E	—	—	—	—	—	—	—	Kurjak and Latin (1979)
Blighted ovum	110300	US +	—	—	—	—	—	—	—	
Blood grouping	—	—	—	—	—	MP (+)E	FBS +	—	—	Teichler-Zallen and Doherty (1983), Simsek et al. (1994)
Bloom syndrome	111700	—	—	—	—	—	—	—	CHR +	Rudiger et al. (1980)
Body stalk anomaly	201900	US +	—	—	—	—	—	—	—	Jauniaux et al. (1990), Abu-Yousef et al. (1987)
BOR syndrome (Branchio-Oto-Renal Dysplasia)	113650	US (+)E	—	—	—	—	—	—	—	Greenberg et al. (1988)
Bradycardia, sinus	—	US +	—	—	—	—	—	—	—	Kleinman et al. (1983)
Bronchial atresia	—	US (+)E	—	—	—	—	—	—	—	McAlister et al. (1987)
Bronchogenic cyst	—	US (+)E	—	—	—	—	—	—	—	Young et al. (1989) (see also Pulmonary cyst)
Bullous erythroderma ichthyosiformis congenita of Brocq (bullous ichthyosiform erythroderma, epidermolytic hyperkeratosis)	113800	—	—	—	—	MP (+)P	—	—	—	Golbus et al. (1980), Anton-Lamprecht (1981), Eady et al. (1986), Rothnagel et al. (1993)
Calcification, ectopic	—	—	—	—	—	—	—	—	FSKB +	Corson et al. (1983)
Calcification, intracranial	—	—	—	—	—	—	—	—	—	See Intracranial calcification
Campomelic dysplasia	211970	US (+)E	—	—	—	—	—	—	—	Cordone et al. (1989)
Canavan's disease (aspartoacylase deficiency)	271900	—	AFC +	CVS +	—	—	—	—	—	Matalon et al. (1992), Kelly (1993)
Carbamoyl-phosphate synthetase deficiency	237300	—	AFS +	—	—	—	—	—	—	See Hyperammonaemia II
Cardiac rhabdomyoma	—	US (+)E	—	—	—	—	—	—	—	Schaffer et al. (1986), Stanford et al. (1987), (see also Tuberous sclerosis)
Cardiomyopathy	—	US (+)E	—	—	—	—	—	—	—	Schmidt et al. (1989)
Cataracts	—	US (+)E	—	—	—	—	—	—	—	Zimmer et al. (1993)
Caudal regression syndrome	—	US (+)E	—	—	—	—	—	—	—	Loewy et al. (1987), Baxi et al. (1990)
Cerebrocostomandibular dysplasia	117650	US (+)E	—	—	—	—	—	—	—	Merlob et al. (1987)
Cerebrohepatorenal (Zellweger syndrome)	214100	—	AFC +	CVS +	—	MP (+)P	—	—	—	Stellaard et al. (1988), Schutgens et al. (1989), Shimozawa et al. (1993)
Cerebrotendinous xanthomatosis	—	—	AFS (+)E	—	—	—	—	—	—	Skrede et al. (1986)
	213700	—	AFC (−)	—	—	—	—	—	—	

Disease	MIM	Imaging	Biochemistry	DNA	Other	References
Charcot–Marie–Tooth disease	118200	—	—	—	—	See Hereditary motor and sensory neuropathy type I
Chediak–Higashi syndrome	214500	—	—	—	—	Diukman et al. (1992), Durandy et al. (1993), Schroeder et al. (1989)
Choledochal cyst	—	US (+)E	—	—	FBS (+)E	Bancroft et al. (1994)
Cholesterol ester storage disease (Wolman disease)	278000	—	AFC +, CVS +	—	—	Gatti et al. (1985), Iavarone et al. (1989)
Chondrodysplasia punctata (Conradi Hunermann type)	118650	US (+)E	—	—	—	Tuck et al. (1990), Pryde et al. (1993)
Chondrodysplasia punctata (rhizomelic type)	215100	US (+)E	AFC +, CVS +	—	—	Schutgens et al. (1989), Duff et al. (1990), Gendall et al. (1994)
Chondroectodermal dysplasia (Ellis–van Creveld syndrome)	225500	US (+)E	—	—	—	Mahoney and Hobbins (1977) Bui et al. (1984)
Chordae tendinae, thickening	—	Other (+)E	—	—	—	Schechter et al. (1987)
Chorioangioma of placenta	—	US (+)E	—	—	—	See Placental tumour
Choroid plexus cyst	—	US +	—	—	—	Gabrielli et al. (1989), Khouzam and Hooker (1989)
Choroid plexus haemorrhage	—	US (+)E	—	—	—	Chambers et al. (1988)
Choroideraemia	303100	—	—	ILP (−), MP (−)	—	Cremers et al. (1987, 1990), Van den Hurk et al. (1992)
Chromosomal aneuploidy	—	—	—	ELP (+)E	CHR +	Hsu (1986)
Chromosomal deletion/duplication	—	—	—	—	CHR +	Hsu (1986)
Chronic granulomatous disease	306400	—	CVS (−)	MP (−)	FBS (+)E	LeVinsky et al. (1986), Huu et al. (1987), Lindlof et al. (1987), Nakamura et al. (1990), De Boer et al. (1992)
Chylothorax	—	US (+)E	—	ELP (+)E	—	Petres et al. (1982), Schmidt et al. (1985), Meizner et al. (1986b)
Citrullinaemia	215700	—	AFC +, AFS +, CVS +	ILP (+)E	—	Northrup et al. (1990)
Cleft lip/palate	119530	US (+)E	—	—	—	Chervenak et al. (1984b); Saltzman et al. (1986)
Cleidocranial dysostosis	119600	US (+)E	—	—	—	Campbell and Pearce (1983)
Cloacal dysgenesis	—	US (+)E	—	—	—	Langer et al. (1992), Petrikovsky et al. (1988), Cilento et al. (1994)

continued on p. 302

Cloverleaf skull (Kleeblattschädel anomaly)	148800	US (+)E	–	–	–	–	–	–	Salvo (1981), Stamm et al. (1987) (see also Thanatophoric dysplasia with cloverleaf skull)
Coarctation of the aorta	120000	US (+)E	–	–	–	–	–	–	Benacerraf et al. (1989a), Hornberger et al. (1994)
Cobalamin E disease	251100	–	–	–	–	–	–	–	See Methylmalonic acidaemia
Coccygeal tail	–	US (+)E	–	–	–	–	–	–	Abbott et al. (1992)
Cockayne syndrome type I	261400	✓	–	–	–	–	–	CHR +	Sugita et al. (1982), Lehmann et al. (1985)
Coffin–Lowry syndrome	303600	–	–	–	–	–	–	–	Hanauer et al. (1988), Biancalana et al. (1992)
Colonic atresia	–	US (+)E	–	ELP (–)	–	–	–	–	Anderson et al. (1993)
Congenital adrenal hyperplasia	201910	–	–	–	–	–	–	–	See Adrenogenital syndrome
Congenital adrenal hypoplasia (autosomal recessive variant)	240200	–	–	–	–	–	–	–	Hensleigh et al. (1978)
Congenital adrenal hypoplasia (X-linked variant)	300200	–	Other +	–	–	–	–	–	Hensleigh et al. (1978), Yates et al. (1987)
Congenital amegakaryocytic thrombocytopenia	–	–	Other +	ELP (–)	–	FBS +	–	–	Mibashan and Rodeck (1984)
Congenital bowing, isolated	–	US (+)E	–	–	–	–	–	–	Kapur and Van Vloten (1986)
Congenital chloridorrhoea (congenital chloride diarrhoea)	214700	US (+)E	–	–	–	–	–	–	Patel et al. (1989)
Congenital coxa vara	122750	US (+)E	–	–	–	–	–	–	Russell (1973)
Congenital dislocation of the knee	–	US (+)E	–	–	–	–	–	–	McFarland (1929), Elchalal et al. (1993)
Congenital dyserythropoietic anaemia type II	224100	Other (+)E	–	–	–	FBS (+)E	–	–	Fukuda et al. (1987)
Congenital heart block	140400	US (+)E	–	–	–	–	–	–	Moodley et al. (1986)
Congenital ichthyosiform erythroderma	242100	–	–	–	–	–	–	–	Holbrook et al. (1988)
Congenital ichthyosiform erythroderma, bullous type (epidermolytic hyperkeratosis)	113800	–	–	–	–	–	–	FSKB +	See Bullous erythroderma ichthyosiformis congenita of Brocq
Congenital muscular dystrophy with arthrogryposis	158810	US (+)E	–	–	–	–	–	–	Socol et al. (1985)

Disease	MIM	Imaging	Biochemistry	DNA	Other	References
Congenital short femur (proximal focal femoral deficiency)	–	US (+)E	–	–	–	Graham (1985), Jeanty and Kleinman (1989)
Conjoined twins	–	US +	–	–	–	Apuzzio et al. (1988), Lituania et al. (1988), Filly et al. (1990)
Conradi disease	215100	–	–	–	–	See Chondrodysplasia punctata
Convulsions, benign familial neonatal	121200	–	–	ELP (–)	–	Leppert et al. (1989)
Copper deficiency (Menkes disease)	309400	–	AFC + CVS +	–	MP (–)	Tonnensen and Horn (1989), Chelly et al. (1993)
Coproporphyria	121300	–	AFS – AFC (–)	–	–	Elder et al. (1976)
Cori disease	232400	–	AFS –	–	–	See Glycogen storage disease III
Cornelia de Lange syndrome	122470	–	Other (+)E	–	–	Westergaard et al. (1983)
Coronal cleft vertebra	–	Other (+)E	–	–	–	Rowley (1955)
Corpus callosum, agenesis	217900	US (+)E	–	–	–	Meizner et al. (1987), Mulligan and Meier (1989), Hilpert and Kurtz (1990)
Corpus callosum, lipoma	–	US (+)E	–	–	–	Mulligan and Meier (1989)
Craniopharyngioma	–	US (+)E	–	–	–	Snyder et al. (1986), Bailey et al. (1990)
Craniosynostosis, sagittal suture	123100	Other (+)E	–	–	–	Campbell and Pearce (1983)
Cranium bifidum	–	US (+)E	–	–	–	Barr et al. (1986)
Crossed renal ectopia	–	US (+)E	–	–	–	Greenblatt et al. (1985)
Crouzon craniofacial dysostosis	123500	US (+)E	–	–	–	Menashe et al. (1989)
Cryptophthalmia syndrome	219000	US (+)E	–	–	–	Feldman et al. (1985)
Cystic adenomatoid malformation	–	US (+)E	–	–	–	Fitzgerald and Toi (1986), Rempen et al. (1987), Heydanus et al. (1993)
Cystic fibrosis (mucoviscidosis)	219700	–	AFS (+)R	ILP + ELP +	MP (+)P	Brock et al. (1988), Feldman et al. (1989), Lemma et al. (1990)
Cystic hygroma	257350	US +	–	–	–	Macken et al. (1989), Thomas (1992)
Cystinosis	219800	–	AFC + CVS +	–	–	Schneider et al. (1974), Steinherz (1985), Patrick et al. (1987)
Cystinuria	220100	–	AFS –	–	–	Komrower (1974)
Cytochrome b_5 reductase deficiency	250800	–	AFS (+)E	–	–	See Methaemoglobinaemia
Cytochrome c oxidase deficiency	220110	–	AFC (+)E CVS (+)E	–	–	Ruitenbeek et al. (1988), Bougeron et al. (1992)

302

Condition	No.	US	AFS	Other	ILP/ELP	MP	CHR	References
Dandy–Walker syndrome	220200	US (+)E	—	—	—	—	—	Russ et al. (1989), Estroff et al. (1992), Cowles et al. (1993)
De la Chapelle dysplasia (neonatal osseous dysplasia I)	256050	US (+)E	—	—	—	—	—	Whitley et al. (1986)
Diaphragmatic hernia/eventration	222400	US (+)E	—	—	—	—	—	Thiagarajah et al. (1990), Manni et al. (1994)
Diastematomyelia	222500	US (+)E	—	—	—	—	—	Pachi et al. (1992), Boulot et al. (1993)
Diastrophic dysplasia	222600	US (+)E	—	—	—	—	—	Gembruch et al. (1988), Hastbacka et al. (1993)
DiGeorge syndrome	188400	—	—	—	ELP (+)E	—	CHR (+)E	Driscoll et al. (1991)
Dihydropteridine reductase deficiency	261630	—	—	—	—	MP (+)E	—	See Phenylketonuria type II
Dihydropyrimidine dehydrogenase deficiency	274270	—	—	—	—	—	—	Jakobs et al. (1991)
Diverticulum, left ventricular	—	—	AFS (+)E	—	—	—	—	Kitchiner et al. (1990)
Double outlet right ventricle	121000	US (+)E	—	—	—	—	—	Stewart et al. (1985)
Duchenne muscular dystrophy	310200	US (+)E	—	—	ILP +	MP (+)P	—	Bakker et al. (1989), Ward et al. (1989), Evans et al. (1991), Benzie et al. (1994), (see also Allelic Becker muscular dystrophy)
Duodenal atresia	223400	US +	—	Other (+)E	ELP +	—	—	Miro and Bard (1988)
Dysautonomia familial (Riley–Day syndrome)	223900	—	—	—	ELP (−)	—	—	Blumenfeld et al. (1993)
Dyskeratosis congenita	305000	—	—	—	ELP (−)	—	—	Connor et al. (1986)
Dyssegmental dwarfism	224400	US (+)E	—	—	—	—	—	Andersen et al. (1988), Izquierdo et al. (1990)
Ebstein anomaly	224700	US (+)E	—	—	—	—	—	Allan et al. (1982), Roberson and Silverman (1989), McIntosh et al. (1992)
Ectodermal dysplasia	305100	—	—	—	—	—	—	See Anhidrotic (hypohidrotic) ectodermal dysplasia
Ectopia cordis	—	US (+)E	—	—	—	—	—	Klingensmith et al. (1988)
Ectopic beat	—	US +	—	—	—	—	—	Steinfeld et al. (1986)
Ectopic fetal liver	—	US (+)E	—	Other +	—	—	—	Mack et al. (1978)
Ectopic pregnancy	—	US (+)R	—	—	—	—	—	Smith et al. (1981)

303

continued on p. 304

Disease	MIM	Imaging	Biochemistry	DNA	Other	References
Ectrodactyly	183600	US (+)E	–	–	–	Henrion et al. (1980)
	225300	–	–	–	–	
Ectrodactyly, ectodermal dysplasia, cleft palate (EEC) syndrome	129900	US (+)E	–	–	–	Anneren et al. (1991), Bronshtein and Gershoni-Baruch (1993)
Ehlers–Danlos syndrome type IV	225350	–	AFC (–)	MP (–)	–	Pope et al. (1989)
	130050	–	–	–	–	
Ehlers–Danlos syndrome Type V	305200	–	AFC (–)	CVS –	–	Di Ferrante et al. (1975)
	–	–	AFS –	–	–	
Ehlers–Danlos syndrome Type VI	225400	–	AFC (+)E	–	–	Dembure et al. (1984)
Elliptocytosis type I (rhesus-linked type, protein 4.1 of erythrocyte membrane defect)	130500	–	–	MP (–)	FBS (+)E	Dhermy et al. (1987)
Elliptocytosis type II (rhesus-unlinked type)	130600	–	–	–	FBS (+)E	Dhermy et al. (1987)
Ellis–van Creveld syndrome	225500	–	–	–	–	See Chondroectodermal dysplasia
Emery–Dreifuss muscular dystrophy	310300	–	–	ELP (–)	–	Yates et al. (1986)
Encephalocele	182940	US +	–	–	–	Chatterjee et al. (1985), Cullen et al. (1990)
Endocardial fibroelastosis	226000	US (+)E	–	–	–	Ben Ami et al. (1986), Achiron et al. (1988)
Epidermolysis bullosa dystrophica (Hallopeau–Siemens type)	305300	–	–	–	FSKB +	Anton-Lamprecht et al. (1981), Heagerty et al. (1986), Bakharev et al. (1990)
	226600	–	–	–	–	
Epidermolysis bullosa dystrophica	131700	–	–	–	FSKB +	Fine et al. (1988)
	–	–	–	–	–	
Epidermolysis bullosa dystrophica inversa	226450	–	–	–	FSKB +	Anton-Lamprecht (1981)
Epidermolysis bullosa herpetiformis (Dowling–Meara type)	131760	–	–	–	FSKB (+)E	Holbrook et al. (1992)
Epidermolysis bullosa lethalis (junctional Herlitz–Pearson type)	226700	–	–	–	FSKB +	Heagerty et al. (1986), Eady et al. (1989), Bakharev et al. (1990), Fine et al. (1990)
Epidermolysis bullosa with pyloric atresia	226730	–	–	–	FSKB +	Nazarro et al. (1990), Dolan et al. (1993)
Exencephaly	–	US (+)E	–	–	–	Hendricks et al. (1988), Kennedy et al. (1990)

Disease	OMIM	US	AFS/AFC	ELP/ILP	MP	FBS	CHR	References
Exomphalos	164750	US +	—	—	—	—	—	Brown et al. (1989), Gray et al. (1989), Pagliano et al. (1990), Morrow et al. (1993)
Extralobar pulmonary sequestration	—	US (+)E	—	—	—	—	—	Mariona et al. (1986), Thomas et al. (1986)
Fabry disease	301500	—	—	—	—	—	—	See Angiokeratoma corporis diffusum
Facioscapulohumeral muscular dystrophy	158900	—	—	—	—	—	—	Wijmenga et al. (1990)
Familial hypercholesterolaemia	143890	—	AFC +	ELP (−) ILP (+)E	MP (+)E	FBS +	—	Martini et al. (1986), Taylor et al. (1988), Reshef et al. (1992)
Familial mediterranean fever	249100	—	—	ELP (−)	—	—	—	Gruberg et al. (1992)
Familial neonatal hyperinsulinemia	—	—	AFS (+)E	—	—	—	—	Aparicio et al. (1993)
Familial polyposis coli	175100	—	—	—	—	—	—	See Intestinal polyposis type I
Fanconi pancytopenia type I	227650	—	—	—	MP (+)P	—	CHR +	Dallapiccola et al. (1985), Auerbach et al. (1986), Murer-Orlando et al. (1993)
Farber disease	228000	—	—	—	—	—	—	See Lipogranulomatosis
Femoral hypoplasia — unusual facies syndrome	134780	US (+)E	—	—	—	—	—	Gamble et al. (1990), Tadmor et al. (1993)
Femur, congenital short (proximal focal femoral deficiency)	—	—	—	—	—	—	—	See Congenital short femur
Femur–fibula–ulna (FFU) syndrome	228200	US (+)E	—	—	—	—	—	Hirose et al. (1989)
Fetal cytomegalovirus infection	—	US (+)R	—	—	—	FBS +	—	Lamy et al. (1992), Donner et al. (1993)
Fetal HIV infection	—	—	AFS +	—	—	FBS +	—	Daffos et al. (1989)
Fetal hydantoin syndrome	—	—	AFC (−)	—	—	—	—	Buehler et al. (1990)
Fetal listeriosis	—	—	—	—	—	FBS +	—	Boucher and Yonekura (1986), Liner (1990)
Fetal parvovirus infection	—	—	AFS (+)E	—	—	FBS +	—	Naides and Weiner (1989), Peters and Nicolaides (1990), Kovacs et al. (1992)
Fetal rubella infection	—	—	—	—	—	FBS +	—	Morgan-Capner et al. (1985), Terry et al. (1986)
Fetal syphillis	—	US (+)R	—	—	—	FBS +	—	Raafat et al. (1993)
Fetal toxoplasmosis infection	—	US (+)R	—	—	—	FBS +	—	Blaakaer (1986), Daffos et al. (1988), Foulon et al. (1990), Cazenave et al. (1992)

continued on p. 306

Disease	MIM	Imaging	Biochemistry	DNA	Other	References
Fetal varicella infection	—	US (+)R	—	—	FBS +	Byrne et al. (1990), Pons et al. (1992)
Fetofetal transfusion syndrome	—	US (+)E	—	—	—	Brennan et al. (1982), Pretorius et al. (1988), Filly et al. (1990) (see also Twin embolization syndrome)
Fetus in fetu	—	US (+)E	—	—	—	Sada et al. (1986)
Fetus papyraceous	—	US (+)E	—	—	—	Kurjak and Latin (1979)
Foramen ovale, premature closure	—	US (+)E	—	—	—	Buis-Liem et al. (1987), Fraser et al. (1989)
Forbe disease	232400	—	—	—	—	See Glycogen storage disease III
Fragile X syndrome	309550	—	—	ILP +	MP +, CHR +	Richards et al. (1991), Murphy et al. (1992), Von Koskull et al. (1992)
Fraser syndrome (cryptophthalmos with other malformations)	219000	US (+)E	—	ELP +	—	Ramsing et al. (1990), Schauer et al. (1990)
Friedreich's ataxia	229300	—	—	—	—	Wallis et al. (1989)
Fryns syndrome	229850	US (+)E	—	ELP (+)E	—	Samueloff et al. (1987), Pellissier et al. (1992)
Fucosidosis	230000	—	AFC +, AFS −, CVS (−)	—	MP (−)	Gatti et al. (1985), Lissens et al. (1987)
Fumarase deficiency (fumarate hydratase deficiency)	136850	—	AFC (−)	—	MP (−)	Petrova-Benedict et al. (1987)
Galactokinase deficiency	230200	—	AFC (−), AFS (−)	—	FBS (−)	Holton et al. (1989)
Galactosaemia	230400	—	AFC +, AFS +, CVS +	—	FBS (−)	Holton et al. (1989)
Galactose epimerase deficiency	230350	—	AFC (−)	—	—	Gillett et al. (1983)
Galactosialidosis (neuraminidase deficiency with β-galactosidase deficiency)	256540	—	AFC (+)E, CVS (−)	—	—	Sewell and Pontz (1988)
Gallbladder agenesis	—	US (+)E	—	—	—	Bronshtein et al. (1993)
Gallstones (fetal)	—	US (+)E	—	—	—	Heijne et al. (1985), Abbitt and McIlhenny (1990)
Gangliosidosis, generalized GM$_1$, types I and II	230500	—	AFC +, CVS +	—	—	Lowden et al. (1973), Warner et al. (1983)
Gangliosidosis, GM$_2$ type I (Tay–Sachs disease)	272800	—	AFC +, AFS (+)E, CVS +	ILP (−)	MP (+)P	Grebner and Jackson (1979, 1985), Triggs-Raine et al. (1990)

Disorder	No.								References
Gangliosidosis, GM₂ type II (Sandhoff disease)	268800	–	AFC +	CVS +	ILP (–)	MP (–)	–	–	Giles et al. (1988)
Gangliosidosis, GM₂ type III (juvenile-onset variant)	230700	–	AFS (+)E	–	–	–	–	–	Zerfowski and Sandhoff (1974)
Gangliosidosis, GM₂ (adult-onset variant)	272800	–	AFC (–)	–	–	–	–	–	Navon et al. (1986)
Gardner syndrome	175300	–	–	–	–	–	–	–	See Intestinal polyposis type III
Gastric obstruction	–	US (+)E	–	–	–	–	–	–	Zimmerman (1978)
Gastroenteric cyst	–	US (+)E	–	–	–	–	–	–	Newnham et al. (1984)
Gastroschisis	230750	US +	–	–	–	–	–	–	Bair et al. (1986), Lindfors et al. (1986), Guzman (1990), Kushnir et al. (1990), Langer et al. (1993)
Gaucher disease	230800	–	–	–	–	–	–	–	See Beta-glucosidase deficiency
Gerstmann–Straussler disease	137440	–	–	–	–	MP (+)P	–	–	Collinge et al. (1989), Brown et al. (1994)
Glanzmann thrombasthenia	187800	–	–	–	–	–	FBS +	–	Kaplan et al. (1985), Seligsohn et al. (1985)
Glioblastoma	273800 137800	US (+)E	AFS –	–	–	–	–	–	Geraghty et al. (1989)
Glucose phosphate isomerase deficiency (phosphohexose isomerase deficiency)	172400	–	AFC +	CVS +	–	–	FBS (–)	–	Dallapiccola et al. (1986)
Glucose-6-phosphate dehydrogenase deficiency	305900	–	AFS –	–	ILP (–)	MP (–)P	FBS (–)	–	Martini et al. (1986), de Vita et al. (1989)
Glutaricaciduria type I (glutaryl-CoA dehyrogenase deficiency)	231670	–	AFS –; AFC +	CVS (–)	ELP (–)	–	–	–	Poenaru (1987), Holme et al. (1989)
Glutaricaciduria type IIA (neonatal form of type II)	305950	–	AFS +; AFC (+)E	–	–	–	–	–	Mitchell et al. (1983)
Glutaricaciduria type IIB (electron transfer flavoprotein dehydrogenase deficiency)	231680	–	AFS (+)E	–	–	–	–	–	Jakobs et al. (1984), Sakuma et al. (1991)
Glycogen storage disease IA (von Gierke disease)	232200	–	AFS –; AFC –	CVS –	–	–	FLB (+)E	Other (+)E	Golbus et al. (1988)

continued on p. 308

Disease	MIM	Imaging	Biochemistry	DNA	Other	References
Glycogen storage disease II (Pompe disease)	232300	–	AFC +, CVS +	–	–	Shin et al. (1989)
Glycogen storage disease III (Forbe or Cori disease)	232400	–	AFC +, CVS (+)E	–	–	Maire et al. (1989), Shin et al. (1989), Yang et al. (1990)
Glycogen storage disease IV (Anderson disease)	232500	–	AFC +, CVS +	–	–	Brown and Brown (1989)
Glycogen storage disease VI (Hers disease)	232700	–	–	ILP (−), MP (−)	–	Newgard et al. (1987)
Glycogen storage disease VII (muscle phosphofructokinase deficiency)	232800	–	–	MP (−)	–	Vora et al. (1987)
Goitre	274600	US (+)E	–	–	–	Kourides et al. (1984)
Goldenhar syndrome	164210	–	–	–	–	See Hemifacial microsomia
Graves disease	–	–	–	–	–	See Thyrotoxicosis
Growth hormone deficiency (one type)	262400	–	–	ILP (−), MP (−)	–	Phillips et al. (1981)
Growth retardation	–	US (+)R	–	–	–	Bruinse et al. (1989), Deter et al. (1989)
GTP cyclohydrolase I deficiency	233910	–	AFS (+)E	–	–	Dhonot et al. (1990)
Gyrate atrophy	258870	–	AFC (−)	ILP (−), MP (−)	–	Mitchell et al. (1989), O'Donnell (1981)
Haemangioma/teratoma	–	US (+)E	–	–	–	Sabbagha et al. (1980), Trecet et al. (1984), Grundy et al. (1985), McGahan and Schneider (1986), Pennel and Baltarowich (1986)
Haematoma, extracranial	–	US (+)E	–	–	–	Harper et al. (1989)
Haematoma, retroplacental	–	US (+)R	–	–	–	Spirt et al. (1987)
Haemoglobin O-Arab	141900	–	–	ILP +, MP +	–	Weatherall et al. (1985)
Haemoglobin Lepore	141900	–	–	ILP +, MP +	–	Weatherall et al. (1985)
Haemoglobin S (sickle cell disease)	142300	–	–	ILP +, ELP +, MP +	FBS +	Kazazian et al. (1978)
Haemoglobin S-O Arab	141900	–	–	ILP +	–	Kazazian et al. (1978)
Haemoglobinopathies	142300	–	–	ILP +, MP (+)P	FBS +	Alter (1984), Kazazian et al. (1985), Old et al. (1986), Kim et al. (1994)
Haemophilia A (factor VIII deficiency)	306700	–	–	ELP +, ILP +, MP (+)P	FBS +	Mibashan et al. (1979), Forestier et al. (1986), Brocker-Vriends et al. (1988)
Haemophilia B (factor IX deficiency)	306900	–	–	ELP +, ILP +, MP (+)P	FBS +	Mibashan et al. (1979), Zeng et al. (1987)
	–	–	–	ELP +	–	–

continued on p. 310

Condition	No.	US/Other	AFC	CVS	ELP/ILP	MP	FBS	Reference
Hair–brain syndrome (Pibids syndrome)	234050	–	AFC (+)E	–	–	–	–	Savary et al. (1991)
Harlequin Ichthyosis	242500	–	–	–	–	–	–	See Ichthyosis congenita, harlequin fetus type
Hemifacial microsomia (Goldenhar syndrome)	164210	US (+)E	–	–	–	–	–	Benacerraf and Frigoletto (1988)
Hemivertebra	257700	US (+)E	–	–	–	–	–	Abrams and Filly (1985), Benacerraf et al. (1986a)
Hepatic adenoma	–	US (+)E	–	–	–	–	–	Marks et al. (1990)
Hepatic cyst	–	US (+)E	–	–	–	–	–	Chung (1986)
Hepatic haemangioma	–	US (+)E	–	–	–	–	–	Nakamoto et al. (1983), Sepulveda et al. (1993)
Hepatic hamartoma	–	US (+)E	–	–	–	–	–	Foucar et al. (1983)
Hepatic necrosis	–	US (+)E	–	–	–	–	–	Nguyen and Leonard (1986)
Hereditary angioedema (C1 esterase inhibitor deficiency)	106100	–	–	–	ILP (-)	MP (-)	–	Cicardi et al. (1987)
Hereditary enlarged parietal foramina	168500	US (+)E	–	–	–	–	–	Fernandez and Hertzberg (1992)
Hereditary motor and sensory neuropathy type I (Charcot–Marie–Tooth disease)	118200	–	–	–	–	–	–	Middleton-Price et al. (1990)
Hereditary motor and sensory neuropathy, X-linked	302800	–	–	–	ELP (-)P	MP (+)E	–	Rozear et al. (1987)
Herrmann–Opitz syndrome	–	US (+)E	–	–	ELP (-)	MP (-)	–	Anyane-Yeboa et al. (1987)
Hirschsprung disease	249200	US (+)E	–	–	–	–	–	Vermesh et al. (1986)
Holoprosencephaly	236100	US (+)E	–	–	–	–	–	McGahan et al. (1990), Toma et al. (1990), Wenstrom et al. (1991)
Holoprosencephaly with hypokinesia	306990	Other (+)E	–	–	–	–	–	Morse et al. (1987b)
Holt–Oram syndrome	142900	US (+)E	–	–	ELP (-)P	–	–	Brons et al. (1988)
Homocystinuria I	236200	–	AFC +	CVS +	ILP (-)	MP (-)	FBS (-)	Fowler et al. (1982), Fensom et al. (1983)
Homocystinuria II (methylenetetrahydrofolate reductase deficiency)	236250	–	AFC (+)E	–	ELP (-)	–	–	Wendel et al. (1983), Christensen and Brandt (1985), Marquet et al. (1994)
Horseshoe kidney	–	US (+)E	–	–	–	–	–	Sherer et al. (1990)
Hunter syndrome	309900	–	–	–	–	–	–	See Mucopolysaccharidosis type II

Disease	MIM	Imaging	Biochemistry	DNA	Other	References
Huntington disease	143100	–	–	–	–	Hayden et al. (1987), Quarrell et al. (1987), Rosser et al. (1994)
Hurler syndrome	252800	–	–	ELP +	MP +	See Mucopolysaccharidosis type IH, IS
Hydatidiform mole	236500	US +	–	–	–	Spirt et al. (1987)
Hydranencephaly	236500	US (+)E	–	–	–	Hadi et al. (1986), Wenstrom et al. (1991)
Hydrocele	–	Other (+)E	–	–	–	Cacchio et al. (1983)
	–	US +	–	–	–	
Hydrocephalus	236600	US (+)L	–	–	–	Benacerraf and Birnholz (1987), Dreazen et al. (1989), Wenstrom et al. (1991)
	–	Other (+)E	–	–	–	
Hydrocephalus and cystic renal disease	–	US (+)E	–	–	–	Reuss et al. (1989)
Hydrocephalus X-linked	307000	US (+)L	–	ELP (+)E	MP (−)	Friedman and Santos-Ramos (1984), Brocard et al. (1993), Ko et al. (1994), Serville et al. (1993)
Hydrolethalus syndrome	236680	US (+)E	–	–	–	Hartikainen-Sorri et al. (1983), Siffring et al. (1991)
Hydrometrocolpos	–	US (+)E	–	–	–	Hill and Hirsch (1985), Mirk et al. (1994)
Hydrometrocolpos, postaxial polydactyly, congenital heart malformation syndrome (Kaufman–McKusick syndrome)	236700	US (+)E	–	–	–	Chitayat et al. (1987)
Hydronephrosis	143400	US +	–	–	–	Grignon et al. (1986a), Quinlan et al. (1986)
Hydrops fetalis	–	US +	–	–	–	Mahony et al. (1984b), Barss et al. (1985)
Hydrosyringomyelia	–	US (+)E	–	–	–	Toma et al. (1991)
Hydrothorax	–	US (+)E	–	–	–	Bovicelli et al. (1981), Peleg et al. (1985)
Hydroureter	–	US (+)E	–	–	–	Grignon et al. (1986b)
Hydroxy-3-methylglutaryl-CoA lyase deficiency (3-hydroxy-3-methylglutaricaciduria)	246450	–	AFC (+)E	CVS (+)E	–	Duran et al. (1979), Chalmers et al. (1989)
	–	–	AFS (+)E	Other (+)L	–	

Disorder	Number	US	AFC/AFS	CVS	ILP/ELP	MP	FLB		References
Hyperammonaemia I (ornithine transcarbamylase deficiency)	311250	—	AFC —	CVS —	ILP +	MP (—)	—	—	Rodeck et al. (1982), Spence et al. (1989)
Hyperammonaemia II (carbamoyl-phosphate synthetase deficiency)	237300	—	AFS — AFC —	— CVS —	ELP + ILP (—)	MP (—)	FLB +	—	Serini et al. (1988)
Hyperammonaemia III (N-acetylglutamate synthetase deficiency)	237310	—	AFS — AFC —	— CVS —	—	—	FLB +	—	Bachmann et al. (1981)
Hypercholesterolaemia, familial	143890	—	AFS — —	—	—	—	FLB +	—	See Familial hypercholesterolaemia
Hyperglycerolaemia	307030	—	AFC (+)E	—	—	MP (+)E	—	—	McCabe et al. (1982), Borresen et al. (1987)
Hyperglycinaemia, ketotic	232000	—	AFS (—)	—	—	—	—	—	See Propionic acidaemia
Hyperglycinaemia (isolated), non-ketotic type I	238300	—	—	CVS (+)E	—	—	—	—	García-Muñoz et al. (1989), Hayasaka et al. (1990), Parvy et al. (1990), Toone et al. (1992), Rolland et al. (1993)
Hyperornithinaemia, hyperammonaemia and homocitrullinuria syndrome	238970	—	AFS (+)R AFC (+)E	CVS (+)E	—	—	—	—	Chadefaux et al. (1989), Shim et al. (1992)
Hyperoxularia type I	259900	—	AFS (+)E	—	—	—	FLB +	—	Danpure et al. (1987, 1989), Illum et al. (1992)
Hyperphenylalanaemia	261600	—	—	—	—	—	—	—	See Phenylketonuria types I and II
Hypertelorism	145400	US (+)E	—	—	—	—	—	—	Pilu et al. (1986a) (see also Opitz G syndrome)
Hypertrophic obstructive cardiomyopathy	192600	—	—	—	—	—	—	—	See Asymmetric septal hypertrophy
Hypertrophic pyloric stenosis	179010	—	—	—	—	—	—	—	See Pyloric stenosis
Hypochondrogenesis	—	US (+)E	—	—	—	—	—	—	Donnenfeld et al. (1986)
Hypochondroplasia	146000	US (+)E	—	—	—	—	—	—	Stoll et al. (1985), Jones et al. (1990)
Hypophosphatasia (severe autosomal recessive variant)	241500	US (+)E	AFC (+)E	CVS (+)E	ILP (+)E	MP (—)	—	—	De Lange and Rouse (1990), Brock and Barron (1991), Kishi et al. (1991)
Hypoplastic left heart	241550	US +	—	—	—	—	—	—	Sahn et al. (1982), Allan et al. (1985), Yagel et al. (1986)

311

continued on p. 312

Disease	MIM	Imaging	Biochemistry	DNA	Other	References
Hypoplastic right ventricle	121000	US (+)E	—	—	—	De Vore and Hobbins (1979)
Hypotelorism	—	US (+)E	—	—	—	Pilu et al. (1986a)
Hypothyroidism	274600	—	—	—	—	Kourides et al. (1984), Hirsch et al. (1990), Perelman et al. (1990) (see also Goitre)
Hypoxanthine guanine phosphoribosyltransferase deficiency (Lesch–Nyhan syndrome)	308000	—	AFS +; AFC +; CVS +	ILP (+)E	MP (+)P; FBS (−)	Gibbs et al. (1986), Zoref-Shani et al. (1989)
I-cell disease	252500	—	—	—	—	See Mucolipidosis type II
Ichthyosis congenita (congenital ichthyosiform erythroderma, lamellar exfoliation of the newborn, collodion fetus)	242300	—	—	—	—	Perry et al. (1987)
Ichthyosis congenita, harlequin fetus type (congenital ichthyosiform erythroderma)	242500	—	—	—	FSKB +	Blanchet-Bardon and Dumez (1984), Suzumori and Kanzaki (1991)
Ichthyosis X-linked (steroid sulphatase deficiency)	308100	—	AFC +; CVS (+)E	ILP (−)	MP (−); FSKB +	Braunstein et al. (1976), Hahnel et al. (1982), Honour et al. (1985), Ballabio et al. (1989)
Illeal atresia	—	US (+)E	AFS (+)E	—	—	Kjoller et al. (1985)
Immunodeficiency disease (T-cell)	164050	—	—	—	—	See Nucleoside phosphorylase deficiency
Immunodeficiency disease, severe combined	102700	—	—	—	FBS +	Durandy et al. (1982, 1987) (see also Adenosine deaminase deficiency)
Immunodeficiency disease, severe combined X-linked variant	300400	—	—	—	FBS (+)E	Goodship et al. (1989), Puck et al. (1990), Noguchi et al. (1993)
Immunodeficiency with increased IgM	308230	—	—	ELP (+)E	MP (−)	Mensink et al. (1987), DiSanto et al. (1994)
Immunodeficiency, X-linked progressive combined variable (Duncan disease, X-linked lymphoproliferative disease)	308240	—	—	ELP (+)E	—	Skare et al. (1987)
	—	—	—	ELP (+)E	—	—

Disorder	No.	US	AFS/AFC	ELP	MP	FBS	References
Imperforate anus	207500	–	–	–	–	–	See Anal atresia
Infantile cortical hyperostosis (Caffey disease)	114000	US (+)E	–	–	–	–	Langer and Kaufmann (1986)
Infantile hereditary agranulocytosis (Kostmann disease)	202700	–	–	–	–	FBS (+)E	Cividalli et al. (1983)
Infantile polycystic disease	263200	US +	–	–	–	–	Morin (1981), Romero et al. (1984), Argubright and Wicks (1987), Zerres et al. (1988), Reuss et al. (1990)
Iniencephaly	–	US +	AFS (+)R	–	–	–	Foderaro et al. (1987), Meizner and Bar-Ziv (1987)
Interrupted aortic arch	107550	US (+)E	–	–	–	–	Allan et al. (1985)
Intestinal duplication	–	US (+)E	–	–	–	–	Van Dam et al. (1984)
Intestinal perforation	–	US (+)E	–	–	–	–	Shalev et al. (1982), Glick et al. (1983)
Intestinal polyposis type I (familial polyposis coli, adenomatous polyposis of the colon)	175100	–	–	ELP (−)	MP (−)	–	Bodmer et al. (1987)
Intestinal polyposis type III (Gardner syndrome)	175300	–	–	ELP (−)	MP (−)	–	Bodmer et al. (1987)
Intestinal volvulus	–	US (+)E	–	–	–	–	Witter and Molteni (1986), Mercado et al. (1993)
Intracerebral haemorrhage	–	US (+)E	–	–	–	–	Mintz et al. (1985)
Intracranial arteriovenous fistula	–	US (+)E	–	–	–	–	See Arteriovenous fistula (brain)
Intracranial calcification	–	US (+)E	–	–	–	–	Ghidini et al. (1989), Koga et al. (1990)
Intracranial haemorrhage (including subdural haematoma)	–	US (+)E	–	–	–	–	Fogarty et al. (1989), Rotmensch et al. (1991)
Intracranial teratoma	–	Other (+)E	–	–	–	–	Vintners et al. (1982)
Intrauterine fetal death	–	US (+)E	–	–	–	–	Bass et al. (1986)
Intrauterine growth retardation	–	US +	–	–	–	–	Rizzo et al. (1987)
Intrauterine membranous cyst	–	US (+)R	–	–	–	–	Kirkinen and Jouppila (1986)
Intraventricular haemorrhage	–	US (+)E	–	–	–	–	McGahan et al. (1984)
Isoimmune thrombocytopenia	–	US (+)E	–	–	MP (+)E	FBS +	Lynch et al. (1988), Johnson et al. (1993)
Isovaleric acidaemia	243500	–	AFC (+)E; AFS +	–	–	–	Hine et al. (1986), Dumoulin et al. (1991)

continued on p. 314

Disease	MIM	Imaging	Biochemistry	DNA	Other	References
Ivemark syndrome (asplenia syndrome)	208530	US (+)E	–	–	–	Chitayat et al. (1988a)
Jarcho–Levin syndrome	277300	US (+)E	–	–	–	Apuzzio et al. (1987), Tolmie et al. (1987a), Romero et al. (1988)
Jejunal atresia	–	US (+)E	–	–	–	Filkins et al. (1985)
Jejunal atresia (apple-peel type)	243600	US (+)E	–	–	–	Fletman et al. (1980)
Jeune syndrome	208500	–	–	–	–	See Asphyxiating thoracic dysplasia
Joubert syndrome	243910	US (+)E	–	–	–	Campbell et al. (1984)
Kennedy disease	313200	–	–	–	–	See Spinal and bulbar muscular atrophy
Kleeblattschädel anomaly	148800	–	–	–	–	See Cloverleaf skull
Klippel–Trenaunay–Weber syndrome	149000	US (+)E	–	–	–	Shalev et al. (1988), Hayashi et al. (1993)
Krabbe disease	245200	–	AFC +	CVS +	–	Giles et al. (1987), Harzer et al. (1987), Zlotogora et al. (1990)
Lacrimal duct cysts	–	US (+)E	–	ELP (–)	–	Davis et al. (1987)
Lacrimoauriculodentodigital syndrome (Ladd syndrome)	149730	US (+)E	–	–	–	Francannet et al. (1994)
Langer–Saldino syndrome	200610	–	–	–	–	See Achondrogenesis type IB
Larsen-like syndrome, lethal type	245650	US (+)E	–	–	–	Mostello et al. (1991)
Laryngeal atresia	–	US (+)E	–	–	–	Dolkart et al. (1992), Weston et al. (1992)
Laurence–Moon–Biedl syndrome	245800	US (+)E	–	–	–	Ritchie et al. (1988)
Leigh disease	–	–	–	–	–	See Mitochondrial complex deficiencies
Leprechaunism	246200	–	AFC (+)E	–	–	Maasen et al. (1990)
Lesch–Nyhan syndrome	308000	–	–	–	–	See Hypoxanthine guanine phosphoribosyl transferase deficiency
Leucocyte adhesion deficiency	116920	–	–	–	MP (–)	FBS (+)E	Liskowska-Grospierre et al. (1986), Kishimoto al. (1989), Weaning et al. (1991)
Leukaemia	–	–	–	–	FBS (+)E	Zerres et al. (1990)
Lipogranulomatosis (Farber disease)	228000	–	AFC + AFS –	CVS –	–	Fensom et al. (1979)
Lipomyelomeningocele	–	US (+)E	–	–	–	Seeds and Powers (1988)
Lissencephaly (Miller–Dieker syndrome)	247200	US (+)L	–	–	–	Saltzman et al. (1991), Okamura et al. (1993)
		Other (+)E	–			
Long chain acyl-CoA dehydrogenase deficiency	201460	–	AFC (–)	CVS (+)E	–	Wanders and Ijlst (1992), Perez-Cerda et al. (1993)

continued on p. 316

Disorder	No.	US	AFC	CVS	ELP/ILP	MP	FBS	References
Lowe oculocerebrorenal syndrome	309000	–	–	–	–	–	–	Silver et al. (1987), Gazit et al. (1990)
Lymphangiomatosis	–	US (+)E	–	–	ELP (–)	–	–	Haeusler et al. (1990)
Lymphoedema	153100	US (+)E	–	–	–	–	–	Adam et al. (1979)
Macrocephaly, benign familial	153470	US (+)E	–	–	–	–	–	Derosa et al. (1989)
Majewski syndrome	263520	–	–	–	–	–	–	See Short rib–polydactyly syndrome type II
Mandibulofacial dysostosis (Treacher Collins syndrome)	154500	US (+)E	–	–	–	–	–	Nicolaides et al. (1984), Crane and Beaver (1986)
Mannosidosis, alpha	248500	Other (+)E	AFC +	CVS +	ELP (–)	–	–	Poenaru et al. (1979), Jones et al. (1984)
Mannosidosis, beta	248510	–	AFC (–)	CVS (–)	–	–	–	Dahl et al. (1986)
Maple syrup urine disease	248600	–	AFC +	CVS +	–	MP (–)	–	Fensom et al. (1978), Wendel and Claussen (1979), Poenaru (1987)
Marfan syndrome	154700	–	AFS –, AFC (–)	–	ILP (–)	MP (+)P	–	Godfrey et al. (1990), Kainulainen et al. (1990), Dietz et al. (1991), Godfrey et al. (1993)
Maroteaux–Lamy disease	253200	–	–	–	ELP (–)	–	–	See Mucopolysaccharidosis type VI
May–Hegglin anomaly	155100	–	–	–	–	–	FBS (+)E	Takashima et al. (1992)
Meckel–Gruber syndrome	249000	US +, Other (+)E	–	–	–	–	–	Pachi et al. (1989), Nyberg et al. (1990a), Dumez et al. (1994)
Meconium ileus	–	US (+)E	–	–	–	–	–	Denholm et al. (1984), Nyberg et al. (1987)
Meconium peritonitis	–	US (+)E	–	–	–	–	–	McGahan and Hanson (1983), Nancarrow et al. (1985)
Meconium plug syndrome	–	US (+)E	–	–	–	–	–	Samuel et al. (1986)
Median cleft face syndrome	136760	US (+)E	–	–	–	–	–	Chervenak et al. (1984b)
Medium chain acyl-CoA dehydrogenase deficiency	201450	–	AFC +	CVS (+)E	–	MP (–)	–	Bennett et al. (1987), Pollitt (1989), Yokota et al. (1990)
Megacystis–microcolon–intestinal hypoperistalsis syndrome	249210	US (+)E	–	–	–	–	–	Garber et al. (1990), Stamm et al. (1991), McNamara et al. (1994)
Megalourethra	–	US (+)E	–	–	–	–	–	Fisk et al. (1990), Sepulveda et al. (1993)
Megaureters	–	US (+)E	–	–	–	–	–	Dunn and Glasier (1985)
Menkes disease	309400	–	–	–	–	–	–	See Copper deficiency
Mesoblastic nephroma	–	US (+)E	–	–	–	–	–	Apuzzio et al. (1986)
Mesomelic dwarfism, Langer type	249700	US (+)E	–	–	–	–	–	Quigg et al. (1985), Evans et al. (1988)

Disease	MIM	Imaging	Biochemistry	DNA	Other	References
Metachromatic leucodystrophy	250100	–	AFC +, CVS +	MP (–)	FBS (–)	Poenaru et al. (1988)
Methaemoglobinaemia (NADH cytochrome b₅ reductase deficiency)	250800	–	AFC +, CVS +	MP (–)	–	Junien et al. (1981)
Methylacetoaceticaciduria (beta-ketothiolase deficiency)	203750	–	AFC (–)	–	–	Hiyama et al. (1986)
Methylglutaconicaciduria (3-methylglutaconyl-CoA hydratase deficiency)	250950	–	AFS (–), AFC (–), CVS (–)	–	–	Narisawa et al. (1986)
Methylmalonic acidaemia (B₁₂ non-responsive)	251000	–	AFS (–), AFC +, CVS +	–	–	Fowler et al. (1988)
Methylmalonic acidaemia (B₁₂ responsive) (cobalamin E disease)	251100	–	AFS +, AFC +, CVS (–)	–	–	Ampola et al. (1975), Rosenblatt et al. (1985)
Mevalonic acidaemia	251170	–	AFS +, AFC (+)E, AFS (+)E, CVS (+)E	–	–	Hoffmann et al. (1992)
Microcephaly	251200	US (+)L	–	–	–	Chervenak et al. (1984a), Tolmie et al. (1987b)
Microcephaly–micromelia syndrome	251230	US (+)E	–	–	–	Ives and Houston (1980)
Micrognathia	–	US (+)E	–	–	–	Pilu et al. (1986a), Majoor-Krakauer et al. (1987)
Microphthalmia	251600	US (+)E	AFS (+)E	–	–	Feldman et al (1985)
Mitochondrial complex I deficiency	–	–	CVS (+)E	–	–	Ruitenbeek et al. (1992)
Mitochondrial complex IV deficiency	–	–	CVS (+)E	–	–	Ruitenbeek et al. (1992)
Mitochondrial complex I and IV deficiency	–	–	CVS (+)E	–	–	Ruitenbeek et al. (1992)
Mitral atresia	121000	US (+)E	–	–	–	Allan (1987)
Molybdenum cofactor deficiency (combined xanthine and sulphite oxidase deficiencies)	252150	–	AFC (+)E, CVS (+)E	–	–	Ogier et al. (1983), Gray et al. (1990)
Morquio disease	253000	–	AFS (+)E	–	–	See Mucopolysaccharidosis type IVA
Mucoid degeneration of cord	–	US (+)E	–	–	–	Iaccarino et al. (1986)
Mucolipidosis type I (sialidosis)	252400	–	AFC +	–	–	Kleijer et al. (1979), Steinman et al. (1980), Sasagasako et al. (1993)
Mucolipidosis type II (I-cell disease)	252500	–	AFC +, AFS +, CVS +	–	–	Ben-Yoseph et al. (1988), Poenaru et al. (1990)

continued on p. 318

Disorder	OMIM		AFS / AFC	CVS	ILP / ELP	MP	FBS	FSKB		Reference
Mucolipidosis type III (pseudo-Hurler polydystrophy)	252600	—	AFC (−)	CVS (−)	—	—	—	—	—	Ben-Yoseph et al. (1988)
Mucolipidosis type IV	252650	—	AFC (+)E	CVS (+)E	—	—	—	—	—	Orney et al. (1987), Zeigler et al. (1992)
Mucopolysaccharidosis type IH, IS (Hurler syndrome, Scheie syndrome)	252800	—	–; AFC +	–; CVS +	—	—	FBS +	FSKB (+)E	—	Kleijer et al. (1983), Rodeck et al. (1983b), Young (1992)
Mucopolysaccharidosis type II (Hunter syndrome)	309900	—	AFS +; AFC +	–; CVS +	ILP (−)	MP (−)	FBS (+)E	—	—	Pannone et al. (1986), Lissens et al. (1988), Flomen et al. (1992), Bunge et al. (1993)
Mucopolysaccharidosis type IIIA (Sanfilippo A disease)	252900	—	AFS +; AFC +	–; CVS +	ELP (−)	—	—	—	—	Kleijer et al. (1986)
Mucopolysaccharidosis type IIIB (Sanfilippo B disease)	252920	—	AFS +; AFC +	CVS +	—	—	—	—	—	Minelli et al. (1988)
Mucopolysaccharidosis type IIIC (Sanfilippo C disease)	252930	—	AFC (−)	CVS +	—	—	—	—	—	Di Natale et al. (1987), He et al. (1994)
Mucopolysaccharidosis type IIID (Sanfilippo D disease)	252940	—	AFS +; AFC (−)	–; CVS (−)	—	MP (−)	—	—	—	Nowakowski et al. (1989)
Mucopolysaccharidosis type IVA (Morquio disease type A)	253000	—	AFC +	CVS +	—	—	—	—	—	Von Figura et al. (1982), Yuen and Fensom (1985), Zhao et al. (1990)
Mucopolysaccharidosis type IVB (Morquio disease type B)	253010	—	AFS +; AFC (−)	–; CVS (−)	—	—	—	—	—	Guigiani et al. (1987)
Mucopolysaccharidosis type V	252800	—	—	—	—	—	—	—	—	See Mucopolysaccharidosis type IH, IS
Mucopolysaccharidosis type VI (Maroteaux–Lamy disease)	253200	—	AFC +	CVS +	—	—	—	—	—	Van Dyke et al. (1981), Rogoyski (1985)
Mucopolysaccharidosis type VII (Sly syndrome)	253220	—	AFS +; AFC (+)E	–; CVS (+)E	—	MP (−)	—	—	—	Maire et al. (1979), Poenaru (1982)
Multiple carboxylase deficiency (late-onset variant, biotinidase deficiency)	253260	—	AFC (+)E; AFS (+)E	—	—	—	—	—	—	Secor McVoy et al. (1984)

317

Disease	MIM	Imaging	Biochemistry	DNA	Other	References
Multiple carboxylase deficiency (neonatal form, holocarboxylase synthase deficiency)	253270	–	AFC (+)E, CVS (–)	–	–	Packman et al. (1982)
Multiple contracture syndrome, Finnish type	253310	US (+)E	AFS (+)E	–	–	Herva et al. (1985), Kirkinen et al. (1987)
Multiple endocrine neoplasia type I	131100	–	–	ELP (–)	–	Bale et al. (1989)
Multiple endocrine neoplasia type IIA	171400	–	–	ELP (–), MP (–)	–	Mathew et al. (1987)
Multiple endocrine neoplasia type IIB	162300	–	–	ELP (–), MP (–)	–	Jackson et al. (1988)
Multiple gestation	–	US +	–	–	–	Neilson et al. (1989), Winn et al. (1989), Filly et al. (1990)
Multiple pterygium syndrome	253290	US (+)E	–	–	–	Lockwood et al. (1988), Zeitune et al. (1988)
Multiple pterygium syndrome with concentric bone fusion	–	US (+)E	–	–	–	van Regemorter et al. (1984)
Multiple pterygium syndrome with spinal fusion	252390	US (+)E	–	–	–	Chen et al. (1984), Zeitune et al. (1988)
Multiple pterygium syndrome, X-linked variant	312150	US (+)E	–	–	–	Tolmie et al. (1987c)
Multiple sulphatase deficiency (mucosulphatidosis)	272200	–	AFC (–), CVS +	–	–	Patrick et al. (1988)
Myasthenia gravis with fetal arthrogryposis	254200	US (+)E	–	–	–	Stoll et al. (1991)
Myotonic dystrophy	160900	–	–	ELP +	–	Myring et al. (1992)
Myotubular myopathy, X-linked	310400	–	–	MP +	–	Bartley and Gies (1990), Liechti-Gallati et al. (1993)
Nail–Patella syndrome	161200	–	–	ELP (+)E	Other (+)E	Gubler and Levy (1993)
Nager acrofacial dysostosis	154400	US (+)E	–	–	–	Benson et al. (1988)
Nephroblastomatosis	267000	US (+)E	–	–	–	Ambrosino et al. (1990)
Nephrogenic diabetes insipidus	304800	–	–	ELP (–)	–	Knoers et al. (1988)
Nephrotic syndrome, congenital (Finnish nephrosis)	256300	–	AFS +	–	–	Morin (1984)
Neu–Laxova syndrome	256520	US (+)E	–	–	–	Mennuti et al. (1990), Gulmezoglu and Ekici (1994)
Neurenteric cyst	–	–	–	–	Other (+)E	Gulrajani et al. (1993)

Disorder	OMIM	US	AFC/AFS	CVS	ELP/ILP	MP	FBS/CHR	Reference
Neuroblastoma, adrenal	256700	US (+)E	—	—	—	—	—	Ferraro et al. (1988)
Neuroblastoma, thoracic	—	US (+)E	—	—	—	—	—	De Filippi et al. (1986)
Neurofibromatosis type I	162200	—	—	—	ILP (+)E	MP (−)	—	Viskochil et al. (1990), Lazaro et al. (1992), Upadhyaya et al. (1992)
Neurofibromatosis type II	101000	—	—	—	—	—	—	Rouleau et al. (1987)
Neuronal ceroid lipofuscinosis (infantile type)	256730	—	—	CVS +	ELP (−)	MP (−)	—	Jarvela et al. (1991), Rapola et al. (1993), Hellsten et al. (1993)
Neuronal ceroid lipofuscinosis (juvenile type, late-onset Batten disease)	204200	—	—	CVS (+)E	ELP (+)E	—	—	Conradi et al. (1989), Gardiner et al. (1990), Uvebrandt et al. (1993)
Neuronal ceroid lipofuscinosis (late infantile type, early-onset Batten disease)	204500	—	—	—	ELP (+)E	—	—	Jarvela et al. (1991)
Niemann–Pick, types A,B	257200	—	AFC +	CVS +	ELP (−)	—	—	Donnai et al. (1981), Vanier et al. (1985)
Niemann–Pick, type C	257220	—	AFS − AFC +	CVS +	ELP (−)	—	—	Vanier et al. (1992), Patterson et al. (1994), Carstea et al. (1993)
Nijmegen breakage syndrome	251260	—	—	—	—	—	CHR (+)E	Jaspers et al. (1990)
Noonan syndrome	163950	US (+)E	—	—	—	—	—	Benacerraf et al. (1989b)
Norrie disease	310600	US (+)E	—	—	—	—	—	Gal et al. (1988), Curtis et al. (1989), Redmond et al. (1993)
Nucleoside phosphorylase deficiency	164050	—	AFC (+)E	CVS (+)E	ELP (+)E ILP (−)	MP (−)	FBS (−)	Linch et al. (1984), Kleijer et al. (1989)
Obstructive uropathy	—	—	AFS (+)E	—	ELP (−)	—	—	Hobbins et al. (1984), Stiller (1989)
Occipital hair	—	US +	—	—	—	—	—	Petrikovsky et al. (1989)
OEIS complex (omphalocele, exstrophy of the bladder, imperforate anus and spinal defects)	—	US (+)E	—	—	—	—	—	Kutzner et al. (1988)
Oesophageal atresia	189960	US (+)R	—	—	—	—	—	Pretorius et al. (1987)
Ohdo syndrome	—	US (+)E	—	—	—	—	—	Ohdo et al. (1987)
Oligodactyly	—	US (+)E	—	—	—	—	—	Russell (1973)

continued on p. 320

319

Disease	MIM	Imaging	Biochemistry	DNA	Other	References
Opitz G syndrome (Opitz BBB syndrome)	145410	US (+)E	—	—	—	Patton et al. (1986), Hogdall et al. (1989)
Oral–facial–digital syndrome type I	311200	US (+)E	—	—	—	Iaccarino et al. (1985)
Ornithinaemia, with gyrate atrophy	258870	—	—	—	—	See Gyrate atrophy
Ornithinine transcarbamylase deficiency	311250	—	—	—	—	See Hyperammonemia I
Oromandibular limb hypogenesis syndrome	—	US (+)E	—	—	—	Shechter et al. (1990)
Orotic aciduria type I	258900	—	—	—	FBS (−)	Suttle et al. (1988)
Osteogenesis imperfecta type I (milder autosomal dominant variant)	166200	US (+)E	—	ILP (+)P	MP (−) MP (+)P	Tsipouras et al. (1987), Pope et al. (1989)
Osteogenesis imperfecta type II (severe congenital form)	166210	US +	CVS (+)E	—	MP (+)P	Constantine et al. (1991), Dimaio et al. (1993)
Osteogenesis imperfecta, other types	259400	US (+)E	—	—	MP (+)P	Carpenter et al. (1986), Robinson et al. (1987), Pope et al. (1989)
Osteopetrosis (milder autosomal dominant variant)	166600	—	—	—	—	Jenkinson et al. (1943), Camera et al. (1989)
	—	Other (+)E	—	—	—	El Khazen et al. (1986), Camera et al. (1989)
Osteopetrosis (severe autosomal recessive variant)	259700	US (+)E	—	—	—	Martini (1952)
Osteopoikilosis	166700	—	—	—	—	
	—	Other (+)E	—	—	—	Cayea et al. (1985)
Otocephaly (synotia)	—	US (+)E	—	—	—	Rizzo et al. (1987), Bagolan et al. (1992)
Ovarian cyst in fetus	—	US (+)E	—	—	—	
Parenti–Fraccaro syndrome	200600	—	—	—	—	See Achondrogensis type IA
Patent urachus	—	US (+)E	—	—	—	Persutte et al. (1988b)
Pelizaeus–Merzbacher disease (myelin protcolipid protein deficiency)	312080	—	—	ILP (+)E	MP (−)	Maenpaa et al. (1990), Bridge et al. (1991), Strautnieks et al. (1992)
Pelvic kidney	—	—	—	ELP (+)E	—	Hill et al. (1994)
Pelvi–ureteric obstruction	143400	US (+)E	—	—	—	See uretero–pelvic junction obstruction
Pena–Shokeir syndrome type I	208150	US (+)E	—	—	—	Ohlsson et al. (1988), Persutte et al. (1988a), Genkins et al. (1989)
Pena–Shokeir syndrome type II	214150	US (+)E	—	—	—	Preus et al. (1977)
Pentalogy of Cantrell	—	US (+)E	—	—	—	Abu-Yousef et al. (1987), Ghidini et al. (1988b)
Pericardial effusion	—	US (+)E	—	—	—	Shenker et al. (1989)
Pericardial tumour	—	US (+)E	—	—	—	Cyr et al. (1988)

Disorder	OMIM	US	AFS/AFC	CVS	ILP	MP	FBS/FLB		References
Peroxisomal 3-oxo-acyl-CoA thiolase deficiency (pseudo-Zellweger syndrome)	261510	—	AFC (+)E	CVS (+)E	—	—	—	—	Schutgens et al. (1989)
Persistent cloaca	—	US (+)E	AFS (+)E	—	—	—	—	—	Holzgreve (1985)
Pfeiffer syndrome (acrocephalosyndactyly type V)	101600	US (+)E	—	—	—	—	—	—	Hill and Grzybek (1994)
Phenylketonuria type I (phenylalanine hydroxylase deficiency)	261600	—	—	—	ILP +	MP (+)P	—	—	Woo et al. (1974), Daiger et al. (1986), Speer et al. (1986), Huang et al. (1990)
Phenylketonuria type II (dihydropteridine reductase deficiency)	261630	—	AFC (+)E	—	ILP (+)E	MP (+)P	—	—	Dahl et al. (1988), Smooker et al. (1993)
Phenylketonuria type III (dihydrobiopterin synthetase deficiency)	261640	—	—	—	—	—	FBS (+)E	—	Firgaira et al. (1983), Niederwieser (1986)
Phenylketonuria with neopterin deficiency	233910	—	AFS (+)E	—	—	—	FLB (−)	—	See GTP cyclohydrolase I deficiency
Phocomelia	223340	US (+)E	—	—	—	—	—	—	Campbell and Pearce (1983)
Phosphoglycerate kinase deficiency	311800	—	—	—	—	MP (−)	—	—	Michelson et al. (1985)
Pierre Robin sequence	261800	US (+)E	—	—	—	—	—	—	Pilu et al. (1986b), Malinger et al. (1987)
Pituitary dysgenesis	262600	AFS (+)E	—	—	—	—	—	—	Stoll et al. (1978)
Placenta, succenturiate lobe	—	US (+)E	—	—	—	—	—	—	Spirt et al. (1987)
Placenta praevia	—	US +	—	—	—	—	—	—	Gottesfeld (1978)
Placental haemangioma	—	US (+)E	—	—	—	—	—	—	Mann et al. (1983)
Placental tumour	—	US (+)E	—	—	—	—	—	—	Kapoor et al. (1989a)
Placentomegaly	—	US +	—	—	—	—	—	—	Quagliarello et al. (1978)
Pleural effusion	—	US (+)E	—	—	—	—	—	—	Bruno et al. (1988), Lien et al. (1990)
Polycystic kidney disease	173900	—	—	—	—	—	—	—	See Infantile polycystic disease and Adult polycystic kidney disease
Polysplenia syndrome	208530	US (+)E	—	—	—	—	—	—	Chitayat et al. (1988a)
Pompe disease	232300	—	—	—	—	—	—	—	See Glycogen storage disease II
Porencephaly	175780	US (+)E	—	—	—	—	—	—	Vintzileos et al. (1987) (see also Schizencephaly)
Porphyria, acute intermittent	176000	—	AFC (+)E	—	ILP (−)	MP (−)	—	—	Sassa et al. (1975), Llewellyn et al. (1987)

continued on p. 322

Disease	MIM	Imaging	Biochemistry	DNA	Other	References
Porphyria, congenital erythropoietic	263700	–	–	MP (–)	–	Nitowsky et al. (1978), Kaiser (1980)
Portal vein aneurysm	–	US (+)E	AFS (+)E	–	–	Gallagher et al. (1993)
Prolidase deficiency (peptidase D deficiency)	170100	–	AFC (–), CVS (–)	–	–	Endo et al. (1990)
Properdin deficiency	312060	–	–	–	–	Goonewardena et al. (1988), Kolble et al. (1993)
Propionic acidaemia (ketotic hyperglycinaemia)	232000	–	AFC +, CVS +	ELP (–)	FBS +	Perez-Cerda et al. (1989), Rolland et al. (1990)
Protein C deficiency	176860	–	AFS +	–	FBS +	Mibashan et al. (1985)
Prune-belly syndrome	100100	US+	–	–	–	Meizner et al. (1985)
Pseudo-Hurler syndrome	252600	–	–	–	–	See Mucolipidosis type III
Pulmonary atresia	178370	US (+)E	–	–	–	Allan et al. (1986)
Pulmonary cyst	–	US (+)E	–	–	–	Lebrun et al. (1985) (see also Bronchogenic cyst)
Pulmonary lymphangiectasia	265300	US (+)E	–	–	–	Wilson et al. (1985)
Pulmonary sequestration	–	US (+)E	–	–	–	Davies et al. (1989)
Pulmonary vein atresia	121000	US (+)E	–	–	–	Samuel et al. (1988)
Pyloric atresia	265950	US (+)E	–	–	–	Peled et al. (1992)
Pyloric stenosis, congenital hypertrophic	179010	US (+)E	–	–	–	Katz et al. (1988)
Pyroglutamic aciduria (glutathione synthetase deficiency)	266130	–	AFC (–), CVS (–)	–	–	Wellner et al. (1974), Erasmus et al. (1993)
Pyropoikilocytosis type II	266140	–	AFS (+)E	–	FBS (+)E	Morris et al. (1986)
Pyruvate carboxylase deficiency	266150	–	AFC +	–	–	Tsuchiyama et al. (1983), Robinson et al. (1985)
Pyruvate dehydrogenase deficiency	208800	–	AFC (–), CVS (–)	–	–	Blass (1980)
Radial aplasia	–	US +	–	–	–	Brons et al. (1990) (see also Holt–Oram syndrome and Thrombocytopenia-absent radius syndrome)
RAG syndrome	–	US (+)E	–	–	–	Saal et al. (1986)
Refsum disease, adult form	266500	–	AFC (–), CVS (–)	–	–	Billimoria et al. (1982)
Refsum disease, infantile form	266510	–	CVS +	–	–	Poll-The et al. (1985), Schutgens et al. (1989)
Renal agenesis (bilateral)	191830	US +	AFS +	–	–	Morse et al. (1987a), Bronshtein et al. (1994)

Condition	OMIM	US	AFC/AFS	CVS	ELP/ILP	MP	FBS	CHR	References
Renal agenesis (unilateral)	—	US +	—	—	—	—	—	—	Jeanty et al. (1990b)
Renal duplication	—	US +	—	—	—	—	—	—	Sherer et al. (1989)
Renal multicystic dysplasia	—	US (+)E	—	—	—	—	—	—	Rizzo et al. (1987), Stiller et al. (1988)
Renal vein thrombosis	—	US (+)E	—	—	—	—	—	—	Patel and Connors (1988)
Retinitis pigmentosa, X-linked types	312600 312610	— —	—	—	ELP (+)E ILP (−)	—	—	—	Wright et al. (1987)
Retinoblastoma	180200	—	—	—	—	MP (−)	—	—	Horsthemke et al. (1987), Mitchell et al. (1988)
Retinoschisis	— 312700	— —	—	—	ELP (−)	—	—	—	Gellert et al. (1988), Sieving et al. (1990)
Rhesus isoimmunization	— —	—	AFS +	—	ELP (−)	—	FBS +	—	—
Roberts syndrome	268300	US (+)E	—	—	—	—	—	CHR (+)R	Romke et al. (1987), Tomkins (1989), Stioui et al. (1992)
Robin anomalad	261800	—	—	—	—	—	—	—	See Pierre Robin sequence
Robinow syndrome	180700	US (+)E	—	—	—	—	—	—	Loverro et al. (1990)
Sacral agenesis	182940	US (+)E	—	—	—	—	—	—	Fellous et al. (1982), Sonek et al. (1990)
Sacrococcygeal teratoma	—	US +	—	—	—	—	—	—	Chervenak et al. (1985), Holzgreve et al. (1985), Gross et al. (1987)
Saldino–Noonan syndrome	263530	—	—	—	—	—	—	—	See Short rib-polydactyly syndrome type I
Salla disease	268740	—	AFC +	CVS (+)E	—	—	—	—	Renlund and Aula (1987)
Sandhoff disease	268800	—	—	—	—	—	—	—	See Gangliosidosis, GM_2 type II
Scheie syndrome	252800	—	—	—	—	—	—	—	See Mucopolysaccharidosis type IS
Schilder disease	300100	—	—	—	—	—	—	—	See Adrenoleucodystrophy
Schindler disease	104170	—	—	—	—	—	—	—	See Acetylgalactosaminidase deficiency
Schinzel–Giedion mid-face retraction, syndrome	269150	US (+)E	—	—	—	—	—	—	Labrune et al. (1994)
Schizencephaly	269250	US (+)E	—	—	—	—	—	—	Lituania et al. (1989), Kormarniski et al. (1990)
Schneckenbecken dysplasia	— 269250	Other (+)E US (+)E	—	—	—	—	—	—	Laxova et al. (1973), Borochowitz et al. (1986)
Schwartz–Jampel syndrome	255800	US (+)E	—	—	—	—	—	—	Hunziker et al. (1989)
Scoliosis	181800	US (+)E	—	—	—	—	—	—	Henry and Norton (1987) (see also Jarcho–Levin syndrome)

continued on p. 324

Disease	MIM	Imaging	Biochemistry	DNA	Other	References
Seckel syndrome	210600	US (+)E	–	–	–	De Elejalde and Elejalde (1984)
Seizures	–	US (+)E	–	–	–	Landy et al. (1989) (see also Convulsions, benign familial neonatal)
Seminal vesicular cyst	–	US (+)E	–	–	–	Hammadeh et al. (1994)
Short chain acyl-CoA dehydrogenase deficiency	201470	–	AFC (–)	CVS (–)	MP (–)	Naito et al. (1989)
Short rib syndrome, Beemer type	269860	US (+)E	–	–	–	Balci et al. (1991), Lungarotti et al. (1993)
Short rib-polydactyly syndrome type I (Saldino–Noonan syndrome)	263530	US (+)E	–	–	–	Meizner and Bar-Ziv (1989)
Short rib-polydactyly syndrome type II (Majewski syndrome)	263520	Other (+)E, US (+)E	–	–	–	Gembruch et al. (1985), Meizner and Bar-Ziv (1985), Benacerraf (1993)
Short rib-polydactyly syndrome type III (Spranger–Verma)	263510	Other (+)E, US (+)E	–	–	–	Verma et al. (1975), De Sierra et al. (1992)
Short rib-polydactyly syndrome type IV (Piepkorn)	–	US (+)E	–	–	–	Piepkorn et al. (1977)
Sialic acid storage disease	269920	–	AFC +, AFS +	CVS +	–	Lake et al. (1989), Vamos et al. (1986)
Sialidosis	252400	–	–	–	–	See Mucolipidosis type I
Sickle cell disease	142300	–	–	–	–	See Haemoglobin S
Simian crease	–	US (+)E	–	–	–	Jeanty et al. (1990) (see also Trisomy 21)
Single umbilical artery	–	US +	–	–	–	Spirt et al. (1987), Jauniaux et al. (1989)
Single ventricle	121000	–	–	–	–	See Univentricular heart
Sirenomelia	–	US (+)E	–	–	–	Fitzmorris-Glass (1989), Sirtori et al. (1989)
Situs inversus	270100	US (+)E	–	–	–	Stoker et al. (1983)
Sjögren–Larsen syndrome	270200	–	AFC (+)E	CVS (+)E	–	Kouseff et al. (1982), Trepeta et al. (1984), Tabsh et al. (1993)
Skull deformation	–	US (+)E	–	–	FSKB (+)E	Romero et al. (1981)
Skull fracture	–	–	–	–	–	Alexander and Davis (1969), McRae et al. (1982)
Sly syndrome	253220	Other (+)E	–	–	–	See Mucopolysaccharidosis VII

continued on p. 326

Disorder	McKusick No.	US	Other	AFS	AFC	ELP	MP	ILP	FBS	References
Smith–Lemli–Opitz syndrome	270400	US (+)E		AFS (+)E						Curry et al. (1987), Irons et al. (1994), Persutte and Hobbins (1994), Johnson et al. (1993)
Spherocytosis	182900		Other (+)E				MP (–)			Lux et al. (1990)
Spina bifida	182940	US +								Nicolaides et al. (1986), Chambers et al. (1989), Van den Hof et al. (1990)
Spinal and bulbar muscular atrophy (Kennedy disease)	313200			AFS (+)R			MP (–)			Fischbeck et al. (1986)
Spinal muscular atrophy type I (Werdnig–Hoffmann disease)	253300					ELP (–)				Melki et al. (1992), Cobben et al. (1994)
Spinal muscular atrophy type II	253550					ELP (+)E				Gilliam et al. (1990)
Spinal muscular atrophy type III (Kugelberg–Welander disease)	253400					ELP (–)				Gilliam et al. (1990)
Splenic cyst		US (+)E								Lichman and Miller (1988)
Spondyloepiphyseal dysplasia congenita	183900	US (+)E				ELP (–)				Donnenfeld and Mennuti (1987), Kirk and Comstock (1990)
Spondylothoracic dysplasia	277300	US (+)E								Marks et al. (1989), see also Jarcho–Levin syndrome
Steroid sulphatase deficiency	308100									See Ichthyosis, X-linked
Stickler syndrome (hereditary progressive arthroophthalmopathy)	108300							ILP (+)P		Zlotogora et al. (1994)
Stomach duplication		US (+)E								Bidwell and Nelson (1986)
Subdural haematoma										See Intracranial haemorrhage
Subdural hygroma		US (+)E								Ghidini et al. (1988a)
Succinic semialdehyde dehydrogenase deficiency	271980				AFC (+)E				FBS (–)	Thorburn et al. (1993), Jakobs et al. (1993)
Supraventricular tachycardia		US (+)E		AFS (+)E						Wiggins et al. (1986), Buiss-Liem et al. (1987)
Takahara disease	115500		Other +							See Acatalasia
Talipes	119800	US (+)E								Bronshtein and Zimmer (1989)
Tangier disease (familial high density lipoprotein deficiency)	205400				AFC (–)					Gebhardt (1979)

Disease	MIM	Imaging	Biochemistry	DNA	Other	References
Tay–Sachs disease	272800	−	−	−	−	See Gangliosidosis GM$_2$, type I
Tay–Sachs variant	272750	−	−	−	−	See Gangliosidosis
Testicular feminization	313700	−	−	−	−	See Androgen insensitivity syndrome
Testicular torsion	−	US (+)E	−	−	−	Hubbard et al. (1984)
Tetralogy of Fallot	185700	US (+)E	−	−	−	Allan et al. (1985)
Thalassaemia, alpha	141800	−	−	ILP +	MP (+)P, FBS +	Zeng and Huang (1985), Wang et al. (1986), Kazazian (1990)
Thalassaemia, beta	141900	−	−	ELP +, ILP +	MP (+)P, FBS +	Cao et al. (1986), Camaschella et al. (1988), Ristaldi et al. (1989), Old et al. (1990), Kazazian (1990)
Thalidomide embryopathy	−	US (+)E	−	ELP +	−	Gollop et al. (1987)
Thanatophoric dysplasia	187600	US (+)E	−	−	−	Pretorius et al. (1986)
Thanatophoric dysplasia with cloverleaf skull	273670	US (+)E	−	−	−	Weiner et al. (1986), Machin and Corsello (1992)
Thoracic dysplasia – hydrocephalus syndrome	273730	US (+)E	−	−	−	Winter et al. (1987)
Thoracic gastroenteric cyst	−	US (+)E	−	−	−	Newnham et al. (1984), Albright et al. (1988)
Thoracoabdominal eventration	−	US (+)E	−	−	−	Seeds et al. (1984)
Thrombocytopenia, neonatal alloimmune	−	−	−	−	FBS +	McFarland et al. (1991)
Thrombocytopenia–absent radius syndrome (TAR syndrome)	274000	US (+)E	−	−	Other (+)E, FBS (+)E	Luthy et al. (1981), Filkins et al. (1984), Donnenfeld et al. (1990)
Thyrotoxicosis (hyperthyroidism)	275000	Other (+)E	AFS (+)E	−	−	Pekonen et al. (1984) (see also Goitre)
Tibial hemimelia	275210	US (+)E	−	−	−	Ramirez et al. (1994)
Tight skin contracture syndrome	189960	−	−	−	FSKB (−)	Hamel et al. (1992)
Tracheo-oesophageal fistula	−	−	−	−	−	See Oesophageal atresia
Transcobalamin II deficiency	275350	−	AFC (−)	−	−	Mayes et al. (1987), Rosenblatt et al. (1987)
Treacher Collins syndrome	154500	−	−	−	−	See Mandibulofacial dysostosis
Tricuspid atresia	121000	US (+)E	−	−	−	De Vore et al. (1987)
Tricuspid incompetence	121000	US (+)E	−	−	−	Brown et al. (1986)
Triose phosphate isomerase deficiency	190450	−	AFC +, CVS +	−	FBS (+)E	Rosa et al. (1986), Dallapiccola et al. (1987), Bellingham et al. (1989)
Triploidy	−	US (+)R	−	−	CHR +	Pircon et al. (1989)
Trisomy 13	−	US (+)R	−	−	CHR +	Benacerraf et al. (1986b)

Condition	No.	US	AFC	AFS	CVS	ELP	MP	CHR	Other	References
Trisomy 18	—	US (+)R	—	—	—	—	—	CHR +	—	Benacerraf et al. (1986b), Bundy et al. (1986)
Trisomy 21	—	US (+)R	—	—	—	—	—	CHR +	—	Benacerraf and Frigoletto (1987), Toi et al. (1987), Nyberg et al. (1990b)
Truncus arteriosus	121000	US (+)E	—	—	—	—	—	—	—	Allan et al. (1985)
Tuberous sclerosis	191100	US (+)E	—	—	—	—	—	—	—	Connor et al. (1987), Chitayat et al. (1988b)
Twin-embolization syndrome	—	US (+)E	—	—	—	ELP (+)P	—	—	—	Patten et al. (1989)
Twin–twin transfusion syndrome	—	—	—	—	—	—	MP (−)P	—	—	See Fetofetal transfusion syndrome
Twins, zygosity	—	—	—	—	—	—	—	—	—	See Multiple pregnancy
Tyrosinaemia, type 1	276700	—	AFC +	AFS +	CVS +	—	—	—	—	Gagne et al. (1982), Kvittingen et al. (1986), Jakobs et al. (1990)
Uhl anomaly	107900	US (+)E	—	—	—	—	—	—	—	Wager et al. (1988)
Umbilical artery aneurysm	—	US (+)E	—	—	—	—	—	—	—	Sidiqi et al. (1992)
Umbilical cord, vesicoallantoic defect	—	US (+)E	—	—	—	—	—	—	—	Donnenfeld et al. (1989)
Umbilical cord angiomyxoma	—	US (+)E	—	—	—	—	—	—	—	Jauniaux et al. (1989)
Umbilical cord cyst	—	US (+)E	—	—	—	—	—	—	—	Rempen (1989)
Umbilical cord elongated	—	US (+)E	—	—	—	—	—	—	—	Collins (1991)
Umbilical cord haemangioma	—	US (+)E	—	—	—	—	—	—	—	Ghidini et al. (1990)
Umbilical cord haematoma	—	US (+)E	—	—	—	—	—	—	—	Sutro et al. (1984)
Umbilical cord thrombosis	—	US (+)E	—	—	—	—	—	—	—	Abrams et al. (1985)
Umbilical vein ectasia	—	US (+)E	—	—	—	—	—	—	—	Vesce et al. (1987)
Univentricular heart	121000	US +	—	—	—	—	—	—	—	Allan et al. (1985)
Urachal cysts	—	US (+)E	—	—	—	—	—	—	—	Hill et al. (1990)
Ureterocele	191650	US (+)E	—	—	—	—	—	—	—	Fitzsimons et al. (1986)
Ureteropelvic junction obstruction	143400	US +	—	—	—	—	—	—	—	Hobbins et al. (1984), Grignon et al. (1986b), Kleiner et al. (1987), Corteville et al. (1991)
Urethral atresia	—	US +	—	—	—	—	—	—	—	Hill et al. (1985), Hayden et al. (1988)
Urethral valves	—	US (+)R	—	—	—	—	—	—	—	Hill et al. (1985), Hayden et al. (1988)
Uterovesical junction obstruction	—	US (+)E	—	—	—	—	—	—	—	Hobbins et al. (1984)
VATER syndrome	192350	US (+)E	—	—	—	—	—	—	—	Claiborne et al. (1986), McGahan et al. (1988)
Ventricular arrhythmia	—	US (+)E	—	—	—	—	—	—	Other +	Lingman et al. (1986)

continued on p. 328

Disease	MIM	Imaging	Biochemistry	DNA	Other	References
Ventricular septal defect	121000	US (+)E	–	–	–	Allan et al. (1985)
Vesicoallantoic abdominal wall defect	–	–	–	–	–	See Umbilical cord, vesicoallantoic defect
Vitamin D-dependent rickets type II	277420	–	AFC (+)E	–	–	Weisman et al. (1990)
von Gierke disease	232200	–	–	–	–	See Glycogen storage disease 1A
von Hippel–Lindau disease	193300	–	–	ELP (–), MP (–)	–	Seizinger et al. (1988)
von Willebrand disease	193400	–	–	ILP (+)E, MP (–)	FBS +	Shelton-Inloes et al. (1987), Bignell et al. (1990)
Walker–Warburg syndrome	236670	US (+)E	–	ELP (–)	–	Vohra et al. (1993)
Weyers syndrome	193530	US (+)E	–	–	–	Elejalde et al. (1983)
Wiedemann–Rautenstrauch syndrome	264090	US (+)E	–	–	–	Castineyra et al. (1992)
Wiskott–Aldrich syndrome	301000	–	–	ELP (+)E	FBS (+)R	Holmberg et al. (1983), Schwartz et al. (1989), Lorenz et al. (1991)
Wilson disease	277900	–	–	ELP (+)E	–	Cossu et al. (1992)
Wolffian duct cyst	–	US (+)E	–	ELP (+)E	–	Kapoor et al. (1989b)
Wolff–Parkinson–White syndrome	194200	Other +	–	–	–	Wiggins et al. (1986)
Wolman disease	278000	–	–	–	–	See Cholesterol ester storage disease
Xanthine oxidase deficiency (xanthinuria)	278300	–	AFC +, CVS +	–	–	Desjacques et al. (1985)
Xeroderma pigmentosum I	278700	–	AFC +, CVS +	–	FBS (–), CHR (+)E	Halley et al. (1979), Arase et al. (1985), Savary et al. (1991)
Xeroderma pigmentosum IV (Trichothiodystrophy with sun sensitivity)	278730	–	CVS (+)E	–	FSKB (+)E	Sarasin et al. (1992)
Zellweger syndrome	214100	–	–	–	–	See Cerebrohepatorenal syndrome
Zellweger-like syndrome	214110	–	AFC (–), CVS (–)	–	–	Schutgens et al. (1989)

REFERENCES

Abbitt, P.L. and McIhenny, J. (1990) Prenatal detection of gallstones. *Journal of Clinical Ultrasound*, 18, 202–204.

Abbott, J.F., Davis, G.H., Endocitt, B., Pfleghaar, K. and Wapner, R.J. (1992) Prenatal diagnosis of vestigial tail. *Journal of Ultrasound in Medicine*, 11, 53–55.

Abrams, S.L., Callen, P.W. and Filly, R.A. (1985) Umbilical vein thrombosis: sonographic detection *in utero*. *Journal of Ultrasound in Medicine*, 4, 283–85.

Abrams, S.L. and Filly, R.A. (1985) Congenital vertebral malformations: prenatal diagnosis using ultrasonography. *Radiology*, 155, 762.

Abu-Yousef, M.M., Wray, A.B., Williamson, R.A. and Bonsib, S.M. (1987) Antenatal ultrasound diagnosis of variant of pentalogy of Cantrell. *Journal of Ultrasound in Medicine*, 6, 535–38.

Achiron, R., Malinger, G., Zaidel, L. and Zakut, H. (1988) Prenatal sonographic diagnosis of endocardial fibroelastosis secondary to aortic stenosis. *Prenatal Diagnosis*, 8, 73–77.

Adam, A.H., Robinson, H.P., Pont, M. *et al.* (1979) Prenatal diagnosis of fetal lymphatic system abnormalities by ultrasound. *Journal of Clinical Ultrasound*, 7, 361–64.

Albright, E.B., Crane, J.P. and Shackelford, G.D. (1988) Prenatal diagnosis of a bronchogenic cyst. *Journal of Ultrasound in Medicine*, 7, 91–95.

Alexander, E. Jr and Davis, C.H. (1969) Intrauterine fracture of the infant's skull. *Journal of Neurosurgery*, 30, 446–54.

Allan, L.D. (1987) Prenatal diagnosis of congenital heart disease. *Hospital Update*, 13, 553–60.

Allan, L.D., Crawford, D.C., Handerson, R. and Tynan, M. (1985) Spectrum of congenital heart disease detected echocardiographically in prenatal life. *British Heart Journal*, 54, 523–26.

Allan, L.D., Crawford, D.C. and Tynan, M.J. (1986) Pulmonary atresia in prenatal life. *Journal of the American College of Cardiology*, 8, 1131–36.

Allan, L.D., Desai, G. and Tynan, M.J. (1982) Prenatal echocardiographic screening for Ebstein's anomaly for mothers on lithium therapy. *Lancet*, ii, 875–76.

Almeida, M.R., Alves, I.L., Sakaki, Y. *et al.* (1990) Prenatal diagnosis of familial amyloidotic polyneuropathy: evidence for an early expression of the associated transthyretin methionine 30. *Human Genetics*, 85, 623–26.

Alter, B.P. (1984) Advances in the prenatal diagnosis of hematologic diseases. *Blood*, 64, 329–40.

Ambrosino, M.M. Hernanz-Schulman, M., Horii, S.C. *et al.* (1990) Prenatal diagnosis of nephroblastomatosis in two siblings. *Journal of Ultrasound in Medicine*, 9, 49–51.

Ampola, M.G., Mahoney, M.J., Nakamura, E. and Tanaka, K. (1975) Prenatal therapy of a patient with vitamin B_{12} responsive methylmalonic acidemia. *New England Journal of Medicine*, 293, 313–17.

Andersen, Jr P.E., Hauge, M. and Bang, J. (1988) Dyssegmental dysplasia in siblings: prenatal ultrasonic diagnosis. *Skeletal Radiology*, 17, 29–31.

Anderson, N., Malpas, T. and Robertson, R. (1993) Prenatal diagnosis of colon atresia. *Pediatric Radiology*, 23, 63–64.

Anneren, G., Andersson, T., Lindgren, P.G. and Kjartansson, S. (1991) Ectodactyly–ectodermal dysplasia–clefting syndrome (EEC), the clinical variation and prenatal diagnosis. *Clinical Genetics*, 40, 257–62.

Anton-Lamprecht, I. (1981) Prenatal diagnosis of genetic disorders of the skin by means of electron microscopy. *Human Genetics*, 59, 392–405.

Anton-Lamprecht, I., Rauskolb, R., Jovanovic, V. *et al.* (1981) Prenatal diagnosis of epidermolysis bullosa dystrophica Hallopeau-Siemens with electron microscopy of fetal skin. *Lancet*, ii, 1077–79.

Anyane-Yeboa, K., Kasznila, J., Malin, J. and Maidman, J. (1987) Herrmann–Optiz syndrome: report of an affected fetus. *American Journal of Medical Genetics*, 27, 467–70.

Aparicio, L., Carpenter, M.W., Schwartz, R. and Gruppuso, P.A. (1993) Prenatal diagnosis of familial neonatal hyperinsulinemia. *Acta Paediatrica, International Journal of Paediatrics*, 82, 683–86.

Apuzzio, J.J., Diamond, N., Ganesh, V. and Desposito, F. (1987) Difficulties in the prenatal diagnosis of Jarcho–Levin syndrome. *American Journal of Obstetrics and Gynecology*, 156, 916–18.

Apuzzio, J.J., Ganesh, V.V., Chervenak, J. and Sama, J.C. (1988) Prenatal diagnosis of dicephalous conjoined twins in a triplet pregnancy. *American Journal of Obstetrics and Gynecology*, 159, 1214–15.

Apuzzio, J.J., Unwin, W., Adhate, A. and Nichols, R. (1986) Prenatal diagnosis of fetal renal mesoblastic nephroma. *American Journal of Obstetrics and Gynecology*, 154, 636–37.

Arase, S., Bohnert, E., Fischer, E. and Jung, E.G. (1985) Prenatal exclusion of xeroderma pigmentosum (XP-D) by amniotic cell analysis. *Photodermatology*, 2, 181–83.

Argubright, K.F. and Wicks, J.D. (1987) Third trimester ultrasonic presentation of infantile polycystic kidney disease. *American Journal of Perinatology*, 4, 1–4.

Arnold, M.L., Rauskolb, R., Anton-Lamprecht, I. *et al.* (1984) Prenatal diagnosis of anhidrotic ectodermal dysplasia. *Prenatal Diagnosis*, 4, 85–98.

Auerbach, A.D., Min, Z., Ghosh, R. *et al.* (1986) Clastogen-induced chromosomal breakage as a marker for first trimester prenatal diagnosis of Fanconi anaemia. *Human Genetics*, 73, 86–88.

Aula, P., Mattila, K., Püroinen, O. *et al.* (1989) First-trimester prenatal diagnosis of aspartylglucosaminuria. *Prenatal Diagnosis*, 9, 617–20.

Bachmann, C., Krahenbuhl, S., Colombo, J.P. *et al.* (1981) N-Acetylglutamate synthetase deficiency: a disorder of ammonia detoxification. *New England Journal of Medicine*, 304, 543.

Bagolan, P., Rivosecchi M., Giorlandino C. *et al.* (1992) Prenatal diagnosis and clinical outcome of ovarian cysts. *Journal of Pediatric Surgery*, 27, 879–81.

Bailey, W., Freidenberg, G.R., James, H.E. *et al.* (1990) Prenatal diagnosis of a craniopharyngioma using ultrasonography and magnetic resonance imaging. *Prenatal Diagnosis*, 10, 623–29.

Bair, J.H., Russ, P.D., Pretorius, D.H. *et al.* (1986) Fetal omphalocele and gastroschisis: a review of 24 cases. *American Journal Roentgenology*, 147, 1047–1051.

Bakharev, V.A., Aivazyan, A.A., Karetnikova, N.A. *et al.* (1990) Fetal skin biopsy in prenatal diagnosis of some genodermatoses. *Prenatal Diagnosis*, **10**, 1–12.

Bakker, E., Bonten, E.J., Veenema, H. *et al.* (1989) Prenatal diagnosis of Duchenne muscular dystrophy: a three-year experience in a rapidly evolving field. *Journal of Inherited Metabolic Disease*, **12** (suppl. 1), 174–90.

Balci, S., Ercal, M.D., Onol, B. *et al.* (1991) Familial short rib syndrome, type Beemer, with pyloric stenosis and short intestine, one case diagnosed prenatally. *Clinical Genetics*, **39**, 298–303.

Bale, S.J., Bale, A.E., Stewart, K. *et al.* (1989) Linkage analysis of multiple endocrine neoplasia type I with INT2 and other markers on chromosome 11. *Genomics*, **4**, 320–22.

Ballabio, A., Carroxxo, R., Parenti, G. *et al.* (1989) Molecular heterogeneity of steroid sulfatase deficiency: a multicentre study on 57 unrelated patients at DNA and protein levels. *Genomics*, **4**, 36–40.

Bancroft, J.D., Bucuvalas, J.C., Ryckman, F.C., Dudgeon, D.L., Saunders, R.C. and Schwarz, K.B. (1994) Antenatal diagnosis of choledochal cyst. *Journal of Pediatric Gastroenterology and Nutrition*, **18**, 142–45.

Barker, D.F., Hostikka, S.L., Zhou, J. *et al.* (1990) Identification of mutations in the COL4A5 collagen gene in Alport syndrome. *Science*, **248**, 1224–27.

Barr, J.T.M., Heidelberger, K.P. and Dorovini-Zis, K. (1986) Scalp neoplasm associated with cranium bifidum in a 24-week human fetus. *Teratology*, **33**, 153–57.

Barss, V.A., Benacerraf, B.R. and Frigoletto, F.D. (1985) Antenatal sonographic diagnosis of fetal gastrointestinal malformations. *Pediatrics*, **76**, 445–49.

Barth, R.A., Filly, R.A. and Sondheimer, F.K. (1990) Prenatal sonographic findings in bladder exstrophy. *Journal of Ultrasound in Medicine*, **9**, 359–61.

Bartley, J.A. and Gies, C.M. (1990) Prenatal diagnosis in X-linked myotubular myopathy (MTM1) with linkage to DXS52. *American Journal of Human Genetics*, **47**, A268.

Bass, H.N., Oliver, J.B., Srinivasan, M. *et al.* (1986) Persistently elevated AFP and AChE in amniotic fluid from a normal fetus following demise of its twin. *Prenatal Diagnosis*, **6**, 33–35.

Baty, B.J., Cubberley, D., Marris, C. and Carey, J. (1988) Prenatal diagnosis of distal arthrogryposis. *American Journal of Medical Genetics*, **29**, 501–10.

Baxi, L., Warren, W., Collins, M.H. and Timor-Tritsch, I.E. (1990) Early detection of caudal regression syndrome with transvaginal scanning. *Obstetrics and Gynecology*, **75**, 486–89.

Bellingham, A.J., Lestas, A.N., Williams, L.H.P. and Nicolaides, K.H. (1989) Prenatal diagnosis of a red cell enzymopathy: triose phosphate isomerase deficiency. *Lancet*, **ii**, 419–21.

Benacerraf, B.R. (1993) Prenatal sonographic diagnosis of short rib polydactyly syndrome type II, Majewski type. *Journal of Ultrasound in Medicine*, **12**, 552–55.

Benacerraf, B.R. and Birnholz, J.C. (1987) The diagnosis of fetal hydrocephalus prior to 22 weeks. *Journal of Clinical Ultrasound*, **15**, 531–36.

Benacerraf, B.R. and Frigoletto, F.D. (1987) Soft tissue nuchal fold in the second-trimester fetus: standards for normal measurements compared with those in Down syndrome. *American Journal of Obstetrics and Gynecology*, **157**, 1146–49.

Benacerraf, B.R. and Frigoletto, F.D. (1988) Prenatal ultra-

sonographic recognition of Goldenhar's syndrome. *American Journal of Obstetrics and Gynecology*, **159**, 950–52.

Benacerraf, B.R., Frigoletto, F.D. and Greene, M.F. (1986b) Abnormal facial features and extremities in human trisomy syndromes: prenatal UK appearance. *Radiology*, **159**, 243–46.

Benacerraf, B.R., Greene, M.F. and Barss, V.A. (1986a) Prenatal sonographic diagnosis of congenital hemivertebra. *Journal of Ultrasound in Medicine*, **5**, 257–59.

Benacerraf, B.R., Greene, M.F. and Holmes, L.B. (1989b) The prenatal sonographic features of Noonan's syndrome. *Journal of Ultrasound in Medicine*, **8**, 59–63.

Benacerraf, B.R., Osathanondh, R. and Bieber, F.R. (1984) Achondrogenesis type I: ultrasound diagnosis *in utero*. *Journal of Clinical Ultrasound*, **12**, 357–59.

Benacerraf, B.R., Saltzman, D.H. and Sanders, S.P. (1989a) Sonographic sign suggesting the prenatal diagnosis of co-arctation of the aorta. *Journal of Ultrasound in Medicine*, **8**, 65–69.

Ben-Ami, A., Shalev, F., Romano, S. and Zuckerman, H. (1986) Mid-trimester diagnosis of endocardial fibroelastosis and atrial septal defect: a case report. *American Journal of Obstetrics and Gynecology*, **155**, 662–63.

Bennett, M.J., Allison, F. and Lowther, G.W. (1987) Prenatal diagnosis of medium-chain acyl coenzyme A dehydrogenase deficiency. *Prenatal Diagnosis*, **7**, 135–41.

Benson, C.B., Pober, B.R., Hirsh, M.P. and Doubilet, P.M. (1988) Sonography of Nager acrofacial dysostosis syndrome *in utero*. *Journal of Ultrasound in Medicine*, **7**, 163–67.

Benson, P.F. and Fensom, A.H. (1985) *Genetic Biochemical Disorders*, Oxford University Press, Oxford, p. 351.

Ben-Yoseph, Y., Mitchell, D.A. and Nadler, H.I. (1988) First trimester prenatal evaluation for I-cell disease by N-acetyl-glucosamine 1-phosphotransferase assay. *Clinical Genetics*, **33**, 38–43.

Benzie, R.J., Ray, P., Thompson, D., Hunter, A.G.W., Ivey, B. and Salvador, L. (1994) Prenatal exclusion of Duchenne muscular dystrophy by fetal muscle biopsy. *Prenatal Diagnosis*, **14**, 235–38.

Berkvens, T.M., Gerritsen, E.J.A., Oldenburg, M. *et al.* (1987) Severe combined immune deficiency due to a homozygous 3.2 kb deletion spanning the promoter and first axon of the adenosine deaminase gene. *Nucleic Acids Research*, **15**, 9365–78.

Besley, G.T.N., Ferguson-Smith, M.E., Frew, C. *et al.* (1988) First trimester diagnosis of Gaucher disease in a fetus with trisomy 21. *Prenatal Diagnosis*, **8**, 471–74.

Biancalana, V., Briard, M.L., David, A. *et al.* (1992) Confirmation and refinement of the genetic localisation of the Coffin-Lowry syndrome locus in Xp22, 1-p22.2. *American Journal of Human Genetics*, **50**, 981–87.

Bick, D.P., Balkite, E.A., Baumgarten, A. *et al.* (1987) The association of congenital skin disorders with acetylcholinesterase in amniotic fluid. *Prenatal Diagnosis*, **7**, 543–49.

Bidwell, J.K. and Nelson, A. (1986) Prenatal ultrasonic diagnosis of congenital duplication of the stomach. *Journal of Ultrasound in Medicine*, **5**, 589–91.

Bignell, P., Standen, G.R., Bowen, D.J. *et al.* (1990) Rapid neonatal diagnosis of von Willebrand's disease by use of the polymerase chain reaction. *Lancet*, **ii**, 638–39.

Billimoria, J.D., Clemens, M.E., Gibberd, F.B. and Whitelaw,

M.N. (1982) Metabolism of phytanic acid in Retsum's disease. *Lancet*, i, 194–96.

Blaakaer, J. (1986) Ultrasonic diagnosis of fetal ascites and toxoplasmosis. *Acta Obstetricia et Gynecologica Scandinavica*, 65, 633–38.

Blagowidow, N., Mennuti, M.T., Huff, D.S. et al. (1986) A possible X-linked lethal disorder characterised by brain, eye and urogenital malformations. *American Journal of Human Genetics*, 39, A53.

Blanchet-Bardon, C. and Dumez, Y. (1984) Prenatal diagnosis of harlequin fetus. *Journal of Dermatology*, 3, 225–28.

Blass, J.P. (1980) Pyruvate dehydrogenase deficiencies. In *Inherited Disorders of Carbohydrate Metabolism*, (eds D. Burman et al.) MTP Press, Lancaster, p. 293.

Blumenfeld, A., Slaugenhaupt, S.A., Axelrod, F.B. et al. (1993) Localization of the gene for familial dysautonomia on chromosome 9 and definition of DNA markers for genetic diagnosis. *Nature Genetics*, 4, 160–64.

Bock, S.C. and Prochownik, E.V. (1987) Molecular genetic survey of 16 kindreds with hereditary antithrombin III deficiency. *Blood*, 70, 1273–78.

Bodmer, W.F., Bailey, C.J., Bodmer, J. et al. (1987) Localisation of the gene for familial adenomatous polyposis on chromosome 5. *Nature*, 328, 614–16.

Boomsa, J.H., Weemhoff, R.A. and Polman, H.A. (1982) Sonographic appearance of annular pancreas *in utero*: a case report. *Diagnostic Imaging*, 51, 288–90.

Borochowitz, Z., Jones, K.L., Silbey, R. et al. (1986) A distinct lethal neonatal chondrodysplasia with snail-like pelvis: Schneckenbecken dysplasia. *American Journal of Medical Genetics*, 25, 47–59.

Borresen, A.L., Hellerud, C., Moller, P. et al. (1987) Prenatal diagnosis of a glycerol kinase deficiency associated with a DNA deletion of the short arm of the X-chromosome. *Clinical Genetics*, 32, 254–59.

Boucher, M. and Yonekura, M.L. (1986) Perinatal listeriosis (early-onset): correlation of antenatal investigations and neonatal outcome. *Obstetrics and Gynecology*, 68, 593–97.

Boue, J., Oberle, I., Heilig, R. et al. (1985) First trimester prenatal diagnosis of adrenoleucodystrophy by determination of very long chain fatty acid levels and by linkage to a DNA probe. *Human Genetics*, 69, 253–54.

Boulot, P., Ferran, J.L., Charlier, C. et al. (1993) Prenatal diagnosis of diastematomyelia. *Pediatric Radiology*, 23, 67–68.

Bourgeron, T., Chretien, D., Rotig, A., Munnich, A. and Rustin, P. (1992) Prenatal diagnosis of cytochrome c oxidase deficiency in cultured amniocytes is hazardous. *Prenatal Diagnosis*, 12, 535–49.

Bovicelli, L., Rizzo, N., Orsini, L.F. and Calderoni, P. (1981) Ultrasonographic real-time diagnosis of fetal hydrothorax and lung hypoplasia. *Journal of Clinical Ultrasound*, 9, 253–54.

Braunstein, G.D., Ziel, F.H., Allen, A. et al. (1976) Prenatal diagnosis of placental steroid sulfatase deficiency. *American Journal of Obstetrics and Gynecology*, 126, 716–19.

Brennan, J.N., Diwan, R.J., Rosen, M.G. and Bellon, E.M. (1982) Fetofetal transfusion syndrome: a prenatal ultrasonographic diagnosis. *Radiology*, 143, 535–36.

Bridge, P.J., MacLeod, P.M. and Lillicrap, D.P. (1991) Carrier

detection and prenatal diagnosis of Pelizaeus–Merzbacher disease using a combination of anonymous DNA polymorphisms and the proteolipid protein (PLP) gene cDNA. *American Journal of Medical Genetics*, 38, 616–21.

Brocard, O., Ragage, C., Vibert, M., Cassier, T. Kowalski, S. and Ragage J.P. (1993) Prenatal diagnosis of X-linked hydrocephalus. *Journal of Clinical Ultrasound*, 21, 211–14.

Brock, D.J.H. and Barron, L. (1991) First-trimester prenatal diagnosis of hypophosphatasia: experience with 16 cases. *Prenatal Diagnosis*, 11, 387–92.

Brock, D.J.H., Clarke, H.A.K. and Barron, L. (1988) Prenatal diagnosis of cystic fibrosis by microvillar enzyme assay on a sequence of 258 pregnancies. *Human Genetics*, 78, 271–75.

Brocker-Vriends, A.H.J.T., Briet, E. et al. (1988) First trimester prenatal diagnosis of haemophilia A: two years' experience. *Prenatal Diagnosis*, 8, 411–21.

Brons, J.T.J., Van der Harten, H.J., van Geijn, H.P. et al. (1990) Prenatal ultrasonographic diagnosis of radial ray reduction malformations. *Prenatal Diagnosis*, 10, 279–88.

Brons, J.T.J., van Geijn, H.P., Wladimiroff, J.W. et al. (1988) Prenatal ultrasound diagnosis of the Holt–Oram syndrome. *Prenatal Diagnosis*, 8, 175–82.

Bronshtein, M. and Gershoni-Baruch, R. (1993) Prenatal transvaginal diagnosis of the ectrodactyly, ectodermal dysplasia, cleft palate (EEC) syndrome. *Prenatal Diagnosis*, 13, 519–22.

Bronshtein, M., Amit, A., Achiron, R., Noyi, I. and Blumenfeld, Z. (1994) The early prenatal sonographic diagnosis of renal agenesis: Techniques and possible pitfalls. *Prenatal Diagnosis*, 14, 291–97.

Bronshtein, M., Weiner, Z., Abramovici, H., Filmar, S., Erlik, Y. and Blumenfeld, Z. (1993) Prenatal diagnosis of gall bladder anomalies — Report of 17 cases. *Prenatal Diagnosis*, 13, 851–61.

Bronshtein, M. and Zimmer, E.Z. (1989) Transvaginal ultrasound diagnosis of fetal club feet at 13 weeks menstrual age. 17, 518–20.

Brown, B.I. and Brown, D.H. (1989) Branching enzyme activity of cultured aminocytes and chorionic villi: prenatal testing for type IV glycogen storage disease. *American Journal of Human Genetics*, 44, 378–81.

Brown, D.L., Emerson, D.S., Shulman, L.P. and Carson, S.A. (1989) Sonographic diagnosis of omphalocele during 10th week of gestation. 153, 825–26.

Brown, J., Gunn, T.R., Mora, J.D. and Mok, P.M. (1986) The prenatal diagnosis of cardiomegaly due to tricuspid incompetence. *Pediatric Radiology*, 16, 440.

Brown, T.R., Lubahn, D.B., Wilson, E.M. et al. (1988) Deletion of the steroid binding domain of the human androgen receptor gene in one family with complete androgen insensitivity syndrome: evidence for further genetic heterogeneity in this syndrome. *Proceedings of the National Academy of Sciences of the USA*, 85, 8151–55.

Bruinse, H.W., Sijmons, E.A. and Reuwer, P.J.H.M. (1989) Clinical value of screening for fetal growth retardation by Doopler ultrasound. *Journal of Ultrasound in Medicine*, 8, 207–209.

Bruno, M., Iskra, L., Dolfin, G. and Farina, D. (1988) Congenital pleural effusion: prenatal ultrasonic diagnosis and therapeutic management. *Prenatal Diagnosis*, 8, 157–59.

Buehler, B.A., Delimont, D., Van Waes, M. and Finnell, R.H. (1990) Prenatal prediction of risk of the fetal hydantoin syndrome. *New England Journal of Medicine*, 322, 1567–71.

Bui, T.H., Lindholm, H., Demir, N. and Thomassen, P. (1992) Prenatal diagnosis of distal arthrogryposis type I by ultrasonography. *Prenatal Diagnosis*, 12, 1047–53.

Bui, T.H., Marsk, L., Eklof, D. and Theorell, K. (1984) Prenatal diagnosis of chondroectodermal dysplasia with fetoscopy. *Prenatal Diagnosis*, 4, 155–59.

Buiss-Liem, T.N., Ottenkamp, J., Meerman, R.H. and Verwey, R. (1987) The concurrence of fetal supraventricular tachycardia and obstruction of the foramen ovale. *Prenatal Diagnosis*, 7, 425–31.

Bundy, A.L., Saltzman, D.H., Pober, B. *et al.* (1986) Antenatal sonographic findings in trisomy 18. *Journal of Ultrasound in Medicine*, 5, 361–64.

Bunge, S., Steglich, C., Zuther, C. *et al.* (1993) Iduronate-2-sulfatase gene mutations in 16 patients with mucopolysaccharidosis type II (Hunter syndrome). *Human Molecular Genetics*, 2, 1871–75.

Byrne, J.L.B., Ward, K., Kochenour, N.K. and Dolcourt, J.L. (1990) Prenatal sonographic diagnosis of fetal varicella syndrome. *American Journal of Human Genetics*, 47, A270.

Cacchio, M., Conti, M. and Plicchi, G. (1983) Anatomo-functional considerations and prenatal ultrasonic diagnosis of fetal cryptorchidism and hydrocele. *Minerva Ginecologica*, 35, 483–88.

Camaschella, C., Serra, A., Saglio, G. *et al.* (1988) Meiotic recombination in the beta globin gene cluster causing an error in prenatal diagnosis of beta thalassaemia. *Journal of Medical Genetics*, 25, 307–310.

Camera, G., Centa, A., Zucchinetti, P. *et al.* (1989) Osteopetrosis: description of 2 cases, non-familial of the fatal infantile form and of a case of the mild adult form. Impossibility of performing early prenatal diagnosis. *Pathologica*, 81, 617–25.

Campbell, S. and Pearce, J.M. (1983) The prenatal diagnosis of fetal structural anomalies by ultrasound. *Clinical Obstetrics and Gynecology*, 10, 475–506.

Campbell, S., Tsannatos, C. and Pearce, J.M. (1984) The prenatal diagnosis of Joubert's syndrome of familial agenesis of the cerebellar vermis. *Prenatal Diagnosis*, 4, 391–95.

Cao, A., Falchi, A.M., Tuveri, T. *et al.* (1986) Prenatal diagnosis of thalassaemia major by fetal blood analysis: experience with 1000 cases. *Prenatal Diagnosis*, 6, 159–67.

Carpenter, M.W., Abuelo, D. and Neave, C. (1986) Midtrimester diagnosis of severe deforming osteogenesis imperfecta with autosomal dominant inheritance. *American Journal of Perinatology*, 3, 80–83.

Carstea, E.D., Polymeropoulos, M.H., Parker, C.C. *et al.* (1993) Linkage of Niemann–Pick disease type C to human chromosome 18. *Proceedings of the National Academy of Sciences (USA)*, 90, 2002–2004.

Castineyra, G., Panal, M., Presas, H.L., Goldschmidt, E. and Sanchez, J.M. (1992) Two sibs with Wiedemann–Rautenstrauch syndrome: possibilities of prenatal diagnosis by ultrasound. *Journal of Medical Genetics*, 29, 434–36.

Cayea, P.D., Bieber, F.R., Ross, M.J. *et al.* (1985) Sonographic findings in otocephaly (synotia). *Journal of Ultrasound in Medicine*, 4, 377–79.

Cazenave J., Forestier, F., Bessieres, M.H., Broussin, B. and Begueret, J. (1992) Contribution of a new PCR assay to the prenatal diagnosis of congenital toxoplasmosis. *Prenatal Diagnosis*, 12, 119–27.

Ceccherini, I., Lituania, M., Cordone, M.S. *et al.* (1989) Autosomal dominant polycystic kidney disease: prenatal diagnosis by DNA analysis and sonography at 14 weeks. *Prenatal Diagnosis*, 9, 751–58.

Chadefaux, B., Bonnefont, J.P., Rabier, D. *et al.* (1989) Potential for the prenatal diagnosis of hyperornithemia, hyperammonemia and homocitrullinuria syndrome. *American Journal of Medical Genetics*, 32, 264.

Chadefaux, B., Ceballos, I., Rabier, D. *et al.* (1990) Prenatal diagnosis of arginosuccinic aciduria by assay of arginosuccinate in amniotic fluid at the 12th week of gestation. *American Journal of Medical Genetics*, 35, 59.

Chalmers, R.A., Tracey, B.M., Mistry, J. *et al.* (1989) Prenatal diagnosis of 3-hydroxy-3-methylglutaric aciduria by GC-MS and enzymology on cultured amniocytes and chorionic villi. *Journal of Inherited Metabolic Disease*, 12, 283–85.

Chambers, J.E., Muir, B.B. and Bell, J.E. (1989) 'Bullet'-shaped head in fetuses with spina bifida: a pointer to the spinal lesion. 16, 25–28.

Chambers, S.E., Johnstone, F.D. and Laing, I.A. (1988) Ultrasound *in utero* diagnosis of choroid plexus haemorrhage. *British Journal of Obstetrics and Gynaecology*, 95, 1317–20.

Chatterjee, M.S., Bondoc, B. and Adhate, A. (1985) Prenatal diagnosis of occipital encephalocele. *American Journal of Obstetrics and Gynecology*, 153, 646–47.

Chelly, J., Tumer, Z., Tonnesen, T. *et al.* (1993) Isolation of a candidate gene for Menkes disease that encodes a potential heavy metal binding protein. *Nature Genetics*, 3, 14–19.

Chen, H., Immken, L. and Lachman, R. (1984) Syndrome of multiple pterygia, camptodactyly, facial anomalies, hypoplastic lungs and heart, cystic hygroma and skeletal anomalies: delineation of a new entity and review of lethal forms of multiple pterygium syndrome. *American Journal of Medical Genetics*, 17, 809–26.

Chervenak, F.A, Berkowitz, R.L., Romero, R. *et al.* (1983) The diagnosis of fetal hydrocephalus. *American Journal of Obstetrics and Gynecology*, 147, 703–16.

Chervenak, F.A., Isaacson, G., Rosenberg, J.C. and Kardon, N.B. (1986) Antenatal diagnosis of frontal cephalocele in a fetus with atelosteogenesis. *Journal of Ultrasound in Medicine*, 5, 111–13.

Chervenak, F.A., Isaacson, G., Touloukian, R. *et al.* (1985) Diagnosis and management of fetal teratomas. *Obstetrics and Gynecology*, 66, 666–71.

Chervenak, F.A., Jeanty, P., Cantraine, F. *et al.* (1984a) The diagnosis of fetal microcephaly. *American Journal of Obstetrics and Gynecology*, 149, 512–17.

Chervenak, F.A., Tortora, M., Mayden, K. *et al.* (1984b) Antenatal diagnosis of median cleft face syndrome: sonographic demonstration of cleft lip and hypertelorism. *American Journal of Obstetrics and Gynecology*, 149, 94–97.

Chitayat, D., Hahm, S.Y.E., Marion, R.W. *et al.* (1987)

Further delineation of the McKusick—Kaufman hydrometrocolpos—polydactyly syndrome. *American Journal of Diseases of Childhood*, **141**, 1133—36.

Chitayat, D., Lao, A., Wilson, D. *et al.* (1988a) Prenatal diagnosis of asplenia/polysplenia syndrome. *American Journal of Obstetrics and Gynecology*, **158**, 1085—87.

Chitayat, D., McGillivray, B.C., Diamant, S. *et al.* (1988b) Role of prenatal detection of cardiac tumours in the diagnosis of tuberous sclerosis — report of two cases. *Prenatal Diagnosis*, **8**, 577—84.

Christensen, E. and Brandt, N.J. (1985) Prenatal diagnosis of 5,10-methylenetetrahydrofolate reductase deficiency. *New England Journal of Medicine*, **313**, 50—51.

Chung, W.M. (1986) Antenatal detection of hepatic cyst. *Journal of Clinical Ultrasound*, **14**, 217—19.

Cicardi, M., Igarashi, T., Rosen, F.S. and Davis, A.E. (1987) Molecular basis for the deficiency of complement 1 in type I hereditary angioneurotic edema. *Journal of Clinical Investigation*, **79**, 698—702.

Cidivalli, G., Yarkoni, S., Dar, H. and Kohn, G. (1983) Can infantile hereditary agranulocytosis be diagnosed prenatally? *Prenatal Diagnosis*, **3**, 157—59.

Cilento, B.G. Jr, Benacerraf, B.R. and Mandell, J. (1994) Prenatal diagnosis of cloacal malformation. *Urology*, **43**, 386—88.

Claiborne, A.K., Blocker, S.H., Martin, C.M. and McAllister, W.H. (1986) Prenatal and postnatal sonographic delineation of gastro-intestinal abnormalities in a case of the VATER syndrome. *Journal of Ultrasound in Medicine*, **5**, 45—47.

Cobben, J.M., Scheffer, H., De Visser, M. *et al.* (1994) Apparent SMA I unlinked to 5q. *Journal of Medical Genetics*, **31**, 242—44.

Cobellis, G., Iannoto, P., Stabile, M. *et al.* (1988) Prenatal ultrasound diagnosis of macroglossia in the Wiedemann—Beckwith syndrome. *Prenatal Diagnosis*, **8**, 79—81.

Collinge, J., Harding, A.E., Owen, F. *et al.* (1989) Diagnosis of Gerstmann—Straussler syndrome in familial dementia with prion protein gene analysis. *Lancet*, **ii**, 15—17.

Collins, J. (1991) First report: Prenatal diagnosis of long cord. *American Journal of Obstetrics and Gynecology*, **165**, 1901.

Connor, J.M., Gatherer, D., Gray, F.C. *et al.* (1986) Assignment of the gene for dyskeratosis congenital to Xq28. *Human Genetics*, **72**, 348—51.

Connor, J.M., Loughlin, S.A.R. and Whittle, M.J. (1987) First trimester prenatal exclusion of tuberous sclerosis. *Lancet*, **i**, 269.

Conradi, N.G., Uvebrandt, P., Hokegard, K.H. *et al.* (1989) First trimester diagnosis of juvenile neuronal ceroid lipofuscinosis by demonstration of finger print inclusions in chorionic villi. *Prenatal Diagnosis*, **9**, 283—87.

Constantine, G., McCormack, J., McHugo, J. and Fowlie, A. (1991) Prenatal diagnosis of severe osteogenesis imperfecta. *Prenatal Diagnosis*, **11**, 103—10.

Cooper, C., Mahony, B.S., Bowie, J.D. and Pope I.I. (1985) Prenatal ultrasound diagnosis of ambiguous genitalia. *Journal of Ultrasound in Medicine*, **4**, 433—36.

Cordone, M., Lituania, M., Zampatti, C. *et al.* (1989) *In utero* ultrasonographic features of campomelic dysplasia. *Prenatal Diagnosis*, **9**, 745—50.

Corney, G., Whitehouse, D.B., Hopkinson, D.A. *et al.* (1987) Prenatal diagnosis of alpha-1-antitrypsin deficiency by fetal blood sampling. *Prenatal Diagnosis*, **7**, 101—108.

Corson, V.L., Sanders, R.C., Johnson, T.R. Jr and Winn, K.J. (1983) Mid-trimester fetal ultrasound: diagnostic dilemmas. *Prenatal Diagnosis*, **3**, 47—51.

Corteville, J.E., Gray, D.L. and Crane, J.P. (1991) Congenital hydronephrosis: correlation of fetal utrasonographic findings with infant outcome. *American Journal of Obstetrics and Gynecology*, **165**, 384—88.

Cossu, P., Pirastu, M., Nucaro, A. *et al.* (1992) Prenatal diagnosis of Wilson's disease by analysis of DNA polymorphism. *New England Journal of Medicine*, **327**, 57.

Cowles, T., Furman, P. and Wilkins, I. (1993) Prenatal diagnosis of Dandy—Walker malformation in a family displaying X-linked inheritance. *Prenatal Diagnosis*, **13**, 87—91.

Crane, J.P. and Beaver, H.A. (1986) Mid-trimester sonographic diagnosis of mandibulofacial dysostosis. *American Journal of Medical Genetics*, **25**, 251—55.

Cremers, F.P.M., Brunsmann, F., Van De Pol, T.J.R. *et al.* (1987) Deletion of the DXS165 locus in patients with classical choroideremia. *Clinical Genetics*, **32**, 421—23.

Cremers, F.P.M., van de Pol, D.J.R. van Kerkhoff, P.M. *et al.* (1990) Cloning of a gene that is rearranged in patients with chorioderemia. *Nature*, **347**, 674—77.

Cullen, M.T., Athanassiadis, A.P. and Romero, R. (1990) Prenatal diagnosis of anterior parietal encephalocele with transvaginal sonography. *Obstetrics and Gynecology*, **75**, 489—91.

Curry, C.J.R., Carey, J.C., Holland, J.S. *et al.* (1987) Smith—Lemli—Opitz syndrome type II. Multiple congenital anomalies with male pseudohermaphroditism and frequent early lethality. *American Journal of Medical Genetics*, **26**, 45—57.

Curtis, D., Blank, C.E., Parsons, M.A. and Hughes, H.N. (1989) Carrier detection and prenatal diagnosis in Norrie disease. *Prenatal Diagnosis*, **9**, 735—40.

Cyr, D.R., Gunteroth, W.G., Nyberg, D.A. *et al.* (1988) Prenatal diagnosis of an intrapericardial teratoma. A cause for non-immune hydrops. *Journal of Ultrasound in Medicine*, **7**, 87—90.

Daffos, F., Forestier, F., Capella-Pavlovsky, M. *et al.* (1988) Prenatal management of 746 pregnancies at risk for congenital toxoplasmosis. *New England Journal of Medicine*, **318**, 271—75.

Daffos, F., Forestier, F., Mandelbrot, L. *et al.* (1989) Prenatal diagnosis of HIV infection: two attempts using fetal blood sampling. *Journal of Acquired Immune Deficiency Syndromes*, **2**, 205—207.

Dahl, D.L., Warren, C.D., Rathke, E.J.S. and Jones, M.Z. (1986) Beta-mannosidosis: prenatal detection of caprine allantoic fluid oligosaccharides with thin layer, gel permeation and HPLC. *Journal of Inherited Metabolic Disease*, **9**, 93—98.

Dahl, H.-H.M., Wake, S., Cotton, R.G.H. and Danks, D.M. (1988) The use of restriction fragment length polymorphisms in prenatal diagnosis of dihydropteridine reductase deficiency. *Journal of Medical Genetics*, **25**, 25—28.

Dahl, K.R., Rouse, G.A. and De Lange, M. (1993) Prenatal sonographic evaluation of Beckwith—Wiedemann syndrome. *Journal of Diagnostic Medical Sonography*, **9**, 249—54.

Dahl, N., Wadelius, C., Anneren, G. and Gustavson, K.H. (1992) Mutation analysis for prenatal diagnosis and heterozygote detection of Gaucher disease type III (Norrbottnian type). *Prenatal Diagnosis*, **12**, 603–608.

Daiger, S.P., Lidsky, A.S., Chakraborty, R. *et al.* (1986) Polymorphic DNA haplotypes at the phenylalanine hydroxylase locus in prenatal diagnosis of phenylketonuria. *Lancet*, **i**, 229–32.

Dallapiccola, B., Carbone, L.D.L., Ferranti, G. *et al.* (1985) Monitoring pregnancies at risk for Fanconi's anaemia by chorionic villi sampling. *Acta Haematologica (Basel)*, **73**, 157–58.

Dallapiccola, B., Novelli, G., Cuoco, C. and Porro, E. (1987) First trimester studies of a fetus at risk for triose phosphate isomerase deficiency. *Prenatal Diagnosis*, **7**, 289–94.

Dallapiccola, B., Novelli, G., Ferranti, G. *et al.* (1986) First trimester monitoring of a pregnancy at risk for glucose phosphate isomerase deficiency. *Prenatal Diagnosis*, **6**, 101–107.

Danpure, C.J., Cooper, P.J., Jennings, P.R. *et al.* (1989) Enzymatic prenatal diagnosis of primary hyperoxaluria type I: potential and limitations. *Journal of Inherited Metabolic Disease*, **12** (suppl. 2), 286–88.

Danpure, C.J., Jennings, P.R. and Watts, R.W.E. (1987) Enzymological diagnosis of primary hyperoxaluria type I by measurement of hepatic alanine: glyoxylate aminotransferase activity. *Lancet*, **i**, 289–91.

Davies, R.P., Ford, W.D.A., Lequesne, G.W. and Orell, S.R. (1989) Ultrasonic detection of subdiaphragmatic pulmonary sequestration *in utero* and postnatal diagnosis by fine needle aspiration biopsy. *Journal of Ultrasound in Medicine*, **8**, 47–49.

Davis, W.K., Mahony, B.S., Carroll, B.A. and Bowie, J.D. (1987) Antenatal sonographic detection of benign dacrocystoceles (lacrimal duct cysts). *Journal of Ultrasound in Medicine*, **6**, 461–65.

De Boer, M., Bolscher, B.G.J.M., Sijmons, R.H., Scheffer, H., Weening, R.S. and Roos, D. (1992) Prenatal diagnosis in a family with X-linked chronic granulomatous disease with the use of the polymerase chain reaction. *Prenatal Diagnosis*, **12**, 773–77.

De Elejalde, M.M. and Elejalde, B.R. (1984) Visualisation of the fetal face by ultrasound. *Journal of Craniofacial Genetics and Developmental Biology*, **4**, 251–57.

De Filippi, G., Canestri, G., Bosio, U. *et al.* (1986) Thoracic neuroblastoma: antenatal detection in a case with unusual postnatal radiographic findings. *British Journal of Radiology*, **59**, 704–706.

De Lange, M. and Rouse, G.A. (1990) Prenatal diagnosis of hypophosphatasia. *Journal of Ultrasound in Medicine*, **9**, 115–17.

Dembure, P.P., Priest, J.H., Snoddy, S.C. and Elsas, L.J. (1984) Genotyping and prenatal assessment of collagen lysyl hydroxylase deficiency in a family with Ehlers–Danlos syndrome type VI. *American Journal of Human Genetics*, **36**, 783–90.

Denholm, T.A., Crow, H.C., Edwards, W.H. *et al.* (1984) Prenatal sonographic appearance of meconium ileus in twins. *American Journal of Roentgenology*, **143**, 371–72.

Derosa, R., Lenke, R.R., Kurczynski, T.W. *et al.* (1989) *In utero* diagnosis of benign fetal macrocephaly. *American Journal of Obstetrics and Gynecology*, **161**, 690–92.

De Sierra, T.M., Ashmead, G. and Bilenker, R. (1992) Prenatal diagnosis of short rib (polydactyly) syndrome with situs inversus. *American Journal of Medical Genetics*, **44**, 555–57.

Desjacques, P., Mousson, B., Vianey-Ziaud, C. *et al.* (1985) Combined deficiency of xanthine oxidase and sulphite oxidase: a diagnosis of a new case followed by an antenatal diagnosis. *Journal of Inherited Metabolic Disease*, **8** (suppl. 2), 117–18.

Deter, R.L., Rossavik, I.K. and Carpenter, R.J. (1989) Development of individual growth standards for estimated fetal weight: II. Weight prediction during the third trimester and at birth. *Journal of Clinical Ultrasound*, **17**, 83–88.

De Vita, G., Alcalay, M., Sampietro, M. *et al.* (1989) Two point mutations are responsible for G6PD polymorphism in Sardinia. *American Journal of Human Genetics*, **44**, 233–40.

De Vore, G.R. and Hobbins, J.C. (1979) Diagnosis of structural abnormalities in the fetus. *Clinical Perinatology*, **6**, 293–319.

De Vore, G.R., Siassi, B. and Platt, L.D. (1987) Fetal echocardiography: the prenatal diagnosis of tricuspid atresia (type 1c) during the second trimester of pregnancy. *Journal of Clinical Ultrasound*, **15**, 317–24.

Dhermy, D., Feo, C., Garbarz, M. *et al.* (1987) Prenatal diagnosis of hereditary elliptocytosis with molecular defect of spectrum. *Prenatal Diagnosis*, **7**, 471–83.

Dhonot, J.L., Tilmont, P., Ringel, J. and Farriaux, J.P. (1990) Pterins analysis in amniotic fluid for the prenatal diagnosis of GTP cyclohydrolase deficiency. *Journal of Inherited Metabolic Disease*, **13**, 879–82.

Dietz, H.C., Cutting, G.R., Pyertiz, R.E. *et al.* (1991) Marfan syndrome caused by a recurrent *de novo* missense mutation in the fibrillin gene. *Nature*, **352**, 337–39.

Di Ferrante, N., Leachman, R.D., Angelini, P. *et al.* (1975) Lysyl oxidase deficiency in Ehlers–Danlos syndrome type V. *Connective Tissue Research*, **3**, 49–53.

Dimaio, M.S., Barth, R., Koprivnikar, K.E. *et al.* (1993) First-trimester prenatal diagnosis of osteogenesis imperfecta type II by DNA analysis and sonography. *Prenatal Diagnosis*, **13**, 589–96.

Di Natale, P., Pannone, N., D'Argenio, G. *et al.* (1987) First trimester prenatal diagnosis of Sanfilippo C disease. *Prenatal Diagnosis*, **7**, 603–605.

DiSanto, J.P., Markiewicz, S., Gauchat, J.F. *et al.* (1994) Brief report: Prenatal diagnosis of X-linked hyper-IgM syndrome. *New England Journal of Medicine*, **330**, 969–73.

Diukman, R., Tanigawara, S., Cowan, M.J. and Golbus, M.S. (1992) Prenatal diagnosis of Chediak–Higashi syndrome. *Prenatal Diagnosis*, **12**, 877–85.

Dolan, C.R., Smith, L.T. and Sybert, V.P. (1993) Prenatal detection of epidemolysis bullosa lethalis with pyloric atresia in a fetus by abnormal ultrasound and elevated alpha-fetoprotein. *American Journal of Medical Genetics*, **47**, 395–400.

Dolkart, L.A., Reimers, B.T., Wertheimer, I.S. and Wilson, B.O. (1992) Prenatal diagnosis of laryngeal atresia. *Journal of Ultrasound in Medicine*, **11**, 496–98.

Donnai, P., Donnai, D., Harris, R. *et al.* (1981) Antenatal diagnosis of Niemann–Pick disease in a twin pregnancy. *Journal of Medical Genetics*, **18**, 359–61.

Donnenfeld, A.E., Gussman, D., Mennuti, M.T. and Zackai, E.H. (1986) Evaluation of an unknown fetal skeletal dysplasia: prenatal findings in hypochondrogenesis. *American Journal of Human Genetics*, 39, A252.

Donnenfeld, A.E. and Mennuti, M.I. (1987) Second trimester diagnosis of fetal skeletal dysplasias. *Obstetrics and Gynecology Survey*, 42, 199–217.

Donnenfeld, A.E., Mennuti, M.T., Templeton, J.M. and Gabbe, G.G. (1989) Prenatal diagnosis of a vesico-allantoic abdominal wall defect. *Journal of Ultrasound in Medicine*, 8, 43–45.

Donnenfeld, A.E., Wiseman, B., Lavi, E. and Weiner, S. (1990) Prenatal diagnosis of thrombocytopenia — absent radius syndrome by ultrasound and cordocentesis. *Prenatal Diagnosis*, 10, 29–35.

Donner, C., Liesnard, C., Content, J., Busine, A., Aderca, J. and Rodesch, F. (1993) Prenatal diagnosis of 52 pregnancies at risk for congenital cytomegalovirus infection. *Obstetrics and Gynecology*, 82, 481–86.

Dooley, T., Fairbanks, L.D., Simmonds, H.A. *et al.* (1987) First trimester diagnosis of adenosine deaminase deficiency. *Prenatal Diagnosis*, 7, 561–65.

Dreazen, E., Tessler, F., Sarti, D. and Crandall, B.F. (1989) Spontaneous resolution of fetal hydrocephalus. *Journal of Ultrasound in Medicine*, 8, 155–57.

Driscoll, D.A., Budarf, M.L. and Emanuel, B.S. (1991) Antenatal diagnosis of DiGeorge syndrome. *Lancet*, 338, 1390–91.

Duff, P., Harlass, F.E. and Milligan, D.A. (1990) Prenatal diagnosis of chondrodysplasia punctata by sonography. *Obstetrics and Gynecology*, 76, 497–500.

Dumez, Y., Dommergues, M., Gubler, M.C. *et al.* (1994) Meckel–Gruber syndrome: Prenatal diagnosis at 10 menstrual weeks using embryoscopy. *Prenatal Diagnosis*, 14, 141–44.

Dumoulin, R., Divry, P., Mandon, G. and Mathieu, M. (1991) A new case of prenatal diagnosis of isovaleric acidaemia. *Prenatal Diagnosis*, 11, 921–22.

Dunn, V. and Glasier, C.M. (1985) Ultrasonographic antenatal demonstration of primary megaureters. *Journal of Ultrasound in Medicine*, 4, 101–103.

Duran, M., Schutgens, R.B.H., Ketel, A. *et al.* (1979) 3-Hydroxy-3-methylglutaryl coenzyme A lyase deficiency: postnatal management following prenatal diagnosis by analysis of maternal urine. *Journal of Pediatrics*, 95, 1004–1007.

Durandy, A., Bretongorius, J. Guy-Grand, D., Dumez, C. and Griscelli C. (1993) Prenatal diagnosis of syndromes associating albinism and immune deficiencies (Chediak–Higashi syndrome and variant). *Prenatal Diagnosis*, 13, 13–20.

Durandy, A., Cerf Bensussan, N., Dumez, Y. and Griscelli, C. (1987) Prenatal diagnosis of severe combined immunodeficiency with defective synthesis of HLA molecules. *Prenatal Diagnosis*, 7, 27–34.

Durandy, A., Griscelli, G., Dumez, Y. *et al.* (1982) Antenatal diagnosis of severe combined immunodeficiency from fetal cord blood. *Lancet*, 7, 852–53.

Eady, R.A.J., Gunner, D.B., Carbone, L.D.L. *et al.* (1986) Prenatal diagnosis of bullous ichthyosiform erythroderma: detection of tonofilament clumps in fetal epidermal and amniotic fluid cells. *Journal of Medical Genetics*, 23, 46–51.

Eady, R.A.J., Gunner, D.B., Garner, A. and Rodeck, C.H.

(1983) Prenatal diagnosis of oculocutaneous albinism by electron microscopy of fetal skin. *Journal of Investigative Dermatology*, 80, 210–12.

Eady, R.A.J., Schofield, O.M.V., Nicolaides, K.H. and Rodeck, C.H. (1989) Prenatal diagnosis of junctional epidermolysis bullosa. *Lancet*, ii, 1453.

Elchalal, U., Itzhak, I.B., BenMeir, G. and Zalel, Y. (1993) Antenatal diagnosis of congenital dislocation of the knee: A case report. *American Journal of Perinatology*, 10, 194–96.

Elder, G.H., Evans, J.O., Thomas, N. *et al.* (1976) The primary enzyme defect in hereditary coproporphyria. *Lancet*, ii, 1217–19.

Elejalde, B.R., De Elejalde, M.M., Booth, C. *et al.* (1983) Prenatal diagnosis of Weyers syndrome (deficient ulnar and fibular rays with bilateral hydronephrosis). *American Journal of Medical Genetics*, 21, 439–44.

Elejalde, B.R., De Elejalde, M.M. and Pansch, D. (1985) Prenatal diagnosis of Jeune syndrome. *American Journal of Medical Genetics*, 21, 433–38.

El Khazen, N., Faverley, D., Vamos, E. *et al.* (1986) Lethal osteopetrosis with multiple fractures *in utero*. *American Journal of Medical Genetics*, 23, 811–19.

Endo, F., Tanoue, A., Kitano, A. *et al.* (1990) Biochemical basis of prolidase deficiency: polypeptide acid RNA phenotypes and relation to clinical phenotypes. *Journal of Clinical Investigation*, 85, 162–69.

Eng, C.M. and Desnick, R.J. (1994) Molecular basis of Fabry disease: Mutations and polymorphisms in the human alpha-galactosidase A gene. *Human Mutation*, 3, 103–111.

Erasmus, E., Mienie, L.J., De Vries, W.N., De Wet, W.J., Carlsson, B. and Larsson, A. (1993) Prenatal analysis in two suspected cases of glutathione synthetase deficiency. *Journal of Inherited Metabolic Disease*, 16, 837–43.

Estroff, J.A., Scott M.R. and Benacerraf, B.R. (1992) Dandy–Walker variant: Prenatal sonographic features and clinical outcome. *Radiology*, 185, 755–58.

Evans, M.I., Greb, A., Kunkel, L.M. *et al.* (1991) *In utero* fetal muscle biopsy for the diagnosis of Duchenne muscular dystrophy. *American Journal of Obstetrics and Gynecology*, 165, 728–32.

Evans, M.I., Zador, I.E., Qureshi, F. *et al.* (1988) Ultrasonographic prenatal diagnosis and fetal pathology of Langer mesomelic dwarfism. *American Journal of Medical Genetics*, 31, 915–20.

Feldman, E., Shalev, E., Weiner, E. *et al.* (1985) Microphthalmia — prenatal ultrasonic diagnosis: a case report. *Prenatal Diagnosis*, 5, 205–207.

Feldman, G.L., Lewiston, N., Fernbach, S.D. *et al.* (1989) Prenatal diagnosis of cystic fibrosis by any linked DNA markers in 138 pregnancies at 1 in 4 risk. *American Journal of Medical Genetics*, 32, 238–41.

Fellous, M., Boue, J., Malbrunot, C. *et al.* (1982) A five-generation family with sacral agenesis and spina bifida: possible similarities with the mouse T-locus. *American Journal of Medical Genetics*, 12, 465–87.

Fensom, A.H., Benson, P.F. and Baker, J.E. (1978) A rapid method for assay of branched-chain ketoacid decarboxylation in cultured cells and its application to prenatal diagnosis of maple syrup urine disease. *Clinica Chimica Acta*, 87, 169–74.

Fensom, A.H., Benson, P.F., Crees, M.J. *et al.* (1983) Prenatal exclusion of homocystinuria (cystathionine beta-synthase deficiency) by assay of phytohaemagglutinin-stimulated fetal lymphocytes. *Prenatal Diagnosis*, 3, 127–30.

Fensom, A.H., Benson, P.F., Neville, B.R.G. *et al.* (1979) Prenatal diagnosis of Farber's disease. *Lancet*, ii, 990–92.

Fernandez, G. and Hertzberg, B.S. (1992) Prenatal sonographic detection of giant parietal foramina. *Journal of Ultrasound in Medicine*, 11, 155–57.

Ferraro, E.M., Fakhry, J., Aruny, J.E. and Bracero, L.A. (1988) Prenatal adrenal neuroblastoma. Case report with review of the literature. *Journal of Ultrasound in Medicine*, 7, 275–78.

Filkins, K., Russo, J., Fikin, W. *et al.* (1985) Third trimester ultrasound diagnosis of intestinal atresia following clinical evidence of diagnosis of polyhydramnios. *Prenatal Diagnosis*, 5, 215–20.

Filkins, K., Russo, J., Bilinki, I. *et al.* (1984) Prenatal diagnosis of thrombocytopenia–absent radius syndrome using ultrasound and fetoscopy. *Prenatal Diagnosis*, 4, 139–42.

Filly, R.A., Goldstein, R.B. and Callen, P.W. (1990) Monochorionic twinning: sonographic assessment. *American Journal of Roentgenology*, 154, 459–69.

Fine, J.D., Eady, R.A.J., Levy, M.L. *et al.* (1988) Prenatal diagnosis of dominant and recessive dystrophic epidermolysis bullosa: application and limitations in the use of KF-1 and LH 7:2 monoclonal antibodies and immunofluorescence techniques. *Journal of Investigative Dermatology*, 91, 465–71.

Fine, J.D., Holbrook, K.A., Elias, S. *et al.* (1990) Applicability of 19-DEJ-1 monoclonal antibody for the prenatal diagnosis or exclusion of junctional epidermolysis bullosa. *Prenatal Diagnosis*, 10, 219–29.

Fink, I.J. and Filly, R.A. (1983) Omphalocele associated with umbilical cord allantoic cyst: sonographic evaluation *in utero*. *Radiology*, 149, 473–76.

Firgaira, F.A., Cotton, R.G.H., Danks, D.M. *et al.* (1983) Prenatal determination of dihydropteridine reductase in a normal fetus at risk for malignant hyperphenylalanemia. *Prenatal Diagnosis*, 3, 7–11.

Fischbeck, K.H., Ionasecu, V., Ritter, A.E. *et al.* (1986) Localisation of the gene for X-linked spinal muscular atrophy. *Neurology*, 36, 1595–98.

Fisk, N.M., Dhillon, H.K., Ellis, C.E. *et al.* (1990) Antenatal diagnosis of megalourethra in a fetus with the prune belly syndrome. *Journal of Clinical Ultrasound*, 18, 124–28.

Fitzgerald, E.J. and Toi, A. (1986) Antenatal ultrasound diagnosis of cystic adenomatoid malformation of the lung. *Journal of the Canadian Association of Radiology*, 37, 48–49.

Fitzmorris-Glass, R., Mattrey, R.F. and Cantrell, C.J. (1989) Magnetic resonance imaging as an adjunct to ultrasound in odigohydramnios. Detection of sirenomelia. *Journal of Ultrasound in Medicine*, 8, 159–62.

Fitzsimons, P.J., Frost, R.A., Millward, S. *et al.* (1986) Prenatal and immediate postnatal ultrasonographic diagnosis of ureteocele. *Journal of the Canadian Association of Radiology*, 337, 189–191.

Fleisher, L.D., Rassin, D.K., Desnick, R.J. *et al.* (1979) Argininosuccinicaciduria: prenatal studies in a family at risk. *American Journal of Human Genetics*, 31, 439–45.

Fletman, D., McQuown, D., Kanchana, Poom, V. and Gyepes, M.I. (1980) 'Apple peel' atresia of the small bowel: prenatal diagnosis of the obstruction by ultrasound. *Pediatric Radiology*, 9, 118–19.

Flomen, R.H., Green, P.M., Bentley, D.R., Giannelli, F. and Green, E.P. (1992) Detection of point mutations and a gross deletion in six Hunter Syndrome patients. *Genomics*, 13, 543–50.

Foderaro, A.E., Abu-Yousef, M.M., Benda, J.A. *et al.* (1987) Antenatal ultrasound diagnosis of iniencephaly. *Journal of Clinical Ultrasound*, 15, 550–54.

Fogarty, K., Cohen, H.L. and Haller, J.O. (1989) Sonography of fetal intracranial hemorrhage: unusual causes and a review of the literature. *Journal of Clinical Ultrasound*, 17, 366–70.

Forestier, F., Daffos, F., Sole, Y. and Rainaut, M. (1986) Prenatal diagnosis of haemophilia by fetal blood sampling under ultrasound guidance. *Haemostasis*, 16, 346–51.

Foucar, E., Williamson, R.A., Yiu-Chiu, V. *et al.* (1983) Mesenchymal hamartoma of the liver identified by fetal sonography. *American Journal of Roentgenology*, 140, 970–72.

Foulon, W., Naessens, A., Mahler, T. *et al.* (1990) Prenatal diagnosis of congenital toxoplasmosis. *Obstetrics and Gynecology*, 76, 769–72.

Fowler, B., Borresen, A.L. and Boman, N. (1982) Prenatal diagnosis of homocystinuria. *Lancet*, ii, 875.

Fowler, B., Giles, L., Sardharwalla, I.B. *et al.* (1988) First trimester diagnosis of methylmalonic aciduria. *Prenatal Diagnosis*, 8, 207–13.

Francannet, C., Vanlieferinghen, P., Dechelotte, P., Urbain, M.F., Campagne, D. and Malpuech, G. (1994) Ladd syndrome in five members of a three-generation family and prenatal diagnosis. *Genetic Counselling*, 5, 85–91.

Fraser, W.D., Nimrod, C., Nicholson, S. and Harder, J. (1989) Antenatal diagnosis of restriction of the foramen ovale. *Journal of Ultrasound in Medicine*, 8, 281–83.

Friedman, J.M. and Santos-Ramos, R. (1984) Natural history of X-linked aqueductal stenosis in the second and third trimesters of pregnancy. *American Journal of Obstetrics and Gynecology*, 150, 104–106.

Fukuda, M.N., Dell, A. and Scartezzini, P. (1987) Primary defect of congenital dyserythropoietic anaemia type II: failure of glycosylation of erythrocyte lactosaminoglycan proteins caused by lowered N-acetylglucosaminyl transferase II. *Journal of Biological Chemistry*, 262, 7195–206.

Gabrielli, S., Reece, E.A., Pilu, G. *et al.* (1989) The clinical significance of prenatally diagnosed choroid plexus cysts. *American Journal of Obstetrics and Gynecology*, 160, 1207–10.

Gagne, R., Lescault, A., Grenier, A. *et al.* (1982) Prenatal diagnosis of hereditary tyrosinaemia: measurement of succinylacetone in amniotic fluid. *Prenatal Diagnosis*, 2, 185–88.

Gal, A., Uhlhass, S., Glaser, D. and Grimm, T. (1988) Prenatal exclusion of Norrie disease with flanking DNA markers. *American Journal of Medical Genetics*, 31, 449–53.

Gallagher, D.M., Leiman, S. and Hux, C.H. (1993) *In utero* diagnosis of a portal vein aneurysm. *Journal of Clinical Ultrasound*, 21, 147–51.

Gamble, C.N., Hershey, D.W. and Schaeffer, C.J. (1990)

Femoral—facial syndrome detected in prenatal ultrasound. *American Journal of Human Genetics*, **47**, 274.

Garber, A., Shohat, M. and Sarti, D. (1990) Megacystis—microcolon—intestinal hypoperistalsis syndrome in two male siblings. *Prenatal Diagnosis*, **10**, 377—88.

Garcia-Munoz, M.J., Belloque, J., Merinero, B. *et al.* (1989) Non-ketotic hyperglycinaemia: glycine/serine ratio in amniotic fluid — an unreliable method for prenatal diagnosis. *Prenatal Diagnosis*, **9**, 473—76.

Gardiner, R.M., Sandford, A., Deadman, M. *et al.* (1990) Batten disease (Spielmeyer—Vogt: juvenile onset neuronal ceroid lipofuscinosis) maps to human chromosome 16. *Genomics*, **8**, 387—90.

Gatti, R.A., Berkel, I., Boder, E. *et al.* (1988) Localisation of an ataxia—telangiectasia gene to chromosome 11q22—23. *Nature*, **336**, 577—80.

Gatti, R., Lombardo, C., Filocamo, M. *et al.* (1985) Comparative study of 15 lysosomal enzymes in chorionic villi and cultured amniotic fluid cells. Early PND in seven pregnancies at risk for lysosomal storage diseases. *Prenatal Diagnosis*, **5**, 329—36.

Gatti, R.A., Peterson, K.L., Novak, J. *et al.* (1993) Prenatal genotyping of ataxia-telangiectasia. *Lancet*, **342**, 376.

Gazit, F., Brand, N., Harel, Y. *et al.* (1990) Prenatal diagnosis of Lowe's syndrome: a case report with evidence of *de novo* mutation. *Prenatal Diagnosis*, **10**, 257—60.

Gebhardt, D.O. (1979) Prenatal detection of Tangier disease. *Lancet*, **ii**, 754—55.

Gellert, G., Petersen, J., Krawczak, M. and Zoll, B. (1988) Linkage relationship between retinoschisis and four marker loci. *Human Genetics*, **79**, 382—84.

Gembruch, U., Chatterjee, M., Bald, R. *et al.* (1990b) Prenatal diagnosis of aortic atresia by colour Doppler flow mapping. *Prenatal Diagnosis*, **10**, 211—18.

Gembruch, U., Hansmann, M. and Fodisch, H.J. (1985) Early prenatal diagnosis of short rib-polydactyly (SRP) syndrome type II (Majewski) by ultrasound in a case at risk. *Prenatal Diagnosis*, **5**, 357—62.

Gembruch, U., Knople, G., Chatterjee, M. *et al.* (1990a) First-trimester diagnosis of fetal congenital heart disease by transvaginal two-dimensional and Doppler echocardiography. *Obstetrics and Gynecology*, **75**, 496—98.

Gembruch, U., Niesen, M., Kehrberg, G. and Hansmann, M. (1988) Diastrophic dysplasia: a specific prenatal diagnosis by ultrasound. *Prenatal Diagnosis*, **8**, 539—46.

Gembruch, U., Steil, E., Redel, D.A. and Hansmann, M. (1990c) Prenatal diagnosis of a left ventricular aneurysm. *Prenatal Diagnosis*, **10**, 203—209.

Gendall, P.W., Baird, C.E. and Becroft, D.M.O. (1994) Rhizomelic chondrodysplasia punctata: Early recognition with antenatal ultrasonography. *Journal of Clinical Ultrasound*, **22**, 271—74.

Genkins, S.M., Hertzberg, B.S., Bowie, J.D. and Blow, O. (1989) Pena—Shokeir type I syndrome: *in utero* sonographic appearance. **17**, 56—61.

Geraghty, A.V., Knott, P.O. and Hanna, H.M. (1989) Prenatal Diagnosis of fetal glioblastoma multiforme. *Prenatal Diagnosis*, **9**, 613—16.

Ghidini, A., Romero, R., Eisen, R.N. *et al.* (1990) Umbilical cord haemangioma. Prenatal identification and review of the literature. *Journal of Ultrasound in Medicine*, **9**, 297—300.

Ghidini, A., Vergani, P., Sirtori, M. *et al.* (1988a) Prenatal diagnosis of subdural hygroma. *Journal of Ultrasound in Medicine*, **7**, 463—65.

Ghidini, A., Sirtori, M., Romero, R. and Hobbins, J.C. (1988b) Prenatal diagnosis of pentalogy of Cantrell. *Journal of Ultrasound in Medicine*, **7**, 567—72.

Ghidini, A., Sirtori, M., Vergani, P. *et al.* (1989) Fetal intracranial calcification. *American Journal of Obstetrics and Gynecology*, **160**, 86—87.

Gibbons, R.J., Suthers, G.K., Wilkie, A.D.M., Buckle, V.J. and Higgs, D.R. (1992) X-linked alpha-thalassemia/mental retardation (ATR-X) syndrome: Localisation to Xq12-q21.31 by X inactivation and linkage analysis. *American Journal of Human Genetics*, **51**, 1136—11.

Gibbs, D.A., Headhouse-Benson, C.M. and Watts, R.W.E. (1986) Family studies of the Lesch—Nyhan syndrome: the use of a restriction fragment length polymorphism (RFLP) closely linked to the disease gene for carrier state and prenatal diagnosis. *Journal of Inherited Metabolic Disease*, **9**, 45—57.

Giles, L., Cooper, A., Fowler, B. *et al.* (1987) Krabbe's disease: first trimester diagnosis confirmed on cultured amniotic fluid cells and fetal tissues. *Prenatal Diagnosis*, **7**, 329—32.

Giles, L., Cooper, A., Fowler, B. *et al.* (1988) First trimester prenatal diagnosis and Sandhoff's disease. *Prenatal Diagnosis*, **8**, 199—205.

Gillett, M.G., Holton, J.B. and MacFaul, R. (1983) Prenatal determination of uridine diphosphate galactose-4-epimerase activity. *Prenatal Diagnosis*, **3**, 57—59.

Glenn, L.W. and Teng, S.S.K. (1985) *In utero* sonographic diagnosis of achondrogenesis. *Journal of Clinical Ultrasound*, **13**, 195—98.

Glick, P.L., Harrison, M.R. and Filly, R.A. (1983) Antepartum diagnosis of meconium peritonitis. *New England Journal of Medicine*, **309**, 1392.

Godfrey, M., Menashe, V., Weleber, R.G. *et al.* (1990) Cosegregation of elastin-associated microfibrillar abnormalities with the Marfan phenotype in families. *American Journal of Human Genetics*, **46**, 652—60.

Godfrey, M., Vandemark, N., Wang, M. *et al.* (1993) Prenatal diagnosis and a donor splice site mutation in fibrillin in a family with Marfan syndrome. *American Journal of Human Genetics*, **53**, 472—80.

Golbus, M.J., Sagebiel, R.W., Filly, R.A. *et al.* (1980) Prenatal diagnosis of congenital bullous ichtyosiform erythroderma (epidermolytic hyperkeratosis) by fetal skin biopsy. *New England Journal of Medicine*, **302**, 93—95.

Golbus, M.S., Simpson, T.J., Koresawa, M. *et al.* (1988) The prenatal determination of glucose-6-phosphatase activity by fetal liver biopsy. *Prenatal Diagnosis*, **8**, 401—404.

Goldstein, R.B., Filly, R.A. and Callen, P.W. (1989) Sonography of anencephaly: pitfalls in early diagnosis. *Journal of Clinical Ultrasound*, **17**, 397—402.

Gollop, T.R., Eigier, A. and Neto, J.G. (1987) Prenatal diagnosis of thalidomide syndrome. *Prenatal Diagnosis*, **7**, 295—98.

Goodship, J., Levinsky, R. and Malcolm, S. (1989) Linkage of PGKL to X-linked severed combined immunodeficiency (IMD4) allows predictive testing in families with no surviving male. *Human Genetics*, **84**, 11—14.

337

Goonewardena, P., Sjoholm, A.G., Nilsson, L.A. and Petters-son, V. (1988) Linkage analysis of the properdin deficiency gene: suggestion of a locus in the proximal part of the short arm of the X chromosome. *Genomics*, **2**, 115–18.

Gorczyca, D.P., McGahan, J.P., Lindfors, K.K. *et al.* (1989) Arthrogryposis multiplex congenita: prenatal ultrasonographic diagnosis. *Journal of Clinical Ultrasound*, **17**, 40–44.

Gotoh, T., Adachi, Y., Nounaka, O. *et al.* (1989) Adrenal hemorrhage in the newborn with evidence of bleeding *in utero*. *Journal of Urology*, **141**, 1145–47.

Gottesfeld, K.R. (1978) Ultrasound in obstetrics. *Clinical Obstetrics and Gynecology*, **21**, 311–27.

Graham, M. (1985) Congenital short femur: prenatal sonographic diagnosis. *Journal of Ultrasound in Medicine*, **4**, 361–63.

Gray, D.L., Martin, C.M. and Crane, J.P. (1989) Differential diagnosis of first trimester ventral wall defect. *Journal of Ultrasound in Medicine*, **8**, 255–58.

Gray, R.G.F., Green, A., Basu, S.N. *et al.* (1990) Antenatal diagnosis of molybdenum cofactor deficiency. *American Journal of Obstetrics and Gynecology*, **163**, 1203–204.

Grebner, E.E. and Jackson, L.G. (1979) Prenatal diagnosis of Tay–Sachs disease: reliability of amniotic fluid. *American Journal of Obstetrics and Gynecology*, **134**, 547–50.

Grebner, E.E. and Jackson, L.G. (1985) Prenatal diagnosis for Tay–Sachs disease using chorionic villus sampling. *Prenatal Diagnosis*, **5**, 313–20.

Greenberg, C.R., Hevenen, C.L. and Evans, J.A. (1988) The BOR syndrome and renal agenesis – prenatal diagnosis and further clinical delineation. *Prenatal Diagnosis*, **8**, 103–108.

Greenblatt, A.M., Beretsky, I., Lankin, D.H. and Phelan, L. (1985) *In utero* diagnosis of crossed ectopia using high-resolution real-time ultrasound. *Journal of Ultrasound in Medicine*, **4**, 105–107.

Grignon, A., Filiatrault, D. and Homsy, Y. *et al.* (1986b) Ureteropelvic junction stenosis: antenatal ultrasonographic diagnosis, postnatal investigation and follow-up. *Radiology*, **160**, 649–51.

Grignon, A., Filion, R., Filiatrault, D. *et al.* (1986a) Urinary tract dilatation *in utero*: classification and clinical applications. *Radiology*, **160**, 645–47.

Gross, S.J., Benzie, R.J., Sermer, M. *et al.* (1987) Sacrococcygeal teratoma: prenatal diagnosis and management. *American Journal of Obstetrics and Gynecology*, **156**, 393–96.

Gruberg, L., Aksentijevich, I., Pras, E., Kastner, D.L. and Pras, M. (1992) Mapping of the familial Mediterranean fever gene to chromosome 16. *American Journal of Reproductive Immunology*, **28**, 241–42.

Gruel, Y., Boizard, B., Daffos, F. *et al.* (1986) Determination of platelet antigens and glycoprotein in the human fetus. *Blood*, **68**, 488–92.

Grundy, H., Glasmann, A., Burlbaw, J. *et al.* (1985) Hemangioma presenting as a cystic mass in the fetal neck. *Journal of Ultrasound in Medicine*, **4**, 147–50.

Gubler, M.C. and Levy, M. (1993) Prenatal diagnosis of Nail–Patella syndrome by intrauterine kidney biopsy. *American Journal of Medical Genetics*, **47**, 122–23.

Guigiani, R., Jackson, M., Skinner, S.J. *et al.* (1987) Progressive mental retardation in siblings with Morquio disease type B (mucopolysaccharidosis IVB). *Clinical Genetics*, **32**, 313–25.

Gulmezoglu, A.M. and Ekici, E. (1994) Sonographic diagnosis of Neu-Laxova syndrome. *Journal of Clinical Ultrasound*, **22**, 48–51.

Gulrajani, M., David, K., Sy, W. and Braithwaite, A. (1993) Prenatal diagnosis of a neurenteric cyst by magnetic resonance imaging. *American Journal of Perinatology*, **10**, 304–306.

Guzman, E.R. (1990) Early prenatal diagnosis of gastroschisis with transvaginal sonography. *American Journal of Obstetrics and Gynecology*, **162**, 1253–54.

Hadi, H.A., Mashini, I.S., Devoe, L.D. *et al.* (1986) Ultrasonographic prenatal diagnosis of hydranencephaly. A case report. *Journal of Reproductive Medicine*, **31**, 254–56.

Haeusler, M.C.H., Hofmann, H.M.H., Hoenigl, W. *et al.* (1990) Congenital generalised cystic lymphangiomatosis diagnosed by prenatal ultrasound. *Prenatal Diagnosis*, **10**, 617–21.

Hahnel, R., Hahnel, E., Wysocki, S.J. *et al.* (1982) Prenatal diagnosis of X-linked ichthyosis. *Clinica Chimica Acta*, **120**, 143–52.

Halley, D.J.J., Kleijler, W., Jaspers, N.G.J. *et al.* (1979) Prenatal diagnosis of xeroderma pigmentosum (group C) using assays of unscheduled DNA synthesis and post replication repair. *Clinical Genetics*, **16**, 137–46.

Hamel, B.C.J., Happle, R., Steylen, P.M. *et al.* (1992) False-negative prenatal diagnosis of restrictive dermopathy. *American Journal of Medical Genetics*, **44**, 824–26.

Hammadeh, M.Y., Dhillon, H.K., Duffy, P.G. and Ransley, P.G. (1994) Antenatally diagnosed seminal vesicular cyst. *Fetal Diagnosis and Therapy*, **9**, 62–64.

Hanauer, A., Alembik, YL, Gilgenkrantz, S. *et al.* (1988) Probable localisation of the Coffin–Lowry locus in Xp.22.2–p22.1 by multipoint linkage analysis. *American Journal of Medical Genetics*, **30**, 523–30.

Harper, A.K., Clark, J.A. and Koontz, W.L. and Holmes, M. (1989) Sonographic appearance of fetal extracranial hematoma. *Journal of Ultrasound in Medicine*, **8**, 693–95.

Hartikainen-Sorri, A.L., Kirkinen, P. and Herva, R. (1983) Prenatal detection of hydrolethalus syndrome. *Prenatal Diagnosis*, **3**, 219–24.

Harzer, K., Hager, H.D. and Tariverdian, G. (1987) Prenatal enzymatic diagnosis and exclusion of Krabbe's disease (globoid cell leucodystrophy) using chorionic villi in five risk pregnancies. *Human Genetics*, **77**, 342–44.

Hastbacka, J., Salonen, R., Laurila, P., De la Chapelle, A. and Kaitila, I. (1993) Prenatal diagnosis of diastrophic dysplasia with polymorphic DNA markers. *Journal of Medical Genetics*, **30**, 265–68.

Hayasaka, K., Iada, K., Fueki, N. and Aikawa, J. (1990) Prenatal diagnosis of nonketotic hyperglycinemia. Enzymatic analysis of the glycine cleavage system in chorionic villi. *Journal of Pediatrics*, **116**, 444–45.

Hayashi, M., Kurishita, M., Sodemodo, T., Kiozu, H., Kumasaka, T. and Saiki, S. (1993) Prenatal ultrasonic appearance of the Klippel–Trenaunay–Weber syndrome mimicking sacrococcygeal teratoma with an elevated level of maternal serum hCG. *Prenatal Diagnosis*, **13**, 1162–63.

Hayden, M.R., Hewitt, J., Kastelein, J.J.P. *et al.* (1987)

First-trimester prenatal diagnosis for Huntington's disease with DNA probes. *Lancet*, **i**, 1284−85.

Hayden, S.A., Russ, P.D., Pretorius, D.H. *et al.* (1988) Posterior urethral obstruction. Prenatal sonographic findings and clinical outcome in fourteen cases. *Journal of Ultrasound in Medicine*, 7, 371−75.

Hayes, M.E. and Robertson, E. (1981) Can oculocutaneous albinism be diagnosed prenatally? *Prenatal Diagnosis*, **1**, 85−89.

He, W., Voznyi, Y.V., Huÿmans, J.G.M., Geilen, G.C. *et al.* (1994) Prenatal diagnosis of Sanfilippo disease type C using a simple fluorometric enzyme assay. *Prenatal Diagnosis*, **14**, 17−22.

Heagerty, A.H.M., Kennedy, A.R., Gunner, D.B. and Eady, R.A.J. (1986) Rapid prenatal diagnosis and exclusion of epidermolysis bullosa using novel antibody probes. *Journal of Investigative Dermatology*, **86**, 603−605.

Heijne, L. *et al.* (1985) The development of fetal gallstones demonstrated by ultrasound. *Radiography*, **51**, 155−56.

Hejtmancik, J.F., Holcomb, J.D., Howard, J. and Vanderford, M. (1989) *In vitro* amplification of the alpha-1-antitrypsin gene: application to prenatal diagnosis. *Prenatal Diagnosis*, 9, 177−86.

Hellsten, E., Vesa, J., Jarvela, I., Makela, T.P., Santavuori, P. and Peltonen, L. (1993) Refined assignment of the infantile neuronal ceroid-lipofuscinosis (INCL) locus at 1p32 and the current status of prenatal and carrier diagnostics. *Journal of Inherited Metabolic Disease*, **16**, 335−38.

Hendricks, S.K., Cyr, D.R., Nyberg, D.A. *et al.* (1988) Exencephaly − Clinical and ultrasonic correlation to anencephaly. *Obstetrics and Gynecology*, 72, 898−901.

Henrion, R., Oury, J.F., Aubry, J.P. and Aubry, M.C. (1980) Prenatal diagnosis of ectrodactyly. *Lancet*, **ii**, 319.

Henry, R.J.W. and Norton, S. (1987) Prenatal ultrasound diagnosis of fetal scoliosis with termination of the pregnancy: case report. *Prenatal Diagnosis*, 7, 663−66.

Hensleigh, P.A., Moore, W.V., Wilson, K. and Tulchinsky, D. (1978) Congenital X-linked adrenal hypoplasia. *Obstetrics and Gynecology*, **52**, 228−32.

Herva, R., Leisti, J., Kirkinen, P. and Sappanen, U. (1985) A lethal autosomal recessive syndrome of multiple congenital contractures. *American Journal of Medical Genetics*, **20**, 431−39.

Heydanus, R., Stewart, P.A., Wladimiroff, J.W. and Los, F.J. (1993) Prenatal diagnosis of congenital cystic adenomatoid lung malformation: A report of seven cases. *Prenatal Diagnosis*, **13**, 65−71.

Hill, L.M., Breckle, R. and Gehrking, W.C. (1985) Prenatal detection of congenital malformations by ultrasonography: Mayo Clinic experience. *American Journal of Obstetrics and Gynecology*, **152**, 44−50.

Hill, L.M. and Grzybek, P.C. (1994) Sonographic findings with Pfeiffer syndrome. *Prenatal Diagnosis*, **14**, 47−49.

Hill, L.M., Grzybek, P., Mills, A. and Hogge, W.A. (1994) Antenatal diagnosis of fetal pelvic kidneys. *Obstetrics and Gynecology*, **83**, 333−36.

Hill, L.M., Kislak, S. and Belfar, H.L. (1990) The sonographic diagnosis of urachal cysts in utero. *JW*, **18**, 434−37.

Hill, L.M., Kislak, S. and Jones, N. (1988) Prenatal ultrasound diagnosis of a forearm constriction band. *Journal*

of Clinical Ultrasound, 7, 293−95.

Hill, L.M., Thomas, M.L. and Peterson, C.S. (1987) The ultrasonic detection of Apert syndrome. *Journal of Ultrasound in Medicine*, 6, 601−604.

Hill, S.J. and Hirsch, J.H. (1985) Sonographic detection of fetal hydrometrocolpos. *Journal of Ultrasound in Medicine*, 4, 323−25.

Hilpert, P.L. and Kurtz, A.B. (1990) Prenatal diagnosis of agenesis of the corpus callosum using transvaginal ultrasound. *Journal of Ultrasound in Medicine*, 9, 363−65.

Hine, D.G., Hack, A.M., Goodman, S.I. and Tanaka, K. (1986) Stable isotope dilution analysis of isovalerylglycine in amniotic fluid and urine and its application for the prenatal diagnosis of isovaleric acidemia. *Pediatric Research*, **20**, 222−26.

Hirose, K., Koyanagi, T., Hara, K. *et al.* (1988) Antenatal ultrasound diagnosis of the femur−fibula−ulna syndrome. *Journal of Clinical Ultrasound*, **16**, 199−203.

Hirsch, M., Josefsberg, Z., Schoenfeld, A. *et al.* (1990) Congenital hereditary hypothyroidism: prenatal diagnosis and treatment. *Prenatal Diagnosis*, **10**, 491−96.

Hiyama, K., Sakura, N., Matsumoto, T. and Kuhara, T. (1986) Deficient beta-ketothiolase activity in a patient with 2-methylacetoacetic aciduria. *Clinica Chimica Acta*, **155**, 189−94.

Hobbins, J.C., Romero, R., Grannum, P. *et al.* (1984) Antenatal diagnosis of renal anomalies with ultrasound. I. Obstructive uropathy. *AJR*, **148**, 868−77.

Hoffman, G.F. *et al.* (1992) Mevalonate kinase assay using DEAE-cellulose column chromatography for first-trimester prenatal diagnosis and complementation analysis in mevalonic aciduria. *Journal of Inherited Metabolic Disease*, **15**, 738−46.

Hogdall, C., Siegl-Bartelt, J., Toi, A. and Ritchie, S. (1989) Prenatal diagnosis of Opitz (BBB) syndrome in the second trimester by ultrasound detection of hypospadias and hypertelorism. *Prenatal Diagnosis*, **9**, 783−93.

Holbrook, K.A., Dale, B.A., Williams, M.L. *et al.* (1988) The expression of congenital ichthyosiform erythroderma in second trimester fetuses of the same family: morphologic and biochemical studies. *Journal of Investigative Dermatology*, **91**, 521−31.

Holbrook, K.A., Wapner, R., Jackson, L. and Zaeri, N. (1992) Diagnosis and prenatal diagnosis of epidermolysis bullosa herpetiformis (Dowling−Meara) in a mother, two affected children, and an affected fetus. *Prenatal Diagnosis*, **12**, 725−39.

Holmberg, L., Gustavi, B. and Johnson, A. (1983) A prenatal study of fetal platelet count and size with application to fetus at risk for Wiskott−Aldrich syndrome. *Journal of Pediatrics*, **102**, 773−76.

Holme, E., Kyllerman, M. and Lindstedt, S. (1989) Early prenatal diagnosis in two pregnancies at risk for glutaryl-CoA-dehydrogenase deficiency. *Journal of Inherited Metabolic Disease*, **12** (suppl. 2), 280−82.

Holton, J.B., Allen, J.T. and Gillett, M.G. (1989) Prenatal diagnosis of disorders of galactose metabolism. *Journal of Inherited Metabolic Disease*, **12** (suppl. 1), 202−206.

Holzgreve, W. (1985) Prenatal diagnosis of persistent common cloaca with prune belly and anencephaly in the second trimester. *American Journal of Medical Genetics*, **20**, 729−32.

Holzgreve, W., Mahony, B.S., Glick, P.L. *et al.* (1985) Sonographic demonstration of fetal sacrococcygeal teratoma. *Prenatal Diagnosis*, 5, 245–57.

Honour, J.W., Goolamali, S.K. and Taylor, N.F. (1985) Prenatal diagnosis and variable presentation of recessive X-linked icthyosis. *British Journal of Dermatology*, 112, 423–30.

Hornberger, L.K., Sahn, D.J., Kleinman, C.S., Copel, J. and Silverman, N.H. (1994) Antenatal diagnosis of coarctation of the aorta: A multicenter experience. *Journal of the American College of Cardiology*, 23, 417–23.

Horsthemke, B., Barnet, H.J., Greger, V. *et al.* (1987) Early diagnosis in hereditary retinoblastoma by detection of molecular deletions at gene locus. *Lancet*, i, 511–12.

Hsu, L.Y.F. (1986) Prenatal diagnosis of chromosome abnormalities, in *Genetics Disorders and the Fetus* 2nd edn (ed. A. Milunsky), Plenum Press, NY, pp. 115–83.

Huang, S.Z., Zhou, X.D., Ren, Z.R. *et al.* (1990) Prenatal detection of an Arg-Ter mutation at codon 111 of the PAH gene using DNA amplification. *Prenatal Diagnosis*, 10, 289–94.

Hubbard, A.E., Ayers, A.B., MacDonald, L.M. and James, C.F. (1984) *In utero* torsion of the testis: antenatal and postnatal ultrasonic appearances. *British Journal of Radiology*, 57, 644–46.

Hughes, I.A., Dyas, J. Riad-Fahmy, D. and Laurence, K.M. (1987) Prenatal diagnosis of congenital adrenal hyperplasia: reliability of amniotic fluid steroid analysis. *Journal of Medical Genetics*, 24, 344–47.

Hunziker, U.A., Savoldelli, G., Bolthauser, E. *et al.* (1989) Prenatal diagnosis of Schwartz–Jampel syndrome with early manifestation. *Prenatal Diagnosis*, 9, 127–31.

Huu, T.P., Dumez, Y., Marquetty, C., Durandy, A. *et al.* (1987) Prenatal diagnosis of chronic granulomatous disease (CGD) in four high risk male fetuses. *Prenatal Diagnosis*, 7, 253–60.

Iaccarino, M., Baldi, F., Persico, D. and Palagiano, A. (1986) Ultrasonographic and pathologic study of mucoid degeneration of umbilical cord. 14, 127–29.

Iaccarino, M., Lonardo, F., Guigliano, M. and Brunna, M.D. (1985) Prenatal diagnosis of Mohr syndrome by ultrasonography. *Prenatal Diagnosis*, 5, 415–18.

Iavarone, A., Dolfin, G., Bracco, G. *et al.* (1989) First trimester prenatal diagnosis of Wolman disease. *Journal of Inherited Metabolic Disease*, 12 (suppl. 2), 299–300.

Illum, N., Lavard, L., Danpure, C.J. *et al.* (1992) Primary hyperoxaluria type 1: Clinical manifestations in infancy and prenatal diagnosis. *Child Nephrology and Urology*, 12, 225–27.

Irons, M., Elias, E.R. and Tint, G.S. (1994) Abnormal cholesterol metabolism in the Smith–Lemli–Opitz syndrome: Report of clinical and biochemical findings in four patients and treatment in one patient. *American Journal of Medical Genetics*, 50, 347–52.

Ives, E.J. and Houston, C.S. (1980) Autosomal recessive microcephaly and micromelia in Cree Indians. *American Journal of Medical Genetics*, 7, 351–60.

Izquierdo, L.A., Kushnir, O., Aase, J. *et al.* (1990) Antenatal ultrasonic diagnosis of dyssegmental dysplasia: a case report. *Prenatal Diagnosis*, 10, 587–92.

Jackson, C.A., Norum, R.A. and O'Neal, J.P. (1988) Linkage between MEN2B and chromosome 10 markers linked to MEN2A. *American Journal of Human Genetics*, 43, A147.

Jacobson, R.L., St John Dignan, P., Miodovnik, M. and Siddiqi, T.A. (1992) Antley–Bixler syndrome. *Journal of Ultrasound in Medicine*, 11, 161–64.

Jaffe, R., Schoenfeld, A. and Ovadia, J. (1990) Sonographic findings in the prenatal diagnosis of bladder exstrophy. *American Journal of Obstetrics and Gynecology*, 162, 675–78.

Jakobs, C., Ogier, H., Rabier, D. and Gibson, K.M. (1993) Prenatal detection of succinic semialdehyde dehydrogenase deficiency (4-hydroxybutyric aciduria). *Prenatal Diagnosis*, 13, 150.

Jakobs, C., Stellaard, F., Kvittingen, E.A. *et al.* (1990) First trimester prenatal diagnosis of tyrosinaemia type I by amniotic fluid succinylacetone determination. *Prenatal Diagnosis*, 10, 133–39.

Jakobs, C., Stellaard, F., Smit, L.M. *et al.* (1991) The first prenatal diagnosis of dihydropyrimidine dehydrogenase deficiency. *European Journal of Pediatrics*, 150, 291.

Jakobs, C., Sweetman, L. and Wadman, S.K. (1984) Prenatal diagnosis of glutaric aciduria type II by direct chemical analysis of dicarboxylic acids in amniotic fluid. *European Journal of Paediatrics*, 141, 153–57.

Jarvela, I., Rapola, J., Peltonen, L. *et al.* (1991) DNA-based prenatal diagnosis of the infantile form of neuronal ceroid lipofuscinosis (INCL, CLN1). *Prenatal Diagnosis*, 11, 323–28.

Jaspers, N.G.J., Van der Kraan, M., Linssen, P.C.M.L. *et al.* (1990) First-trimester prenatal diagnosis of the Nijmegen breakage syndrome and ataxia telangiectasia using an assay of radioresistant DNA synthesis. *Prenatal Diagnosis*, 10, 667–74.

Jauniaux, E., Campbell, S. and Vyas, S. (1989) The use of color Doppler imaging for prenatal diagnosis of umbilical cord anomalies: report of three cases. *American Journal of Obstetrics and Gynecology*, 161, 1195–97.

Jauniaux, E., Vyas, S., Finlayson, C. *et al.* (1990) Early sonographic diagnosis of body stalk anomaly. *Prenatal Diagnosis*, 10, 127–32.

Jeanty, P. (1990) Prenatal detection of Simian crease. *Journal of Ultrasound in Medicine*, 9, 131–36.

Jeanty, P., Kepple, D., Roussis, P. and Shah, D. (1990a) *In utero* detection of cardiac failure from an aneurysm of the vein of Galen. *American Journal of Obstetrics and Gynecology*, 163, 50–51.

Jeanty, P. and Kleinman, G. (1989) Proximal femoral focal deficiency. *Journal of Ultrasound in Medicine*, 8, 639–42.

Jeanty, P., Romero, R., Kepple, D. *et al.* (1990b) Prenatal diagnosis in unilateral ampty renal fossa. *Journal of Ultrasound in Medicine*, 9, 651–54.

Jenkinson, E.L., Pfisterer, W.H., Latteier, K.K. and Martin, H. (1943) A prenatal diagnosis of osteopetrosis. *American Journal of Roentgenology*, 49, 455–61.

Johnson, J.A., McFarland, J.G., Blanchette, V.S., Freedman, J. and Siegel-Bartelt, J. (1993) Prenatal diagnosis of neonatal alloimmune thrombocytopenia using an allele-specific oligonucleotide probe. *Prenatal Diagnosis*, 13, 1037–42.

Johnson, M.L., Dunne, M.G., Mack, L.A. and Rashbaum, C.L. (1980) Evaluation of fetal intracranial anatomy by static and real-time ultrasound. *Journal of Clinical Ultrasound*, 8, 311–12.

Jones, M.Z., Rathke, E.J.S., Cavanagh, K. and Hancock,

L.W. (1984) Beta-mannosidosis: prenatal biochemical and morphological characteristics. *Journal of Inherited Metabolic Disorders*, 7, 80–85.

Jones, S.M., Robinson, L.K. and Sperrazza, R. (1990) Prenatal diagnosis of a skeletal dysplasia identified postnatally as hypochondroplasia. *American Journal of Medical Genetics*, 36, 404–407.

Journel, H., Guyot, C., Barc, R.M. *et al.* (1989) Unexpected ultrasonographic prenatal diagnosis of autosomal dominant polycystic kidney disease. *Prenatal Diagnosis*, 9, 663–71.

Journet, D., Durandy, A., Doussau, M. *et al.* (1992) Carrier detection and prenatal diagnosis of X-linked agammaglobulinemia. *American Journal of Medical Genetics*, 43, 885–87.

Junien, C., Leroux, A., Lostanlen, D. *et al.* (1981) Prenatal diagnosis of congenital enzymopenic methemoglobinaemia with mental retardation due to generalized cytochrome B_5 reductase deficiency: first report of two cases. *Prenatal Diagnosis*, 1, 17–24.

Juul, S., Ledbetter, D., Wight, T.N. and Woodrum, D. (1990) New insights into idiopathic infantile arterial calcinosis. *American Journal of Diseases of Children*, 144, 229–33.

Kainulainen, K., Pulkkinen, L., Savolainen, A. *et al.* (1990) Location on chromosome 15 of the gene defect causing Marfan syndrome. *New England Journal of Medicine*, 323, 935–39.

Kaiser, I.H. (1980) Brown amniotic fluid in congenital erythropoietic porphyria. *Obstetrics and Gynecology*, 56, 383.

Kalugdan, R.G., Satoh, S., Koyanagi, T. *et al.* (1989) Antenatal diagnosis of pulmonary arteriovenous fistula using real-time ultrasound and color Doppler flow imaging. *Journal of Clinical Ultrasound*, 17, 607–14.

Kaplan, C., Patereau, C., Reznikoff-Etievant, M.F. *et al.* (1985) Antenatal PL AI typing and detection of GP IIb–IIIa complex. *British Journal of Haematology*, 60, 586–88.

Kapoor, R., Gupta, A.K., Sing, S. *et al.* (1989a) Antenatal sonographic diagnosis of chorioangioma of placenta. *Australasian Radiology*, 33, 288–89.

Kapoor, R., Saha, M.M. and Mandal, A.K. (1989b) Antenatal sonographic detection of Wolffian duct cyst. *Journal of Clinical Ultrasound*, 17, 515–17.

Kapur, S. and Van Vloten, A. (1986) Isolated congenital bowed long bones. *Clinical Genetics*, 29, 165–67.

Katz, S., Basel, D. and Branski, D. (1988) Prenatal gastric dilatation and infantile hypertrophic pyloric stenosis. *Journal of Pediatric Surgery*, 23, 1021–22.

Kazazian, Jr, H.H. (1990) The thalassemia syndromes: molecular basis and prenatal diagnosis in 1990. *Seminars in Hematology*, 27, 209–28.

Kazazian, Jr, H.H., Boehm, C.D. and Dowling, C.E. (1985) Prenatal diagnosis of hemoglobinopathies by DNA analysis. *Annals of the New York Academy of Sciences*, 445, 337–48.

Kazazian, Jr, H.H., Dover, G.L., Lightbody, K.L. and Park, I.J. (1978) Prenatal diagnosis in a fetus at risk for haemoglobin S–O Arab disease. *Journal of Pediatrics*, 93, 502–504.

Kazazian, Jr, H.H., Phillips, D.G., Dowling, C.E. and Boehm, C.D. (1988) Prenatal diagnosis of sickle cell anaemia.

Annals of the New York Academy of Sciences, 565, 44–47.

Keller, E., Andreas, A., Scholz, S. *et al.* (1991) Prenatal diagnosis of 21-hydroxylase deficiency by RFLP analysis of the 21-hydroxylase, complement C4 and HLA class II genes. *Prenatal Diagnosis*, 11, 827–40.

Kelley, R.I. (1993) Prenatal detection of Canavan disease by measurement of N-acetyl-L-aspartate in amniotic fluid. *Journal of Inherited Metabolic Disease*, 16, 918–19.

Kennedy, K.A., Flick, K.J. and Thurmond, A.S. (1990) First trimester diagnosis of exencephaly. *American Journal of Obstetrics and Gynecology*, 162, 461–63.

Khouzam, M.N. and Hooker, J.G. (1989) The significance of prenatal diagnosis of choroid plexus cysts. *Prenatal Diagnosis*, 9, 213–16.

Kim, J.H., Lebo, R.V., Cai, S.P. *et al.* (1994) Prenatal diagnosis of unusual hemoglobinopathies. *American Journal of Medical Genetics*, 50, 15–20.

Kirk, J.S. and Comstock, C.H. (1990) Antenatal sonographic appearance of spondyloepiphyseal dysplasia congenita. *Journal of Ultrasound in Medicine*, 9, 173–75.

Kirkinen, P., Herva, R. and Leisti, J. (1987) Prenatal diagnosis of a lethal syndrome of multiple congenital contractures. *Prenatal Diagnosis*, 7, 189–96.

Kirkinen, P. and Jouppila, P. (1986) Intrauterine membranous cyst: a report of antenatal diagnosis of obstetric aspects in two cases. *Obstetrics and Gynecology*, 67, 265–305.

Kishi, F., Matsuura, S., Murano, I. *et al.* (1991) Prenatal diagnosis of infantile hypophosphatasia. *Prenatal Diagnosis*, 11, 305–309.

Kishimoto, T.K., O'Connor, K. and Springer, T.A. (1989) Leucocyte deficiency. Aberrant splicing of a conceived integrin sequence causes a moderate deficiency phenotype. *Journal of Biological Chemistry*, 264, 3588–95.

Kitchiner, D., Leung, M.P. and Arnold, R. (1990) Isolated congenital left ventricular diverticulum: echocardiographic features in a fetus. *American Heart Journal*, 119, 1435–37.

Kjoller, M., Holm-Nielsen, G., Meiland, H. *et al.* (1985) Prenatal obstruction of the ileum diagnosed by ultrasound. *Prenatal Diagnosis*, 5, 427–30.

Kleijer, W.J., Hoogeveen, A., Verheijen, F.W. *et al.* (1979) Prenatal diagnosis of sialidosis with combined neuraminidase and beta-galactosidase deficiency. *Clinical Genetics*, 16, 60–61.

Kleijer, W.J., Hussarts-Odijk, L.M., Los, F.J. *et al.* (1989) Prenatal diagnosis of purine nucleoside phosphorylase deficiency in the first and second trimesters of pregnancy. *Prenatal Diagnosis*, 9, 401–407.

Kleijer, W.J., Hussarts-Odijk, L.M., Sachs, E.S. *et al.* (1987) Prenatal diagnosis of Fabry's disease by direct analysis of chorionic villi. *Prenatal Diagnosis*, 7, 283–87.

Kleijer, W.J., Janse, H.C., Vosters, R.P.L. *et al.* (1986) First trimester diagnosis of mucopolysaccharidosis IIIA (Sanfilippo A disease). *New England Journal of Medicine*, 314, 185–86.

Kleijer, W.J., Thompson, E.J. and Niermeijer, M.F. (1983) Prenatal diagnosis of the Hurler syndrome: report on 40 pregnancies at risk. *Prenatal Diagnosis*, 3, 179–86.

Kleiner, B., Callen, P.H. and Filly, R.A. (1987) Sonographic analysis of the fetus with ureteropelvic junction obstruction. 148, 359–63.

Kleinman, C.S., Donnerstein, R.L., Devore, G.V. *et al.* (1982) Fetal echocardiography for evaluation of *in utero*, congestive heart failure. *New England Journal of Medicine*, **306**, 568−75.

Kleinman, C.S., Donnerstein, R.L., Jaffe, C.C. *et al.* (1983) Fetal echocardiography. A tool for evaluation of *in utero* cardiac arrythmias and monitoring of *in utero* therapy: analysis of 71 patients. *American Journal of Cardiology*, **51**, 237−43.

Klingensmith, W.C., Cioffi-Ragan, D.T. and Harvey, D.E. (1988) Diagnosis of ectopia cordis in the second trimester. *Journal of Clinical Ultrasound*, **16**, 204−206.

Knoers, N., Van der Heyden, H., Van Oost, B.A. *et al.* (1988) Nephrogenic diabetes insipidus-close linkage with markers from the distal long arm of the human X chromosome. *Human Genetics*, **80**, 31−38.

Ko, T.M., Hwa, H.L., Tseng, L.H., Hsieh, F.J., Huang, S.F. and Lee, T.Y. (1994) Prenatal diagnosis of X-linked hydrocephalus in a Chinese family with four successive affected pregnancies. *Prenatal Diagnosis*, **14**, 57−60.

Koga, Y., Mizumot, M., Matsumoto, M.D. *et al.* (1990) Prenatal diagnosis of fetal intracranial calcifications. *American Journal of Obstetrics and Gynecology*, **163**, 1543−45.

Kolble, K., Cant, A.J., Fay, A.C. Whaley, K., Scholesinger, M. and Reid, K.B.M. (1993) Carrier detection in families with properdin deficiency by microsatellite haplotyping. *Journal of Clinical Investigation*, **91**, 99−102.

Komrower, G.M. (1974) The philosophy and practice of screening for inherited diseases. *Pediatrics*, **53**, 182−89.

Kourides, L.A., Berkowitz, R.L., Pang, S. *et al.* (1984) Antepartum diagnosis of goitrous hypothyroidism by fetal ultrasonography and amniotic fluid thyrotrophin concentration. *Journal of Clinical Endocrinology and Metabolism*, **59**, 1016−18.

Kormarniski, C.A., Cyr, D.R., Mack, L.A. and Weinberger, E. (1990) Prenatal diagnosis of schizencephaly. *Journal of Ultrasound in Medicine*, **9**, 305−307.

Kousseff, B.G., Matsuoka, L.Y., Stenn, K.S. *et al.* (1982) Prenatal diagnosis of Sjögren−Larsen syndrome. *Journal of Pediatrics*, **101**, 998−1001.

Kovacs, B.W., Carlson, D.E., Shahbahrami, B. and Platt, L.D. (1992) Prenatal diagnosis of human parvovirus B19 in nonimmune hydrops fetalis by polymerase chain reaction. *American Journal of Obstetrics and Gynecology*, **167**, 461−66.

Kurjak, A. and Latin, V. (1979) Ultrasound diagnosis of fetal abnormalities in multiple pregnancy. *Acta Obstetricia et Gynecologica Scandinavica*, **58**, 153−61.

Kurtz, A.B., Filly, R.A, Wapner, R.J. *et al.* (1986) *In utero* analysis of heterozygous achondroplasia: variable time of onset as detected by femur length measurements. *Journal of Ultrasound in Medicine*, **5**, 137−40.

Kushnir, O., Izquierdo, L., Vigil, D. and Curet, L.B. (1990) Early transvaginal sonographic diagnosis of gastroschisis. *Journal of Clinical Ultrasound*, **18**, 194−97.

Kutzner, D.K., Wilson, W.G. and Hogge, W.A. (1988) DETS complex (cloacal exstrophy): prenatal diagnosis in the second trimester. *Prenatal Diagnosis*, **8**, 247−53.

Kvittingen, E.A., Guibaud, P.P., Divry, P. *et al.* (1986) Prenatal diagnosis of hereditary tyrosinaemia type I by determination of fumarylacetoacetase in chorionic villus

material. *European Journal of Pediatrics*, **144**, 597−98.

Labrune, P., Lyonnet, S., Zupan, V. *et al.* (1994) Three new cases of the Schinzel−Giedion syndrome and review of the literature. *American Journal of Medical Genetics*, **50**, 90−93.

Lake, B.D., Young, E.P. and Nicolaides, K. (1989) Prenatal diagnosis of infantile sialic acid storage disease in a twin pregnancy. *Journal of Inherited Metabolic Disease*, **12**, 152−56.

Lamy, M.E., Mulongo, K.N., Gadisseux, J.F. *et al.* (1992) Prenatal diagnosis of fetal cytomegalovirus infection. *American Journal of Obstetrics and Gynecology*, **166**, 91−94.

Landy, H.J., Khoury, A.N. and Heyl, P.S. (1989) Antenatal ultrasonographic diagnosis of fetal seizure activity. *American Journal of Obstetrics and Gynecology*, **161**, 308.

Langer, J.C., Brennan, B. Lappalainen, R.E. *et al.* (1992) Cloacal extrophy: Prenatal diagnosis before rupture of the cloacal membrane. *Journal of Pediatric Surgery*, **27**, 1352−55.

Langer, J.C., Khanna, J., Caco, C., Dykes, E.H. and Nicolaides, K.H. (1993) Prenatal diagnosis of gastroschisis: Development of objective sonographic criteria for predicting outcome. *Obstetrics and Gynecology*, **81**, 53−56.

Langer, R. and Kaufmann, H.J. (1986) Case report 363. Infantile cortical hyperostosis (Caffey disease ICH) of iliac bones, femora, tibiae and left fibula. *Skeletal Radiology*, **15**, 377−82.

Lau, Y.L., Levinsky, R.J., Malcolm, S. *et al.* (1988) Genetic prediction in X-linked agammaglobulinemia. *American Journal of Medical Genetics*, **31**, 437−48.

Laxova, R., O'Hara, P.T., Ridler, M.A.C. and Timothy, J.A.D. (1973) Family with probable achondrogenesis and lipid inclusions in fibroblasts. *Archives of Disease in Childhood*, **48**, 212−16.

Lazaro, C., Ravella, A., Casals, T. *et al.* (1992) Prenatal diagnosis of sporadic neurofibromatosis 1. *Lancet*, **339**, 119−20.

Lebo, R.V., Martelli, L., Su, Y. *et al.* (1993) Prenatal diagnosis of Charcot−Marie−Tooth disease type 1A by multicolor *in situ* hybridization. *American Journal of Medical Genetics*, **47**, 441−50.

Lebrun, D., Avni, E.F., Goolaerts, J.P. *et al.* (1985) Prenatal diagnosis of a pulmonary cyst by ultrasonography. *European Journal of Pediatrics*, **144**, 399−402.

Lee, W., Comstock, C.H. and Jurcak-Zaleski, S. (1992) Prenatal diagnosis of adrenal hemorrhage by ultrasonography. *Journal of Ultrasound in Medicine*, **11**, 369−71.

Lehmann, A.R., Francis, A.J. and Gianelli, F. (1985) Prenatal diagnosis of Cockayne's syndrome. *Lancet*, **i**, 486−88.

Leithiser, Jr, R.E., Fyfe, D., Weatherby, E. *et al.* (1986) Prenatal sonographic diagnosis of atrial hemangioma. *American Journal of Roentgenology*, **147**, 1207−208.

Lemna, W.K., Reldman, G.L., Kerem, B.-S. *et al.* (1990) Mutation analysis for heterozygote detection and the prenatal diagnosis of cystic fibrosis. *New England Journal of Medicine*, **322**, 291−96.

Leppert, M., Anderson, V.E., Quattlebaum, T. *et al.* (1989) Benign familial neonatal convulsions linked to genetic markers on chromosome 20. *Nature*, **337**, 647−48.

LeVinsky, R., Harvey, B., Nicolaides, K. and Rodeck, C. (1986) Antenatal diagnosis of chronic granulomatous disease. *Lancet*, i, 504.

Lichman, J.P. and Miller, E.I. (1988) Prenatal ultrasonic diagnosis of a splenic cyst. *Journal of Ultrasound in Medicine*, 7, 637–38.

Liechti-Gallati, S., Wolff, G., Ketelsen, U.P. and Braga, S. (1993) Prenatal diagnosis of X-linked centronuclear myopathy by linkage analysis. *Pediatric Research*, 33, 201–204.

Lien, J.M., Colmorgen, G.H.C., Gehret, J.F. and Evantash, A.B. (1990) Spontaneous resolution of fetal pleural effusion diagnosed during the second trimester. *Journal of Clinical Ultrasound*, 18, 54–56.

Linch, D.C., Beverley, P.C.L., Levinsky, R.J. *et al.* (1984) Prenatal diagram of three cases of severe combined immunodeficiency disease: severe T cell deficiency during the first hall of gestation in fetuses with ADA deficiency. *Clinical and Experimental Immunology*, 56, 223–32.

Lindfors, K.K., McGahan, J.P. and Walter, J.P. (1986) Fetal omphalocele and gastroschisis: pitfalls in sonographic diagnosis. *American Journal of Roentgenology*, 147, 797–800.

Lindlof, M., Kele, J., Ristola, M. *et al.* (1987) Prenatal diagnosis of X-linked chronic granulomatous disease using restriction fragment length polymorphism analysis. *Genomics*, 1, 87–92.

Liner, R.I. (1990) Intrauterine listeria infection: prenatal diagnosis by biophysical assessment and amniocentesis. *American Journal of Obstetrics and Gynecology*, 163, 1596–97.

Lingman, G., Lundstrom, N.R., Marsal, K. and Ohrlander, S. (1986) Fetal cardiac arrhythmia. Clinical outcome in 113 cases. *Acta Obstetricia et Gynecologica Scandinavica*, 65, 263–67.

Liskowska-Grospierre, B., Bohler, M.-C., Fisher, A. *et al.* (1986) Defective membrane expression of the LFA-1 complex may be secondary to the absence of the beta chain in a child with recurrent bacterial infection. *European Journal of Immunology*, 16, 205–208.

Lissens, W., Bril, T., Vercammen, M. *et al.* (1987) First trimester prenatal diagnosis of lysosomal storage disease. Study of alpha-L-fucosidase isoenzyme patterns in fetal and maternal tissue. *Annales de Biologie Clinique*, 45, 464–68.

Lissens, W., Van Lierde, M., Decaluwe, J. *et al.* (1988) Prenatal diagnosis of Hunter syndrome using fetal plasma. *Prenatal Diagnosis*, 8, 59–62.

Lituania, M., Cordone, M., Zampatti, C. *et al.* (1988) Prenatal diagnosis of a rare heteropagus. *Prenatal Diagnosis*, 8, 547–51.

Lituania, M., Passamonti, U., Cordone, M.S. *et al.* (1989) Schizencephaly: prenatal diagnosis by computed tomography and magnetic resonance imaging. *Prenatal Diagnosis*, 9, 649–55.

Llewellyn, D.H., Elder, G.H., Kalsheker, N.A. *et al.* (1987) DNA polymorphism of human porphobilinogen deaminase gene in acute intermittent porphyria. *Lancet*, ii, 706–708.

Lobaccaro, J.M., Lumbroso, S., Carre Pigeon, F. *et al.* (1992) Prenatal prediction of androgen insensitivity syndrome using exon 1 polymorphism of the androgen receptor gene. *Journal of Steroid Biochemistry and Molecular Biology*, 43, 659–63.

Lockwood, C., Irons, M., Troiani, J. *et al.* (1988) The pre-

natal sonographic diagnosis of lethal multiple pterygium syndrome: a heritable cause of recurrent abortion. *American Journal of Obstetrics and Gynecology*, 159, 474–76.

Loewy, J.A., Richards, D.G. and Toi, A. (1987) In-utero diagnosis of the caudal regression syndrome: report of three cases. *Journal of Clinical Ultrasound*, 15, 469–74.

Lonenz, P., Bollmann, R., Hinkel, G.K. *et al.* (1991) False-negative prenatal exclusion of Wiskott–Aldrich syndrome by measurement of fetal platelet count and size. *Prenatal Diagnosis*, 11, 819–25.

Loverro, G., Guanti, G., Carso, G. and Selvaggi, L. (1990) Robinow's syndrome: prenatal diagnosis. *Prenatal Diagnosis*, 10, 121–26.

Lowden, J.A., Cutz, E., Conen, P.F. *et al.* (1973) Prenatal diagnosis of GML-gangliosidosis. *New England Journal of Medicine*, 288, 225–28.

Lungarotti, M.S., Martello, C., Marinelli, I. and Falasca, L. (1993) Lethal short rib syndrome of the Beemer type without polydactyly. *Pediatric Radiology*, 23, 325–26.

Luthy, D.A., Mack, I., Hirsch, J. *et al.* (1981) Prenatal ultrasound diagnosis of thrombocytopenia with absent radii. *American Journal of Obstetrics and Gynecology*, 141, 3350–51.

Lux, S.E., Tse, W.T., Menninger, J.C. *et al.* (1990) Hereditary spherocytosis associated with deletion of human erythrocyte ankyrin gene on chromosome 8. *Nature*, 345, 736–39.

Lynch, L., Bussel, J., Goldberg, J.D. *et al.* (1988) The *in utero* diagnosis and management of autoimmune thrombocytopenia. *Prenatal Diagnosis*, 8, 329–31.

Maasen, J.A., Lindhout, D., Reuss, A. and Kleijer, W.J. (1990) Prenatal analysis of insulin receptor autophosphorylation in a family with leprechaunism. *Prenatal Diagnosis*, 10, 13–16.

McAlister, W.H., Wright, Jr, J.R. and Crane, J.P. (1987) Main-stem bronchial atresia: intrauterine sonographic diagnosis. *American Journal of Roentgenology*, 148, 364–66.

McCabe, E., Sadava, P., Bullen, W. *et al.* (1982) Human glycerol kinase deficiency: enzyme kinetics and fibroblast hybridisation. *Journal of Inherited Metabolic Disease*, 5, 177–82.

MacDermot, K.D., Morgan, S.H., Cheshire, J.K. and Wilson, T.M. (1987) Anderson–Fabry disease, a close linkage with highly polymorphic DNA markers DXS17, DXS87 and DXS88. *Human Genetics*, 77, 263–66.

McFarland, J.G., Aster, R.H., Bussel, J.B. *et al.* (1991) Prenatal diagnosis of neonatal alloimmune thrombocytopenia using allele-specific oligonucleotide probes. *Blood*, 78, 2276–82.

McFarland, S.L. (1929) Congenital dislocation of the knee. *Journal of Bone and Joint Surgery*, 11, 281.

McGahan, J.P., Ellis, W., Lindfors, K.K. *et al.* (1988) Prenatal sonographic diagnosis of VATER association. *JW*, 16, 588–91.

McGahan, J.P., Haesslein, H.C., Meyers, M. and Ford, K.B. (1984) Sonographic recognition of *in utero* intraventricular hemorrhage. *American Journal of Roentgenology*, 142, 171–73.

McGahan, J.P. and Hanson, J. (1983) Meconium peritonitis with accompanying pseudocyst: prenatal sonographic diagnosis. *Radiology*, **148**, 125–26.

McGahan, J.P., Nyberg, D.A. and Mack, L.A. (1990) Sonography of facial features of alobar and senilobar holoprosencephaly. *American Journal of Roentgenology*, **154**, 143–48.

McGahan, J.P. and Schneider, J.M. (1986) Fetal neck hemangiondothelioma with secondary hydrops fetalis: sonographic diagnosis. *Journal of Clinical Ultrasound*, **14**, 384–88.

McIntosh, N., Chitayat, D., Bardanis, M. and Fouron, J.C. (1992) Ebstein anomaly: Report of a familial occurrence and prenatal diagnosis. *American Journal of Medical Genetics*, **42**, No. 3, 307–309.

McNamara, H.M., Onwude, J.L. and Thornton, J.G. (1994) Megacystis–microcolon–intestinal hypoperistalsis syndrome: A case report supporting autosomal recessive inheritance. *Prenatal Diagnosis*, **14**, 153–54.

Machin, G.A. and Corsello, G. (1992) Thanatophoric dysplasia in monozygotic twins discordant for cloverleaf skull: Prenatal diagnosis, clinical and pathological findings. *American Journal of Medical Genetics*, **44**, 842–43.

Mack, L., Gottesfeld, K. and Johnson, M.L. (1978) Antenatal detection of ectopic fetal liver by ultrasound. *Journal of Clinical Ultrasound*, **6**, 226–27.

Macken, M.B., Grantmyre, E.B. and Vincer, M.L. (1989) Regression of nuchal cystic hygroma *in utero*. *Journal of Ultrasound in Medicine*, **8**, 101–103.

McKusick, V.A. (1990) *Mendelian Inheritance in Man. Catalogs of Autosomal Dominant, Autosomal Recessive and X-linked Traits*, 9th edn, Johns Hopkins University Press, Baltimore.

McRae, S.M., Speed, R.A. and Sommerville, A.J. (1982) Intrauterine skull fracture diagnosed by ultrasound. *Australian and New Zealand Journal of Obstetrics and Gynaecology*, **22**, 159–60.

Maenpaa, J., Lindahl, E., Aula, P. and Savontaus, M.-L. (1990) Prenatal diagnosis in Pelizaeus–Merzbacher disease using RFLP analysis. *Clinical Genetics*, **37**, 141–46.

Mahoney, M.J. and Hobbins, J.C. (1977) Prenatal diagnosis of chondroectodermal dysplasia (Ellis–Van Creveld syndrome) with fetoscopy and ultrasound. *New England Journal of Medicine*, **297**, 258–60.

Mahony, B.S., Filly, R.A, Callen, P.W. and Golbus, M.S. (1985) The amniotic band syndrome: antenatal sonographic diagnosis and potential pitfalls. *American Journal of Obstetrics and Gynecology*, **152**, 63–68.

Mahony, B.S., Filly, R.A., Callen, P.W. *et al.* (1984b) Severe nonimmune hydrops fetalis: sonographic evaluation. *Radiology*, **151**, 757–61.

Mahony, B.S., Filly, R.A. and Cooperberg, P.L. (1984a) Antenatal sonographic diagnosis of achondrogenesis. *Journal of Ultrasound in Medicine*, **3**, 333–35.

Maire, I., Mandon, G. and Mathieu, M. (1989) First trimester prenatal diagnosis of glycogen storage disease type III. *Journal of Inherited Metabolic Disease*, **12** (suppl. 2), 292–94.

Maire, I., Mandon, G., Zabot, M.T. *et al.* (1979) Beta-Glucuronidase deficiency: enzyme studies in an affected family and prenatal diagnosis. *Journal of Inherited Metabolic Disease*, **2**, 29–34.

Majoor-Krakauer, D.F., Waldimiroff, J.W., Stewart, P.A. *et al.* (1987) Microcephaly, micrognathia, and bird-headed

dwarfism: prenatal diagnosis of a Seckel-like syndrome. *American Journal of Medical Genetics*, **27**, 183–88.

Malinger, G., Rosen, N., Achiron, R. and Zakut, H. (1987) Pierre Robin sequence associated with amniotic band syndrome. Ultrasonographic diagnosis and pathogenesis. *Prenatal Diagnosis*, **7**, 455–59.

Mann, L., Alroomi, L., McNay, M. and Ferguson-Smith, M.A. (1983) Placental haemangioma: case report. *British Journal of Obstetrics and Gynaecology*, **90**, 983–86.

Manni, M., Heydanus, R., Den Hollander, N.S., Stewart, P.A., De Vogelaere, C. and Wladimiroff, J.W. (1994) Prenatal diagnosis of congenital diaphragmatic hernia: A retrospective analysis of 28 cases. *Prenatal Diagnosis*, **14**, 187–90.

Mao, K. and Adams, J. (1983) Antenatal diagnosis of intracranial arteriovenous fistula by ultrasonography. Case report. *British Journal of Obstetrics and Gynaecology*, **90**, 872–73.

Marino, J., Martinez-Urrutia, M.J., Hawkins, F. and Gonzalez, A. (1990) Encysted adrenal haemorrhage. Prenatal diagnosis. *Acta Paediatrica Scandinavica*, **79**, 230–31.

Mariona, F., McAlpin, G., Zador, I. *et al.* (1986) Sonographic detection of fetal extrathoracic pulmonary sequestration. *Journal of Ultrasound in Medicine*, **5**, 283–85.

Marks, F., Hernanz-Schulman, M., Horri, S. *et al.* (1989) Spondylthoracic dysplasia. Clinical and sonographic diagnosis. *Journal of Ultrasound in Medicine*, **8**, 1–5.

Marks, F., Thomas, P., Lustig, I. *et al.* (1990) *In utero* sonographic description of a fetal liver adenoma. *Journal of Ultrasound in Medicine*, **9**, 119–22.

Marquet, J., Chadefaux, B., Bonnefont, J.P. Saudubray, J.M. and Zittoun, J. (1994) Methylenetetrahydrofolate reductase deficiency: Prenatal diagnosis and family studies. *Prenatal Diagnosis*, **14**, 29–33.

Martini, G., Toniolo, D., Vulliamy, T. *et al.* (1986) Structural analysis of the X-linked gene encoding human glucose-6-phosphate dehydrogenase. *European Molecular Biology Organisation Journal*, **5**, 1849–55.

Martini, N. (1952) Case reports: osteopoikilosis (spotted bones) *British Journal of Radiology*, **25**, 612–14.

Matalon, R., Michals, K. and Gashkoff, P. (1992). Prenatal diagnosis of Canavan's disease. *Journal of Inherited Metabolic Disease*, **15**, 392–94.

Mathew, C.G.P., Chin, K.S., Easton, D.F. *et al.* (1987) A linked genetic marker for multiple endocrine neoplasia type 2a on chromosome 10. *Nature*, **328**, 528–30.

Mayes, J.S., Say, B. and Marcus, D.L. (1987) Prenatal studies in a family with transcobalamin II deficiency. *American Journal of Human Genetics*, **41**, 686–87.

Meizner, I., Barki, Y. and Hertzanu, Y. (1987) Prenatal sonographic diagnosis of agenesis of corpus callosum. *Journal of Clinical Ultrasound*, **15**, 262–64.

Meizner, I. and Bar-Ziv, J. (1985) Prenatal ultrasonic diagnosis of short-rib polydactyly syndrome (SRPS) type III: a case report and a proposed approach to the diagnosis of SRPS and related conditions. *Journal of Clinical Ultrasound*, **13**, 284–87.

Meizner, I. and Bar-Ziv, J. (1989) Prenatal ultrasonic detection of short rib polydactyly syndrome type I. A case report. *Journal of Reproductive Medicine*, **34**, 668–72.

Meizner, I. and Bar-Ziv, J. (1987) Prenatal ultrasonic diagnosis of a rare case of iniencephaly apertus. *Journal of*

Clinical Ultrasound, 15, 200–203.

Meizner, I., Bar-Ziv, J., Barki and Abellovich D. (1986a) Prenatal ultrasonic diagnosis of radial-ray apiasa and renal anomalies (acrorenal syndrome). Prenatal Diagnosis, 6, 223–25.

Meizner, I., Bar-Ziv, J. and Katz, M. (1985) Prenatal ultrasonic diagnosis of the extreme form of prune belly syndrome. Journal of Clinical Ultrasound, 13, 581–83.

Meizner, I., Carmi, R. and Bar-Ziv, J. (1986b) Congenital chylothorax: prenatal ultrasonic diagnosis and successful post partum management. Prenatal Diagnosis, 6, 217–21.

Melki, J., Abdelhak, S., Burlet, P. et al. (1992) Prenatal prediction of Werdnig–Hoffman disease using linked polymorphic DNA probes. Journal of Medical Genetics, 29, 171–74.

Menashe, Y., Baruch, G.B., Rabinovitch, O. et al. (1989) Exophthalmos: prenatal ultrasonic features for diagnosis of Crouzon syndrome. Prenatal Diagnosis, 9, 805–808.

Mennuti, M.T., Zackai, E.H., Curtis, M.T. et al. (1990) Early ultrasound diagnosis of Neu–Laxova syndrome. American Journal of Human Genetics, 47, A281.

Mensink, E.J.B.M., Thompson, A., Sandkuyl, L.A. et al. (1987) X-linked immunodeficiency with hyperimmunoglobulinaemia M appears to be linked to DXS42 restriction fragment length polymorphism locus. Human Genetics, 76, 96–99.

Mercado, M.G., Bulas, D.I. and Chandra, R. (1993) Prenatal diagnosis and management of congenital volvulus. Pediatric Radiology, 23, 601–602.

Merlob, P., Schonfeld, A., Grunebaum, M. et al. (1987) Autosomal dominant cerebro-costo-mandibular syndrome: ultrasonographic and clinical findings. American Journal of Medical Genetics, 26, 195–202.

Mibashan, R.S., Millar, D.S., Rodeck, C.H. et al. (1985) Prenatal diagnosis of hereditary protein C deficiency. New England Journal of Medicine, 313, 1607.

Mibashan, R.S. and Rodeck, C.H. (1984) Haemophilia and other genetic defects of haemostasis, in Prenatal Diagnosis, Proceedings of the 11th RCOG Study Group (eds C.H. Rodeck and K.H. Nicolaides), Wiley Chichester.

Mibashan, R.S., Rodeck, C.H., Thumpston, J.K. et al. (1979) Plasma assay of fetal factors VIIIC and IX for prenatal diagnosis of haemophilia. Lancet, i, 1309–11.

Michelson, A.M., Blake, C.C.F., Evans, S.T. and Orkin, S.H. (1985) Structure of the human phosphoglycerate kinase gene and the intron-mediated evolution and dispersal of the nucleotide binding domain. Proceedings of the National Academy of Sciences of the USA, 82, 6965–69.

Middleton-Price, H.R., Harding, A.E., Monteiro, O. et al. (1990) Linkage of hereditary motor and sensory neuropathy type I to the pericentromeric region of chromosome 17. American Journal of Human Genetics, 46, 92–94.

Minelli, A., Danesino, C., Curto, F.L. et al. (1988) First trimester prenatal diagnosis of Sanfilippo disease (MPS III) type B. Prenatal Diagnosis, 8, 47–52.

Mintz, M.C., Arger, P.H. and Coleman, B.G. (1985) In utero sonographic diagnosis of intracerebral haemorrhage. Journal of Ultrasound in Medicine, 4, 375–76.

Mirk, P., Pintus, C. and Speca, S. (1994) Ultrasound diagnosis of hydrocolpos: Prenatal findings and postnatal follow-up. Journal of Clinical Ultrasound, 22, 55–58.

Miro, J. and Bard, H. (1988) Congenital atresia and stenosis of the duodenum: the impact of a prenatal diagnosis. American Journal of Obstetrics and Gynecology, 158, 555–59.

Mitchell, C., Nicolaides, K., Kingston, J. et al. (1988) Prenatal exclusion of hereditary retinoblastoma. Lancet, i, 826.

Mitchell, G.A., Brody, L. C., Sipila, I. et al. (1989) At least two mutant alleles of ornithine delta-aminotransferase cause gyrate atrophy of the choriod and retina in Finns. Proceedings of the National Academy of Sciences of the USA, 86, 197–201.

Mitchell, G., Saudubray, J.M., Benoit, Y. et al. (1983) Antenatal diagnosis of glutaric aciduria type II. Lancet, i, 1099.

Moodley, T.R., Vaughan, J.E., Chuntapursat, I. et al. (1986) Congenital heart block detected in utero. A case report. South African Medical Journal, 70, 433–34.

Morgan-Capner, P., Rodeck, C.H., Nicolaides, K.H. and Cradock-Watson, J.E. (1985) Prenatal detection of rubella-specific IgM in fetal sera. Prenatal Diagnosis, 5, 21–26.

Morin, P.R. (1981) Prenatal detection of the autosomal recessive type of polycystic kidney disease by trenalase assay in amniotic fluid. Prenatal Diagnosis, 1, 5–9.

Morin, P.R. (1984) Prenatal detection of the congenital nephrotic syndrome (Finnish type) by trenalase assay in amniotic fluid. Prenatal Diagnosis, 4, 257–60.

Morris, M., Nichols, W. and Benson, M. (1991) Prenatal diagnosis of hereditary amyloidosis in a Portuguese family. American Journal of Medical Genetics, 39, 123–24.

Morris, S.A., Ohanian, V., Lewis, M.L. et al. (1986) Prenatal diagnosis of hereditary red cell membrane defect. British Journal of Haematology, 62, 763–72.

Morrow, R.J., Whittle, M.J., McNay, M.B., Raine, P.A.M., Gibson, A.A.M. and Crossley, J. (1993) Prenatal diagnosis and management of anterior abdominal wall defects in the West of Scotland. Prenatal Diagnosis, 13, 111–15.

Morse, R.P., Rawnsley, E., Crowe, H.C. et al. (1987a) Bilateral renal agenesis in three consecutive siblings. Prenatal Diagnosis, 7, 573–79.

Morse, R.P., Rawnsley, E., Sargent, S.K. and Graham, J.M. (1987b) Prenatal diagnosis of a new syndrome: holoprosencephaly with hypokinesia. Prenatal Diagnosis, 7, 631–38.

Mostello, D., Hoechstetter, L., Bendon, R.W. et al. (1991) Prenatal diagnosis of recurrent Larsen syndrome: further definition of a lethal variant. Prenatal Diagnosis, 11, 215–25.

Mulligan, G. and Meier, P. (1989) Lipoma and agenesis of the corpus callosum with associated choroid plexus lipomas. In utero diagnosis. Journal of Ultrasound in Medicine, 8, 583–88.

Murer-Orlando, M., Llerena, J.C. Jr, Birjandi, F., Gibson, R.A. and Mathew, C.G. (1993) FACC gene mutations and early prenatal diagnosis of Fanconi's anaemia. Lancet, 342, 686.

Murphy, P.D., Wilmot, P.L. and Shapiro, J.R. (1992) Prenatal diagnosis of fragile X syndrome: Results from parallel molecular and cytogenetic studies. American Journal of Medical Genetics, 43, 181–86.

Myring, J., Meredith, A.L., Harley, H.G. et al. (1992) Specific molecular prenatal diagnosis for the CTG mutation in myotonic dystrophy. Journal of Medical Genetics, 29, 785–88.

Nadler, H.L. and Egan, T.J. (1970) Deficiency of lysosomal acid phosphatase. A new familial metabolic disorder. *New England Journal of Medicine*, 282, 302–307.

Naides, S.J. and Weiner, C.P. (1989) Antenatal diagnosis and palliative treatment of non-immune hydrops fetalis secondary to fetal parvovirus B19 infection. *Prenatal Diagnosis*, 9, 105–114.

Naito, E., Ozasa, H., Ikeda, Y. and Tanaka, K. (1989) Molecular cloning and nucleotide sequence of complementary DNAs encoding human short chain acyl coenzyme A dehydrogenase and the study of the molecular basis of human short chain acyl-coenzyme A dehydrogenase deficiency. *Journal of Clinical Investigation*, 83, 1605–13.

Nakamoto, S.K., Dreilinger, A., Dattel, B. *et al.* (1983) The sonographic appearance of hepatic hemangioma *in utero*. *Journal of Ultrasound in Medicine*, 2, 239–41.

Nakamura, M., Imajoh-Ohmi, S., Kanegasaki, S. *et al.* (1990) Prenatal diagnosis of cytochrome-deficient chronic granulomatous disease. *Lancet*, 336, 118–19.

Nancarrow, P.A., Mattrey, R.F., Edwards, D.K. and Skram, C. (1985) Fibroadhesive meconium peritonitis: *in utero* sonographic diagnosis. *Journal of Ultrasound in Medicine*, 4, 213–15.

Narayan, H. and Scott I.V. (1991) Prenatal ultrasound diagnosis of Apert's syndrome. *Prenatal Diagnosis*, 10, 187–92.

Narisawa, K., Gibson, K.M., Sweetman, L. *et al.* (1986) Deficiency of 3-methyl-glutaconyl-coenzyme A hydratase in two siblings with 3-methylglutaconic I aciduria. *Journal of Clinical Investigation*, 77, 1148–52.

Navon, R., Sandbank, U., Frisch, A. *et al.* (1986) Adult-onset GM$_2$ gangliosidosis diagnosed in a fetus. *Prenatal Diagnosis*, 6, 169–76.

Nazzaro, V., Nicolini, U., Deluca, L. *et al.* (1990) Prenatal diagnosis of junctional epidermolysis bullosa associated with pyloric atresia. *Journal of Medical Genetics*, 27, 244–48.

Neilson, J.P., Danskin, F. and Hastie, S.J. (1989) Monozygotic twin pregnancy: diagnostic and Doppler ultrasound studies. *British Journal of Obstetrics and Gynaecology*, 96, 1413–18.

Newgard, C.B., Fletterick, R.J., Anderson, L.A. and Lebo, R.V. (1987) The polymorphic locus for glycogen storage disease VI (liver glycogen phosphorylase) maps to chromosome 14. *American Journal of Human Genetics*, 40, 351–64.

Newnham, J.P., Crues, J.V. III, Vinstein, A.L. and Medeatis, A.L. (1984) Sonographic diagnosis of thoracic gastroenteric cyst *in utero*. *Prenatal Diagnosis*, 4, 467–71.

Nguyen, D.L. and Leonard, J.C. (1986) Ischemic hepatic necrosis: a cause of fetal liver calcification. *American Journal of Roentgenology*, 147, 596–97.

Nichols, W.C. and Benson, M.D. (1990) Hereditary amyloidosis: detection of variant prealbumin genes by restriction enzyme analysis of amplified genomic DNA sequences. *Clinical Genetics*, 37, 44–53.

Nichols, W.C., Padilla, L.-M. and Benson, M.D. (1989) Prenatal detection of a gene for hereditary amyloidosis. *American Journal of Medical Genetics*, 34, 520–24.

Nicolaides, K.H., Campbell, S., Gabbe, S.G. and Guidetti, R. (1986) Ultrasound screening for spina bifida: cranial and cerebellar signs. *Lancet*, ii, 72–74.

Nicolaides, K.H., Johansson, D., Donnai, D. and Rodeck, C.H. (1984) Prenatal diagnosis of mandibulofacial dysostosis. *Prenatal Diagnosis*, 4, 201–205.

Niederwieser, A. (1986) Prenatal diagnosis of dihydrobiopterin synthetase deficiency: a variant form of phenylketonuria. *European Journal of Pediatrics*, 145, 176–78.

Nishi, T. and Nakano, R. (1994) Amniotic band syndrome: Serial ultrasonographic observations in the first trimester. *Journal of Clinical Ultrasound*, 2, 275–78.

Nitowsky, H.M., Sassa, S., Nakagawa, M. and Jagani, B. (1978) Prenatal diagnosis of congenital erythropoietic porphyria. *Pediatric Research*, 12, 455.

Noguchi, M., Yi, H., Rosenblatt H.M. *et al.* (1993) Interleukin-2 receptor gamma chain mutation results in X-linked severe combined immunodeficiency in humans. *Cell*, 73, 147–57.

Northrup, H., Beaudet, A.L. and O'Brien, E.W. (1990) Prenatal diagnosis of citrullinaemia: review of a 10-year experience including recent use of DNA analysis. *Prenatal Diagnosis*, 10, 771–79.

Novelli, G., Frontali, M., Baldini, D. *et al.* (1989) Prenatal diagnosis of adult polycystic kidney disease with DNA markers on chromosome 16 and the genetic heterogeneity problem. *Prenatal Diagnosis*, 9, 759–67.

Nowakowski, R.W., Thompson, J.N. and Taylor, K.B. (1989) Sanfilippo syndrome, type D: a spectrophotometric assay with prenatal diagnostic potential. *Pediatric Research*, 26, 462–66.

Nyberg, D.A., Hallesy, D., Mahony, B.S. *et al.* (1990a) Meckel–Gruber syndrome. Importance of prenatal diagnosis. *Journal of Ultrasound in Medicine*, 9, 691–96.

Nyberg, D.A., Hastrup, W., Watts, H. and Mack, L.A. (1987) Dilated fetal bowel. A sonographic sign of cystic fibrosis. *Journal of Ultrasound in Medicine*, 6, 257–60.

Nyberg, D.A., Resta, R.G., Luthy, D.A. *et al.* (1990b) Prenatal sonographic findings of Down syndrome: review of 94 cases. *Obstetrics and Gynecology*, 76, 370–77.

O'Donnell, J. (1981) Gyrate atrophy of the retina and choroid. *International Ophthalmology*, 4, 33–36.

Ogier, H., Wadman, S.K., Johnson, J.L. *et al.* (1983) Antenatal diagnosis of combined xanthine and sulphite oxidase deficiencies. *Lancet*, ii, 1363–64.

Ohdo, S., Madokoro, H., Sonoda, T. *et al.* (1987) Association of tetra-amelia, octodermal dysplasia, hypoplastic lacrimal ducts and sacs opening towards the exterior, peculiar face and developmental retardation. *Journal of Medical Genetics*, 24, 609–12.

Ohlsson, A., Fong, K.W., Rose, T.H. and Moore, D.C. (1988) Prenatal sonographic diagnosis of Pena–Shokeir syndrome type I, or fetal akinesia deformation sequence. *American Journal of Medical Genetics*, 29, 59–65.

Okamura, K., Murotsuki, J., Sakai, T., Matsumoto, K., Shirane, R. and Yajima, A. (1993) Prenatal diagnosis of lissencephaly by magnetic resonance image. *Fetal Diagnosis and Therapy* 8, 56–59.

Old, J.M., Fitches, A., Heath, C. *et al.* (1986) First trimester fetal diagnosis for haemoglobinopathies: report on 200 cases. *Lancet*, ii, 763–67.

Old, J.M., Varawalla, N.Y. and Weatherall, D.J. (1990) Rapid detection and prenatal diagnosis of beta-thalassaemia in Indian and Cypriot populations in the UK. *Lancet*, ii, 834–37.

Ordorica, S.A., Marks, F., Frieden, F.J. *et al.* (1990) Aneurysm of the vein of Galen: a new cause for Ballantyne syndrome. *American Journal of Obstetrics and Gynecology*, **162**, 1166–67.

Orney, A., Arnon, J., Grebner, E. *et al.* (1987) Early prenatal diagnosis of mucolipidosis IV. *American Journal of Medical Genetics*, **27**, 983–85.

Owerbach, D., Draznin, M.B., Carpenter, R.J. and Greenberg, F. (1992) Prenatal diagnosis of 21-hydroxylase deficiency congenital adrenal hyperplasia using the polymerase chain reaction. *Human Genetics*, **89**, 109–110.

Pachi, A., Giancotti, A., Torci, F. *et al.* (1989) Meckel–Gruber syndrome. *Prenatal Diagnosis*, **9**, 187–90.

Pachi, A., Maggi E., Giancotti, A. *et al.* (1992) Prenatal diagnosis of diastematomyelia in a diabetic woman. *Prenatal Diagnosis*, **12**, 535–39.

Packman, S., Cowan, M.J., Golbus, M.S. *et al.* (1982) Prenatal treatment of biotin-responsive multiple carboxylase deficiency. *Lancet*, i, 1435–39.

Pagliano, M., Mossetti, M. and Ragno, P. (1990) Echographic diagnoses of omphalocele in the first trimester of pregnancy. *Journal of Clinical Ultrasound*, **18**, 658–60.

Pannone, N., Gatti, R., Lombardo, C. *et al.* (1986) Prenatal diagnosis of Hunter syndrome. *Prenatal Diagnosis*, **6**, 107–10.

Parvy, P., Rabier, D., Boue, J. *et al.* (1990) Glycine/serine ratio and prenatal diagnosis of non-ketotic hyperglycaemia. *Prenatal Diagnosis*, **10**, 303–305.

Patel, P., Kolawole, T., Ba'Aguiel, H. *et al.* (1989) Antenatal sonographic findings in congenital chloride diarrhea. *Journal of Clinical Ultrasound*, **17**, 115–18.

Patrick, A., Young, E., Ellis, C. *et al.* (1988) Multiple sulphatase deficiency. *Prenatal Diagnosis*, **8**, 303–306.

Patrick, A., Young, R., Mossman, J. *et al.* (1987) First trimester diagnosis of cystinosis. *Prenatal Diagnosis*, **7**, 71–74.

Patterson, M.C., Pentchev, P.G., Lake, B.D. and Kelly, D.A. (1994) Diagnosis of Niemann–Pick disease type C. *Journal of Pediatrics*, **124**, 655–56.

Patten, R.M., Mack, L.A., Nyberg, D.A. and Filly, R.A. (1989) Twin embolisation syndrome: prenatal sonographic detection and significance. *Radiology*, **173**, 685–89.

Patti, G., Fiocca, G., Latini, T., Celli, E., Bellussi, A. and Nazzicone, P. (1993) Prenatal diagnosis of bilateral adrenal cysts. *Journal of Urology*, **150**(4), 1189–91.

Patton, M., Baraister, M., Nicolaides, K. *et al.* (1986) Prenatal treatment of hydrops (Opitz-G syndrome). *Prenatal Diagnosis*, **6**, 109–15.

Pekonen, F., Tetamo, K., Makinen, T. *et al.* (1984) Prenatal diagnosis and treatment of fetal thyrotoxicosis. *American Journal of Obstetrics and Gynecology*, **150**, 893–94.

Peled, Y., Hod, M., Friedman, S., Mashiach, R., Greenberg, N. and Ovadia, J. (1992) Prenatal diagnosis of familial congenital pyloric atresia. *Prenatal Diagnosis*, **12**, 151–54.

Peleg, D., Golichowski, A.M. and Ragan, W.D. (1985) Fetal hydrothorax and bilateral pulmonary hypoplasia. Ultrasonic diagnosis. *Acta Obstetricia and Gynecologica Scandinavica*, **64**, 451–53.

Pellissier, M.C., Philip, N., Potier, A. *et al.* (1992) Prenatal diagnosis of Fryns' syndrome. *Prenatal Diagnosis*, **12**, 299–303.

Pennel, R.G. and Baltatowich, O.H. (1986) Prenatal sonographic diagnosis of a fetal facial haemangioma. *Journal of Ultrasound in Medicine*, 5, 523–25.

Perelman, A.H., Johnson, R.H., Clemons, R.D. *et al.* (1990) Intrauterine diagnosis and treatment of fetal goitrous hypothyroidism. *Journal of Clinical Endocrinology and Metabolism*, **71**, 618–21.

Perez-Cerda, C., Merinero, B. and Jimenez, A. (1993) First report of prenatal diagnosis of long-chain 3-hydroxyacyl-CoA dehydrogenase deficiency in a pregnancy at risk. *Prenatal Diagnosis*, **13**, 529–33.

Perez-Cerda, C., Merinero, B., Sanz, P. *et al.* (1989) Successful first trimester diagnosis in a pregnancy at risk for propionic acidemia. *Journal of Inherited Metabolic Disease*, **12** (suppl. 2), 274–76.

Perry, T.B., Holbrook, K.A., Hoff, M.S. *et al.* (1987) Prenatal diagnosis of congenital non-bullous ichthyosiform erythroderma (lamellar ichthyosis). *Prenatal Diagnosis*, 7, 145–55.

Persutte, W.H. and Hobbins, J.C. (1994) First trimester prenatal sonographic diagnosis of Smith–Lemli–Opitz syndrome, type II with a prototypic flexible embryoscope. *Journal of Diagnostic Medical Sonography*, **10**, 39–40.

Persutte, W.H., Lenke, R.R and Derosa, R.T. (1990) Prenatal ultrasonographic appearance of the agnatnia malformation complex. *Journal of Ultrasound in Medicine*, 9, 725–28.

Persutte, W.H., Lenke, R.R., Kropp, K. and Ghareeb, C. (1988b) Antenatal diagnosis of fetal patent uracus. *Journal of Ultrasound in Medicine*, 7, 399–403.

Persutte, W.H., Lenke, R.R., Krczynski, T.W. and Brinker, R.A. (1988a) Antenatal diagnosis of Pena–Skokeir syndrome (type I) with ultrasonography and magnetic resonance imaging. *Obstetrics and Gynecology*, **72**, 472–75.

Peters, M.T. and Nicolaides, K.H. (1990) Cordocentesis for the diagnosis and treatment of human fetal parvovirus infection. *Obstetrics and Gynecology*, **75**, 501–504.

Petres, R.E., Redwine, F.O. and Cruikshank, D.P. (1982) Congenital bilateral chylothorax. Antepartum diagnosis and successful intrauterine surgical management. *JAMA*, **248**, 1360–61.

Petrikovsky, B.M., Vintzileos, A.M. and Rodis, J.F. (1989) Sonographic appearance of occipital fetal hair. *Journal of Clinical Ultrasound*, **17**, 425–27.

Petrikovsky, B.M., Walzak, M.P. and D'Addario, P.F. (1988) Fetal cloacal anomalies: prenatal sonographic findings and differential diagnosis. *Obstetrics and Gynecology*, **72**, 464–69.

Petrova-Benedict, R., Robinson, B.H., Stacey, T.E. *et al.* (1987) Deficient fumarase activity in an infant with fumaricacidemia and its distribution between different forms of the enzyme seen on isoelectric focussing. *American Journal of Human Genetics*, **40**, 257–266.

Phillips, J.A., Hjelle, B.L., Seeburg, P.H. and Zachmann, M. (1981) Molecular basis for familial isolated growth hormone deficiency. *Proceedings of the National Academy of Sciences of the USA*, **78**, 6372–75.

Piepkorn, M., Karp, L.E., Hickok, D. *et al.* (1977) A lethal neonatal dwarfing condition with short ribs, polysyndactyly, cranial synostosis, cleft palate, cardiovascular and urogenital anomalies and severe ossification defect. *Teratology*, **16**, 345–50.

Pilu, G., Reece, A., Romero, R. *et al.* (1986a) Prenatal diagnosis of craniofacial malformations with ultrasonography. *American Journal of Obstetrics and Gynecology*, **155**, 45–50.

Pilu, G., Romero, R., Reece, A. *et al.* (1986b) The prenatal diagnosis of Robin anomalad. *American Journal of Obstetrics and Gynecology*, **154**, 630–32.

Pircon, R.A., Porto, M., Towers, C.V. *et al.* (1989) Ultrasound findings in pregnancies complicated by fetal triploidy. *Journal of Ultrasound in Medicine*, **8**, 507–11.

Poenaru, I. (1982) Prenatal diagnosis of a heterozygote for mucopolysaccharidosis type VII (beta-glucuronidase deficiency). *Prenatal Diagnosis*, **2**, 251–56.

Poenaru, L. (1987) First trimester prenatal diagnosis of metabolic diseases: a survey in countries from the European community. *Prenatal Diagnosis*, **7**, 333–41.

Poenaru, L., Castelnau, L., Besancon, A.-M. *et al.* (1988) First trimester prenatal diagnosis of metachromatic leucodystrophy on chorionic villi by 'immunoprecipitation electrophoresis'. *Journal of Inherited Metabolic Disease*, **11**, 123–30.

Poenaru, L., Girard, S., Thepot, F. *et al.* (1979) Antenatal diagnosis in three pregnancies at risk for mannosidosis. *Clinical Genetics*, **16**, 428–32.

Poenaru, I., Mezard, C., Akli, S. *et al.* (1990) Prenatal diagnosis of mucolipidosis type II on first-trimester amniotic fluid. *Prenatal Diagnosis*, **10**, 231–35.

Pollitt, R.J. (1989) Disorders of mitochondrial beta-oxidation: prenatal and early postnatal diagnosis and their relevance to Reye's syndrome and sudden infant death. *Journal of Inherited Metabolic Disease*, **12** (suppl. 1), 215–30.

Poll-The, B.T., Poulos, A., Sharp, P. *et al.* (1985) Antenatal diagnosis of infantile Refsum's disease. *Clinical Genetics*, **27**, 524–26.

Pons, J.C., Rozenberg, F., Imbert MC. *et al.* (1992) Prenatal diagnosis of second-trimester congenital varicella syndrome. *Prenatal Diagnosis*, **12**, 975–76.

Pope, F.M., Daw, S.C.M., Narcisi, P. *et al.* (1989) Prenatal diagnosis and prevention of inherited disorders of collagen. *Journal of Inherited Metabolic Disease*, **12** (suppl.), 135–73.

Pretorius, D.H., Drose, J.A., Dennis, M.A. *et al.* (1987) Tracheoesophageal fistula *in utero*: twenty-two cases. *Journal of Ultrasound in Medicine*, **6**, 509–13.

Pretorius, D., Manchester, D., Barkin, S. *et al.* (1988) Doppler ultrasound of twin transfusion syndrome. *Journal of Ultrasound in Medicine*, **7**, 117–24.

Pretorius, D.H., Rumack, C.M., Manco-Johnson, M.L. (1986) Specific skeletal dysplasia *in utero*: sonographic diagnosis. *Radiology*, **159**, 237–42.

Preus, M., Kaplan, P. and Kirkham, T.H. (1977) Renal anomalies and oligohydramnios in the cerebro-oculofacio-skeletal syndrome. *American Journal of Diseases of Children*, **131**, 62–64.

Pryde, P.G., Bawle, E., Brandt, F., Romero, R., Treadwell, M.C. and Evans, M.I. (1993) Prenatal diagnosis of nonrhizomelic chondrodysplasia punctata (Conradi–Hunermann syndrome). *American Journal of Medical Genetics*, **47**, 426–31.

Puck, J.M., Kraus, C.M., Puck, S.M. *et al.* (1990) Prenatal test for X-linked severe combined immunodeficiency by analysis of maternal X-chromosome inactivation and linkage analysis. *New England Journal of Medicine*, **322**, 1063–66.

Quagliatello, J.R., Passalaqua, A.M., Greco, M.A. *et al.* (1978) Ballantyne's triple edema syndrome: prenatal diagnosis with ultrasound and maternal renal biopsy findings. *American Journal of Obstetrics and Gynecology*, **132**, 580–81.

Quan, F., Korneluk, R.G., Tropak, M.B. and Gravel, R.A. (1986) Isolation and characterisation of the human catalase gene. *Nucleic Acids Research*, **14**, 5321–35.

Quarrell, O.W.J., Meredith, A.L., Tyler, A. *et al.* (1987) Exclusion tasting for Huntington's disease in pregnancy with a closely linked DNA marker. *Lancet*, **i**, 1281–83.

Quigg, M.H., Evans, M.I., Zador, I. *et al.* (1985) Ultrasonographic prenatal diagnosis of Langer-type mesomelic dwarfism. *American Journal of Human Genetics*, **37**, A225.

Quinlan, R.W., Cruz, A.C. and Huddleston, J.F. (1986) Sonographic detection of fetal urinary tract anomalies. *Obstetrics and Gynecology*, **67**, 558–65.

Raafat, N.A., Birch, A.A., Altieri, L.A., Felker, R.E., Smith, W.C. and Emerson, D.S. (1993) Sonographic osseous manifestations of fetal syphilis: A case report. *Journal of Ultrasound in Medicine*, **12**, 783–85.

Ramirez, M., Hecht, J.T., Taylor, S. and Wilkins, I. (1994) Tibial hemimelia syndrome: Prenatal diagnosis by real-time ultrasound. *Prenatal Diagnosis*, **14**, 167–71.

Ramsing, M., Rehd, H., Holzgreve, W. *et al.* (1990) Fraser syndrome (cryptopthalmos with syndactyly) in the fetus and newborn. *Clinical Genetics*, **37**, 84–96.

Rapola, J., Salonen, R., Ammala, P. and Santavuori, P. (1993) Prenatal diagnosis of infantile neuronal ceroid-lipofuscinosis, INCL: Morphological aspects. *Journal of Inherited Metabolic Disease*, **16**, 349–52.

Redmond, R.M., Vaughan, J.I., Jay, M. and Jay B. (1993) *In utero* diagnosis of Norrie disease by ultrasonography. *Ophthalmic Paediatrics and Genetics*, **14**, 1–3.

Reiter, A.A., Hunta, J.C., Carpenter, R.J. *et al.* (1986) Prenatal diagnosis of arteriovenous malformation of the vein of Galen. *Journal of Clinical Ultrasound*, **14**, 623–28.

Rempen, A. (1989) Sonographic first-trimester diagnosis of umbilical cord cyst. *Journal of Clinical Ultrasound*, **17**, 53–55.

Rempen, A., Feige, A. and Wunsch, P. (1987) Prenatal diagnosis of bilateral cystic adenomatoid malformation of the lung. *Journal of Clinical Ultrasound*, **15**, 3–8.

Renlund M., and Aula, P. (1987) Prenatal detection of Salla disease based upon increased free sialic acid in amniocytes. *American Journal of Medical Genetics*, **28**, 377–84.

Reshef, A., Meiner, V., Dann, E.J., Granat, M. and Leitersdorf, E. (1992) Prenatal diagnosis of familial hypercholesterolemia caused by the 'Lebanese' mutation at the low density lipoprotein receptor locus. *Human Genetics*, **89**, 237–39.

Reuss, A., Den Hollander, J.C., Niermeijer, M.F. *et al.* (1989) Prenatal diagnosis of cystic renal disease with ventriculomegaly: a report of six cases in two related sibships. *American Journal of Medical Genetics*, **33**, 385–89.

Reuss, A., Waldimiroff, J.W. and Stewart, P.A. (1990) Prenatal diagnosis by ultrasound in pregnancies at risk for autosomal recessive polycystic kidney disease. *Ultrasound*

348

in Medicine and Biology, **16**, 355–59.

Richards, R.L., Holman, K., Kozman, H. *et al.* (1991) Fragile X syndome: genetic localisation by linkage mapping of two microsatellite repeats FRAXAC1 and FRAXAC2 which immediately flank the fragile site. *Journal of Medical Genetics*, **28**, 818–23.

Ristaldi, M.S., Piratsu, M., Rosatelli, C. *et al.* (1989) Prenatal diagnosis of beta-thalassaemia in Mediterranean populations by dot-blot analysis with DNA amplification and allele specific oligonucleotide probes. *Prenatal Diagnosis*, **9**, 629–38.

Ritchie, G., Jequier, S. and Lussier-Lazaroff, J. (1988) Prenatal renal ultrasound of Laurence–Moon–Biedl syndrome. *Pediatric Radiology*, **19**, 65–66.

Rizzo, G., Arduini, D., Pennestri, F. *et al.* (1987) Fetal behaviour in growth retardation: its relationship to fetal blood flow. *Prenatal Diagnosis*, **7**, 229.

Rizzo, N., Gabrielli, S., Perolo, A. *et al.* (1987) Prenatal diagnosis and management of fetal ovarian cysts. *Prenatal Diagnosis*, **7**, 97–108.

Rizzo, N., Gabrielli S., Pilu, G. *et al.* (1987) Prenatal diagnosis and obstetrical management of multicystic dysplastic kidney disease. *Prenatal Diagnosis*, **7**, 109–18.

Roberson, D.A. and Silverman, N.H. (1989) Ebstein's anomaly: echocardiographic and clinical features in the fetus and neonate. *Journal of the American College of Cardiology*, **14**, 1300–307.

Robinson, B.H., Toone, J.R., Benedict, R.P. *et al.* (1985) Prenatal diagnosis of pyruvate carboxylase deficiency. *Prenatal Diagnosis*, **5**, 67–71.

Robinson, I.P., Worthen, N.J., Lachman, R.S. *et al.* (1987) Prenatal diagnosis of osteogenesis imperfecta type III. *Prenatal Diagnosis*, **7**, 7–15.

Rodeck, C.H., Patrick, A.D., Pembrey, P.F. *et al.* (1982) Fetal liver biopsy for prenatal diagnosis of ornithine carbamyl transferase deficiency. *Lancet*, **ii**, 297–300.

Rodeck, C.H., Tansley, I.R., Benson, P.F. *et al.* (1983b) Prenatal exclusion of Hurler's disease by leucocyte alpha-L-iduronidase assay. *Prenatal Diagnosis*, **3**, 61–63.

Rogoyski, A. (1985) Postnatal and prenatal diagnosis of Maroteaux–Lamy syndrome. *Acta Anthropogenetica*, **9**, 109–16.

Rolland, M.O., Divry, P., Mandon, G. *et al.* (1990) Early prenatal diagnosis of propionic acidaemia with simultaneous sampling of chorionic villus and amniotic fluid. *Journal of Inherited Metabolic Disease*, **13**, 345–48.

Rolland, M., Sarramon, M.F., and Bloom, M.C. (1991) Astomia-agnathia-holoprosencephaly association. Prenatal diagnosis of a new case. *Prenatal Diagnosis*, **11**, 199–203.

Rolland, M.O., Mandon, G. and Mathieu, M. (1993) First-trimester prenatal diagnosis of non-ketotic hyperglycinaemia by a microassay of glycine cleavage enzyme *Prenatal Diagnosis*, **13**, 771–72.

Romero, R., Chevenak, I.A., Devore, G. *et al.* (1981) Fetal head deformation and congenital torticollis associated with a uterine tumour. *American Journal of Obstetrics and Gynecology*, **141**, 839–40.

Romero, R., Cullen, M., Jeanty, P. *et al.* (1984) The diagnosis of congenital renal anomalies with ultrasound. II. Infantile polycystic kidney disease. *American Journal of Obstetrics*

and Gynecology, **150**, 259–62.

Romero, R., Ghindi, A., Eswara, M.S. *et al.* (1988) Prenatal findings in a case of spondylocostal dysplasia type I (Jarcho–Levin syndrome). *Obstetrics and Gynecology*, **71**, 988–91.

Romke, C., Froster-Iskenius, U., Heyne, K. *et al.* (1987) Roberts syndrome and SC phocomelia: a single genetic entity. *Clinical Genetic*, **31**, 170–77.

Rosa, R., Prehu, M.O., Calvin, M.C. *et al.* (1986) Possibility of prenatal diagnosis of hereditary triose phosphate isomerase deficiency. *Prenatal Diagnosis*, **6**, 231–34.

Rosenblatt, D.S. (1987) Expression of transcobalamin II by amniocytes. *Prenatal Diagnosis*, **7**, 35–39.

Rosenblatt, D.S., Cooper, B.A., Schmutz, S.M. *et al.* (1985) Prenatal vitamin B12 therapy of a fetus with methylcobalamin deficiency (cobalamin E disease) *Lancet*, **i**, 1127–29.

Rosler, A., Lieberman, E., Rosenmann, A. *et al.* (1979) Prenatal diagnosis of 11 beta-hyroxylase deficiency congenital adrenal hyperplasia. *Journal of Clinical Endocrinology and Metabolism*, **49**, 546–51.

Rosser, E., Huson, S.M. and Norbury, G. (1994) Prenatal, presymptomatic, and diagnostic testing with direct mutation analysis in Huntington's disease. *Lancet*, **343**, 487–88.

Rothnagel, J.A., Longley, M.A., Holder, R.A., Kuster, W. and Roop, D.R. (1994) Prenatal diagnosis of epidermolytic hyperkeratosis by direct gene sequencing. *Journal of Investigative Dermatology*, **102**, 13–16.

Rotmensch, S., Grannum, P.A., Nores, J.A. *et al.* (1991) *In utero* diagnosis and management of fetal subdural haematoma. *American Journal of Obstetrics and Gynecology*, **164**, 1246–48.

Rouleau, G.A., Wertelecki, W., Haines, J.L. *et al.* (1987) Genetic linkage of bilateral acoustic neurofibromatosis to a DNA marker on chromosome 22. *Nature*, **329**, 246–48.

Rowley, K.A. (1955) Coronal cleft vertebra. *Journal of the Faculty of Radiologists*, **6**, 267.

Rozear, M.P., Pericak-Vance, M.A., Fischbeck, K. *et al.* (1987) Hereditary motor and sensory neuropathy, X-linked: a half century follow-up. *Neurology*, **37**, 1460–65.

Rudiger, H.W., Bartram, C.R., Harder, W. and Passarge, E. (1980) Rate of sister chromatid exchanges in Bloom syndrome fibroblasts reduced by co-cultivation with normal fibroblasts. *American Journal of Human Genetics*, **32**, 150–57.

Ruitenbeek, W., Sengers, R., Albani, M. *et al.* (1988) Prenatal diagnosis of cytochrome C oxidase deficiency by biopsy of chorionic villi. *New England Journal of Medicine*, **319**, 1095.

Ruitenbeek, W., Sengers, R.C.A., Trijbels, J.M.F. *et al.* (1992) The use of chorionic villi in prenatal diagnosis of mitochondropathies. *Journal of Inherited Metabolic Disease*, **15**, 303–306.

Russ, P.D., Pretorius, P.M. and Johnson, M.J. (1989) Dandy–Walker syndrome: a review of fifteen cases evaluated by prenatal sonography. *American Journal of Obstetrics and Gynecology*, **161**, 401–406.

Russell, J.G.B. (1973) *Radiology in Obstetrics and Antenatal Paediatrics*, Butterworth, London, pp. 79–80.

Saal, H.M., Deutsch, L., Herson V. *et al.* (1986) The RAG syndrome: a new autosomal recessive syndrome with Robin sequence, ancreolia and profound growth and developmental delays. *American Journal of Human Genetics*, **39**, A78.

Sabbagha, R.E., Tamura, R.K., Compo, S.D. *et al.* (1980) Fetal cranial and craniocervical masses: ultrasound characteristics and differential diagnosis. *American Journal of Obstetrics and Gynecology*, **138**, 511–17.

Sada, I., Shiratori, H. and Nakamura, Y. (1986) Antenatal diagnosis of fetus *in fetu*. *Asia–Oceania Journal of Obstetrics and Gynaecology*, **12**, 353–56.

Sahn, D.J., Shenker, L., Reed, K.L. *et al.* (1982) Prenatal ultrasound diagnosis of hypoplastic left heart syndrome *in utero* associated with hydrops fetalis. *American Heart Journal*, **104**, 1368–72.

Sakuma, T., Sugiyama, N., Ichiki, T. *et al.* (1991) Analysis of acylcarnitines in maternal urine for prenatal diagnosis of glutaric aciduria type 2. *Prenatal Diagnosis*, **11**, 77–82.

Saltzman, D.H., Benacerraf, B.R. and Frigoletto, F.D. (1986) Diagnosis and management of fetal facial clefts. *American Journal of Obstetrics and Gynecology*, **155**, 377–79.

Saltzman, D.H., Krauss, C.M., Goldman, J.M. and Benacerraf, B.R. (1991) Prenatal diagnosis of lissencephaly. *Prenatal Diagnosis*, **11**, 139–43.

Salvo, A.F. (1981) *In utero* diagnosis of Kleeblattschadel (cloverleaf skull). *Prenatal Diagnosis*, **1**, 141–45.

Samuel, N., Dicker, D., Landman, J. *et al.* (1986) Early diagnosis and intrauterine therapy of meconium plug syndrome in the fetus: risks and benefits. *Journal of Ultrasound in Medicine*, **5**, 425–28.

Samuel, N., Sirotta, L., Bar-Ziv, J. *et al.* (1988) The ultrasonic appearance of common pulmonary vein atresia *in utero*. *Journal of Ultrasound in Medicine*, **7**, 25–28.

Samueloff, A., Navot, D., Bickenfeld, A. and Schenker, J.G. (1987) Fryns syndrome: a predictable, lethal pattern of multiple-congenital anomalies. *American Journal of Obstetrics and Gynecology*, **156**, 86–88.

Sarasin, A., Blanchet Bardon, C., Renault, G., Lehmann, A., Arlett, C. and Dumez, Y. (1992) Prenatal diagnosis in a subset of trichothiodystrophy patients defective in DNA repair. *Journal of Dermatology*, **127**, 485–91.

Sasagasako, N., Miyahara, S., Saito, N., Shinnoh, N., Kobayashi, T. and Goto, I. (1993) Prenatal diagnosis of congenital sialidosis. *Clinical Genetics*, **44**, 8–11.

Sassa, S., Solish, G., Levere, R.D. and Kappas, A. (1975) Studies in porphyria IV. Expression of the gene defect of acute intermittent porphyria in cultured human skin fibroblasts and amniotic fluid cells: PND of the porphyric trait. *Journal of Experimental Medicine*, **142**, 722–31.

Savary, J.B., Vasseur, F. and Deminatti, M.M. (1991) Routine autoradiographic analysis of DNA excision repair. Report of prenatal and postnatal diagnosis in eleven families. *Annales de Génétique*, **34**, 76–81.

Savary, J.B., Vasseur, F., Vinatier, D. *et al.* (1991) Prenatal diagnosis of PIBIDS. *Prenatal Diagnosis*, **11**, 859–66.

Savodelli, G. and Schinzel, A. (1983) Prenatal ultrasound detection of humero-radial synostosis in a case of Antley–Bixler syndrome. *Prenatal Diagnosis*, **2**, 219–33.

Schaffer, R.M., Cabbad, M., Minkoff, H. *et al.* (1986) Sonographic diagnosis of fetal cardiac rhabdomyoma. *Journal of Ultrasound in Medicine*, **5**, 531–33.

Schauer, G.M., Dunn, L.K., Godmilow, L. *et al.* (1990) Prenatal diagnosis of Fraser syndrome at 18.5 weeks gestation with autopsy findings at 19 weeks. *American Journal of Medical Genetics*, **37**, 583–91.

Schechter, A.G., Fakhry, J., Shapiro, L.R. and Gewitz, M.H. (1987) *In utero* thickening of the chordae tendenae: a cause of intracardiac echogenic foci. *Journal of Ultrasound in Medicine*, **6**, 691–95.

Schindler, D., Bishop, D.F., Wolfe, D.E. *et al.* (1989) Neuro-axonal dystrophy due to lysosomal α-N-acetylgalacto-saminidase deficiency. *New England Journal of Medicine*, **320**, 1735–40.

Schinzel, A., Savodelli, G., Briner, J. and Schubiger, G. (1985) Prenatal sonographic diagnosis of Jeune syndrome. *Radiology*, **154**, 777–78.

Schinzel, A., Savodelli, G., Briner, J. *et al.* (1983) Antley–Bixler syndrome in sisters: a term newborn and a prenatally diagnosed fetus. *American Journal of Medical Genetics*, **14**, 139–47.

Schmidt, K.G., Birk, E., Silverman, N.H. and Scagnelli, S.A. (1989) Echocardiographic evaluation of dilated cardiomyopathy in the human fetus. *American Journal of Cardiology*, **63**, 599–605.

Schmidt, W., Harms, E. and Wolf, D. (1985) Successful prenatal treatment of non-immune hydrops fetalis due to congenital chylothorax. Case report. *British Journal of Obstetrics and Gynaecology*, **92**, 685–87.

Schneider, J.A., Verroust, F.M., Kroll, W.A. *et al.* (1974) Prenatal diagnosis of cystinosis. *New England Journal of Medicine*, **290**, 878–82.

Schroeder, D., Smith, L. and Prain, H.C. (1989) Antenatal diagnosis of choledochal cyst at 15 weeks' gestation: etiologic implications and management. *Journal of Pediatric Surgery*, **24**, 936–38.

Schumert, Z., Rosenmann, A., Landau, H. and Rosler, A. (1980) 11-Deoxycortisol in amniotic fluid: prenatal diagnosis of congenital adrenal hyperplasia due to 11 beta-hydroxylase deficiency. *Clinical Endocrinology*, **12**, 257–60.

Schutgens, R.B.H., Schrakamp, G., Wanders, R.J.A. *et al.* (1989) Prenatal and perinatal diagnosis of peroxisomal disorders. *Journal of Inherited Metabolic Disease*, **12** (suppl. 1), 118–34.

Schuurman, H.J., Huber, J., Zegers, B.J.M. and Roord, J.J. (1985) Placental diagnosis of bare lymphocyte syndrome. *New England Journal of Medicine*, **313**, 757.

Schwartz, M., Mibashan, R. and Nicolaides, K.H. (1989) First-trimester diagnosis of Wiskott–Aldrich syndrome by DNA markers. *Lancet*, **ii**, 1405.

Schwartz, S., Flannery, D.B. and Cohen, M.M. (1985) Tests appropriate for prenatal diagnosis of ataxia telangiectasia. *Prenatal Diagnosis*, **5**, 9–14.

Secor McVoy, J.R., Heard, G.S. and Wolf, B. (1984) Potential for prenatal diagnosis of biotinidase deficiency. *Prenatal Diagnosis*, **4**, 317–18.

Seeds, J.W., Cefalo, R.C., Lies, S.C. and Koontz, W.I. (1984) Early prenatal sonographic appearance of rare thoraco-abdominal eventration. *Prenatal Diagnosis*, **4**, 437–41.

Seeds, J.W. and Powers, S.K. (1988) Early prenatal diagnosis of familial lipomyelomeningocele. *Obstetrics and Gynecology*, **72**, 469–71.

Seizinger, B.R., Rouleau, G.A., Ozelius, L.J. *et al.* (1988) Von Hippel—Lindau disease maps to the region of chromosome 3 associated with renal cell carcinoma. *Nature*, **332**, 268—69.

Seligsohn, V., Mibashan, R.S., Rodeck, C.H. (1985) Prenatal diagnosis of Glanzmann's thrombasthenia. *Lancet*, **ii**, 1419.

Sepulveda, W., Berry, S.M., Romero, R., King, M.E., Johnson, M.P. and Cotton, D.B. (1993) Prenatal diagnosis of congenital megalourethra. *Journal of Ultrasound in Medicine*, **12**, 761—66.

Serini, I.P., Bachmann, C., Pfister, U. *et al.* (1988) Prenatal diagnosis of carbamoyl-phosphate synthetase deficiency by fetal liver biopsy. *Prenatal Diagnosis*, **8**, 307—309.

Serville, F., Benit, P., Saugier, P. *et al.* (1993) Prenatal exclusion of X-linked hydrocephalus — stenosis of the aqueduct of sylvius sequence using closely linked DNA markers. *Prenatal Diagnosis*, **13**, 435—39.

Sewell, A.C. and Pontz, B.F. (1988) Prenatal diagnosis of galactosialidosis. *Prenatal Diagnosis*, **8**, 151—55.

Shah, Y.G. and Metlay, L. (1990) Prenatal ultrasound diagnosis of Beckwith—Wiedemann syndrome. *Journal of Clinical Ultrasound*, **18**, 597—600.

Shalev, E. (1983) Prenatal ultrasound diagnosis of intestinal calcification with imperforate anus. *Acta Obstetricia et Gynecologica Scandinavica*, **62**, 95—96.

Shalev, E., Romano, S., Nseit, T. and Zuckerman, H. (1988) Klippel—Trenaunay syndrome: ultrasonic prenatal diagnosis. *Journal of Clinical Ultrasound*, **16**, 268—70.

Shalev, J., Frankel, Y., Avigad, I. and Mashiach, S. (1982) Spontaneous intestinal perforation *in utero*: ultrasonic diagnostic criteria. *American Journal of Obstetrics and Gynecology*, **144**, 855—57.

Shechter, S.A., Sherer, D.M., Geilfuss, C.J. *et al.* (1990) Prenatal sonographic appearance and subsequent management of a fetus with cromandibular limb hypogenesis syndrome associated with pulmonary hypoplasia. *Journal of Clinical Ultrasound*, **18**, 661—65.

Shelton-Inloes, B.B., Chehab, F.F., Mannucci, P.M. *et al.* (1987) Gene deletions correlate with the development of alloantibodies in von Willebrand disease. *Journal of Clinical Investigation*, **79**, 1459—65.

Shenker, L., Reed, K.L., Anderson, C.F. and Kern, W. (1989) Fetal pericardial effusion. *American Journal of Obstetrics and Gynecology*, **160**, 1505—508.

Sherer, D.M., Cullen, J.B.H., Thompson, H.O. *et al.* (1990) Prenatal sonographic findings associated with a fetal horseshoe kidney. *Journal of Ultrasound in Medicine*, **9**, 477—79.

Sherer, D.M., Menashe, M., Lebensart, P. *et al.* (1989) Sonographic diagnosis of unilateral fetal renal duplication with associated ectopic ureterocele. *Journal of Clinical Ultrasound*, **17**, 371—73.

Shim, V.E., Laframboise, R., Mandell, R., Pichette, J. (1992) Neonatal form of the hyperornithinaemia, hyperammonaemia, and homocitrullinuria (HHH) syndrome and prenatal diagnosis. *Prenatal Diagnosis*, **12**, 717—23.

Shimizu, H., Ishiko, A., Kikuchi, A., Akiyama, M., Suzumori, K., Nishikawa, T. (1992) Prenatal diagnosis of tyrosinase-negative oculocutaneous albinism. *Lancet*, **340**, 739—40.

Shimozawa, Y., Suzuki, Y., Orii, T., Tsukamoto, T. and Fujiki, Y. (1993) Prenatal diagnosis of Zellweger syndrome using DNA analysis. *Prenatal Diagnosis*, **13**, 149.

Shin, Y.S., Rieth, M., Tausenfreund, J. and Endres, W. (1989) First trimester diagnosis of glycogen storage disease type II and type III. *Journal of Inherited Metabolic Disease*, **12** (suppl. 2), 289—91.

Shintaku, H., Hsiao, K.J., Liu, T.T. *et al.* (1994) Prenatal diagnosis of 6-pyruvoyl tetrahydropterin synthase deficiency in seven subjects. *Journal of Inherited Metabolic Disease*, **17**, 163—66.

Sidiqi, T.A., Bendon, R., Schultz, D.M. and Miodovnik, M. (1992) Umbilical artery aneurysm: Prenatal diagnosis and management. *Obstetrics and Gynecology*, **80**, 530—33.

Siebert, J.R., Warkany, J. and Lemire, R.J. (1986) Atelencephalic microcephaly in a 21-week human fetus. *Teratology*, **34**, 9—19.

Sieck, U.V. and Ohlsson, A. (1984) Fetal polyuria and hydramnics associated with Bartter's syndrome. *Obstetrics and Gynecology*, **63**, 226—45.

Sieving, P.A., Bingham, E.L., Roth, M.S. *et al.* (1990) Linkage relationships of X-linked juvenile retinoschisis with Xp. 22.1—p. 22.3 probes. *American Journal of Human Genetics*, **47**, 616—21.

Siffring, P.A., Forrest, T.S. and Frick, M.P. (1991) Sonographic detection of hydrolethalus syndrome. *Journal of Clinical Ultrasound*, **19**, 43—47.

Silver, D.N., Lewis, R.A. and Nussbaum, R.L. (1987) Mapping the Lowe oculocerebro-renal syndrome to Xq24—q26 by use of restriction fragment length polymorphisms. *Journal of Clinical Investigation*, **79**, 282—85.

Silverman, N.H., Enderlein, M.A. and Golbus, M.S. (1984) Ultrasonic recognition of aortic valve atresia *in utero*. *American Journal of Cardiology*, **53**, 391—92.

Simsek, S., Bleeker, P.M.M., Von dem Borne, A.E.G.K., Bennett, P., Warwick, R. and Cartron, J.P. (1994) Prenatal determination of fetal RhD type (9). *New England Journal of Medicine*, **330**, 795—96.

Sirtori, M., Ghidini, A., Romero, R. and Robbins, J.C. (1989) Prenatal diagnosis of sirenomelia. *Journal of Ultrasound in Medicine*, **8**, 83—88.

Skare, J.C., Milunsky, A., Byron, K.S. and Sullivan, J.L. (1987) Mapping the X-linked lymphoproliferative syndrome. *Proceedings of the National Academy of Sciences of the USA*, **84**, 2015—18.

Skrede, S., Bjorkhem, I., Kvittingen, E.A. *et al.* (1986) Demonstrations of 26-hydroxylation of C-27 steroids in human skin fibroblasts and a deficiency of this activity in cerebrotendinous xanthomatosis. *Journal of Clinical Investigation*, **78**, 729—35.

Smith, H.J., Hanken, H. and Brundelet, P.J. (1981) Ultrasound diagnosis of interstitial pregnancy. *Acta Obstetricia Gynecologica Scandinavia*, **60**, 413—16.

Smooker, P.M., Cotton, R.G.H. and Lipson, A. (1993) Prenatal diagnosis of DHPR deficiency by direct detection of mutation. *Prenatal Diagnosis*, **13**, 881—84.

Snyder, J.R., Lustig-Gillman, I., Milio, L. *et al.* (1986) Antenatal ultrasound diagnosis of an intracranial neoplasm (craniopharyngioma). *Journal of Clinical Ultrasound*, **14**, 304—306.

Socol, M.L., Sabbagha, R.E., Elias, S. *et al.* (1985) Prenatal diagnosis of congenital muscular dystrophy producing arthrogryposis. *New England Journal of Medicine*, **313**, 1230.

351

Sonek, J.D., Gabbe, S.G., Landon, M.B. (1990) Antenatal diagnosis of sacral agenesis syndrome in a pregnancy complicated by diabetes mellitus. *American Journal of Obstetrics and Gynecology*, **162**, 806–808.

Spear, R., Mack, L.A., Benedetti, T.J. and Cole, R.E. (1990) Idiopathic infantile arterial calcification: *in utero* diagnosis. *Journal of Ultrasound in Medicine*, **9**, 473–76.

Spector, E.B., Kiernan, M., Bernard, B. and Cederbaum, S.D. (1980) Properties of fetal and adult red blood cell arginase deficiency. *American Journal of Human Genetics*, **32**, 79–97.

Speer, A., Bollman, R., Michel, A. *et al.* (1986) Prenatal diagnosis of classical phenylketonuria by linked restriction fragment length polymorphism analysis. *Prenatal Diagnosis*, **6**, 447–50.

Speiser, P.W., Laforgia, N., Kato, K. *et al.* (1990) First trimester prenatal treatment and molecular genetic diagnosis of congenital adrenal hyperplasia (21-hydroxylase deficiency). *Journal of Clinical Endocrinology and Metabolism*, **70**, 838–48.

Speiser, P.W., White, P.C., Dupont, J., Zhu, D., Mercado, A.B. and New, M.I. (1994) Prenatal diagnosis of congenital adrenal hyperplasia due to 21-hydroxylase deficiency by allele-specific hybridization and Southern blot. *Human Genetics*, **93**, 424–28.

Spence, J.E., Maddalena, A., O'Brien, W.E. *et al.* (1989) Prenatal diagnosis and heterozygote detection by DNA analysis in ornithine transcarbamylase deficiency. *Journal of Pediatrics*, **114**, 582–88.

Spirt, B.A., Gordon, L.P. and Oliphant, M. (1987) *Prenatal Ultrasound: A Colour Atlas with Anatomic and Pathologic Correlation*, Churchill Livingstone, Edinburgh.

Spritz, R.A., Strunk, K.M., Giebel, I.B. and King, R.A. (1990) Detection of mutations in the tyrosinase gene in a patient with type IA oculocutaneous albinism. *New England Journal of Medicine*, **322**, 1724–28.

Stamm, E., King, G. and Thickman, D. (1991) Megacystic–microcolon–intestinal hypoperistalsis syndrome: prenatal identification in siblings and review of the literature. *Journal of Ultrasound in Medicine*, **10**, 599–602.

Stamm, E.R., Pretorius, D.H., Rumack, C.M. and Manco-Johnson, M.I. (1987) Kleeblattschadel anomaly. *In utero* sonographic appearance. *Journal of Ultrasound in Medicine*, **6**, 319–24.

Stanford, W., Abu-Yousef, M. and Smith, W. (1987) Intra-cardiac tumour (rhabdomyoma) diagnosed by *in utero* ultrasound: a case report. *Journal of Clinical Ultrasound*, **15**, 337–41.

Steinfeld, L., Rappaport, H.L., Rossbach, H.C. and Martinez, E. (1986) Diagnosis of fetal arrhythmias using echocardiographic and Doppler techniques. *Journal of the American College of Cardiology*, **9**, 1425–33.

Steinherz, R. (1985) Prenatal diagnosis of cystinosis upon exposure of amniotic cells to cystine dimethyl ester. *Israeli Journal of Medical Science*, **21**, 537–39.

Steinman, L., Tharp, B.R., Dorfman, L.J. *et al.* (1980) Peripheral neuropathy in the cherry-red spot myoclonus syndrome (sialidosis type I). *Annals of Neurology*, **7**, 450–56.

Stellaard, F., Langelaar, S.A., Kok, R.M. *et al.* (1988) Prenatal diagnosis of Zellweger syndrome by determination of trihydroxycoprostanic acid in amniotic fluid. *European*

Journal of Pediatrics, **148**, 175–76.

Stephens, J.D. (1984) Prenatal diagnosis of testicular feminisation. *Lancet*, **ii**, 1038.

Stewart, P.A., Buis-Liem, T., Verwey, R.A. and Wladimiroff, J.W. (1986) Prenatal ultrasonic diagnosis of familial asymmetric septal hypertrophy. *Prenatal Diagnosis*, **6**, 249–56.

Stewart, P.A., Wladimiroff, J.W. and Becker, A.E. (1985) Early prenatal detection of double outlet right ventricle by echocardiography. *British Heart Journal*, **54**, 340–42.

Stiller, R.J., Pinto, M., Heller, C. and Hobbins, J.C. (1988) Oligohydramnios associated with bilateral multicystic dysplastic kidneys: prenatal diagnosis at 15 weeks gestation. *Journal of Clinical Ultrasound*, **16**, 436–39.

Stiller, R.J. (1989) Early ultrasonic appearance of fetal bladder outlet obstruction. *American Journal of Obstetrics and Gynecology*, **160**, 584–85.

Stiou, S, Privitera, O., Brambati, B., Zuliani, G., Lalatta F. and Simoni, G. (1992) First trimester prenatal diagnosis of Roberts syndrome. *Prenatal Diagnosis*, **12**, 145–49.

Stoker, A.F., Jonnes, S.V. and Spence, J. (1983) Ultrasound diagnosis of situs inversus *in utero*. A case report. *South African Medical Journal*, **64**, 832–34.

Stoll, C., Ehret-Mentre, M.-C., Treisser, A. and Tranchant, C. (1991) Prenatal diagnosis of congenital myasthenia with arthrogryposis in a myasthenic mother. *Prenatal Diagnosis*, **11**, 17–22.

Stoll, C., Willard, D., Czernichow, P. and Boue, J. (1978) Prenatal diagnosis of primary pituitary dysgenesis. *Lancet*, **i**, 932.

Stoll, C., Willard, D., Czernichow, P. and Boue, J. (1985) Prenatal diagnosis of hypochondroplasia. *Prenatal Diagnosis*, **5**, 423–26.

Strautnieks, S., Rutland, P., Winter, R.M., Baraitser, M. and Malcolm, S. (1992) Pelizaeus–Merzbacher disease: Detection of mutations Thr181-)Pro and Leu 223-)Pro in the proteolipid protein gene. *American Journal of Human Genetics*, **51**, 871–78.

Sugita, T., Ikenaga, M., Suchara, N. *et al.* (1982) Prenatal diagnosis of Cockayne syndrome using assay of colony-forming ability in ultraviolet light irradiated cells. *Clinical Genetics*, **22**, 137–42.

Sutro, W.H., Tuck, S.M., Loesevitz, A. *et al.* (1984) Prenatal observation of umbilical cord hematoma. *American Journal of Roentgenology*, **142**, 801–802.

Suttle, D.P., Bugg, B.Y., Winkler, J.K. and Kanalas, J.J. (1988) Molecular cloning and nucleotide sequence for the complete coding region of human UMP synthase. *Proceedings of the National Academy of Sciences of the USA*, **85**, 1754–58.

Suzumori, K. and Kanzaki, T. (1991) Prenatal diagnosis of harlequin ichthyosis by total skin biopsy, report of two cases. *Prenatal Diagnosis*, **11**, 451–57.

Tabsh, K., Rizzo, W.B., Holbrook, K. and Theroux, N. (1993) Sjögren-Larsson syndrome: Technique and timing of prenatal diagnosis. *Obstetrics and Gynecology*, **82**, 700–703.

Tadmor, O.P., Hammerman, C., Rabinowitz, R. *et al.* (1993) Femoral hypoplasia – Unusual facies syndrome: Prenatal ultrasonographic observations. *Fetal Diagnosis and Therapy*, **8**, 279–84.

Takashima, T., Maeda, H., Koyanagi, T., Nishimura, J. and Nakano, H. (1992) Prenatal diagnosis and obstetrical management of May-Hegglin anomaly: A case report. *Fetal Diagnosis and Therapy*, 7, 186–89.

Taylor, R., Jeenah, M., Seed, M. and Humphries, S. (1988) Four DNA polymorphisms in the LDL receptor gene: their genetic relationship and use in the study of variation at LDL receptor locus. *Journal of Medical Genetics*, 25, 653–59.

Teichler-Zallen, D. and Doherty, R.A. (1983) Fetal ABO blood group typing using amniotic fluid. *Clinical Genetics*, 23, 120–24.

Terry, G.M., Ho-Terry, L., Warten, R.C. *et al.* (1986) First trimester prenatal diagnosis of congenital rubella: a laboratory investigation. *BMJ*, 292, 930–33.

Thiagarajah, S., Abbitt, P.L., Hogge, W.A. and Leason, S.H. (1990) Prenatal diagnosis of eventration of the diaphragm. *Journal of Clinical Ultrasound*, 18, 46–49.

Thomas, C.S., Leopold, G.R., Hitton, S. *et al.* (1986) Fetal hydrops associated with extralobar pulmonary sequestration. *Journal of Ultrasound in Medicine*, 5, 668–71.

Thomas, R.L. (1992) Prenatal diagnosis of giant cystic hygroma: Prognosis, counselling, and management; case presentation and review of the recent literature. *Prenatal Diagnosis*, 12, 919–23.

Thorburn, D.R., Thompson, G.N. and Howells, D.W. (1993) A fluorimetric assay for succinic semialdehyde dehydrogenase activity suitable for prenatal diagnosis of the enzyme deficiency. *Journal of Inherited Metabolic Disease*, 16, 942–49.

Toi, A., Simpson, G.F. and Filly, R.A. (1987) Ultrasonically evident fetal nuchal skin thickening: is it specific for Down syndrome? *American Journal of Obstetrics and Gynecology*, 156, 150–53.

Tolmie, J.L., McNay, M.B. and Connor, J.M. (1987a) Prenatal diagnosis of severe autosomal recessive spondylothoracic dysplasia (Jarcho–Levin type). *Prenatal Diagnosis*, 7, 129–34.

Tolmie, J.L., McNay, M.B., Stephenson, J.B.P. *et al.* (1987b) Microcephaly: genetic counselling and antenatal diagnosis. *American Journal of Medical Genetics*, 27, 583–94.

Tolmie, J.L., Patrick, A. and Yates, J.R.W. (1987c) A lethal multiple pterygium syndrome with apparent X-linked recessive inheritance. *American Journal of Medical Genetics*, 27, 913–19.

Toma, P., Costa, A., Magnano, G.M. *et al.* (1990) Holoprosencephaly: prenatal diagnosis by sonography and magnetic resonance imaging. *Prenatal Diagnosis*, 10, 429–36.

Toma, P., Dell'Acqua, A., Cordone, M. *et al.* (1991) Prenatal diagnosis of hydrosyringomyelia by high-resolution ultrasonography. *Journal of Clinical Ultrasound*, 19, 51–54.

Tomkins, D.J. (1989) Premature centromere separation and the prenatal diagnosis of Roberts syndrome. *Prenatal Diagnosis*, 9, 450–51.

Tonnensen, T. and Horn, N. (1989) Prenatal and postnatal diagnosis of Menkes disease, an inherited disorder of copper metabolism. *Journal of Inherited Metabolic Disease*, 12 (suppl. 1), 207–14.

Toone, J.R., Applegarth, D.A. and Levy, H.L. (1992) Prenatal diagnosis of non-ketotic hyperglycinaemia. *Journal of Inherited Metabolic Disease*, 15, 713–19.

Trecet, J.C., Claramunt, V., Larraz, J. *et al.* (1984) Prenatal ultrasound diagnosis of fetal teratoma of the neck. *Journal of Clinical Ultrasound*, 12, 509–11.

Trepeta, R., Stenn, K.S. and Mahoney, M.J. (1984) Prenatal diagnosis of Sjögren–Larsson syndrome. *Seminars in Dermatology*, 3, 221–24.

Triggs-Raine, B.L., Archibald, A., Gravel, R.A. and Clarke, J.T.R. (1990) Prenatal exclusion of Tay-Sachs disease by DNA analysis. *Lancet*, i, 1164.

Tsipouras, P., Schwartz, R.C., Goldberg, J.D. *et al.* (1987) Prenatal prediction of osteogenesis imperfecta (OI type IV): exclusion of inheritance using a collagen gene probe. *Journal of Medical Genetics*, 24, 406–409.

Tsuchiyama, A., Oyanagi, K., Hirano, S. *et al.* (1983) A case of pyruvate carboxylase deficiency with later prenatal diagnosis of an unaffected sibling. *Journal of Inherited Metabolic Disease*, 6, 85–88.

Tuck, S.M., Slack, J. and Buckland, G. (1990) Prenatal diagnosis of Conradi's syndrome. Case report. *Prenatal Diagnosis*, 10, 195–98.

Turco, A., Peissel, B., Quaia, P., Morandi, R., Bovicelli, L. and Pignatti, P.F. (1992) Prenatal diagnosis of autosomal dominant polycystic kidney disease using flanking DNA markers and the polymerase chain reaction. *Prenatal Diagnosis*, 12, 513–24.

Upadhyaya, M., Fryer, A., MacMillan, J., Broadhead, W., Huson, S.M. and Harper, P.S. (1992) Prenatal diagnosis and presymptomatic detection of neurofibromatosis type 1. *Journal of Medical Genetics*, 29, 180–83.

Uvebrant, P., Bjorck, E., Conradi, N., Hokegard, K.H., Martinsson, T. and Wahlstrom, J. (1993) Successful DNA-based prenatal exclusion of juvenile neuronal ceroid lipofuscinosis. *Prenatal Diagnosis*, 13, 651–57.

Vamos, E., Libert, J., Elkhazen, N. *et al.* (1986) Prenatal diagnosis and confirmation of infantile sialic acid storage disease. *Prenatal Diagnosis*, 6 437–46.

Van Dam, L.J., de Groot, C.J., Hazebroek, F.W. and Waldimiroff, J.W. (1984) Case report. Intrauterine demonstration of bowel duplication by ultrasound. *European Journal of Obstetrics, Gynecology and Reproductive Biology*, 18, 229–32.

Van den Hof, M.C., Nicolaides, K.H., Campbell, J. and Campbell, S. (1990) Evaluation of the lemon and banana signs in one hundred and thirty fetuses with open spina bifida. *American Journal of Obstetrics and Gynecology*, 162, 322–27.

Van den Hurk, J.A.J.M., Van Zandvoort, P.M., Brunsmann, F. *et al.* (1992) Prenatal exclusion of choroideremia. *American Journal of Medical Genetics*, 44, 822–23.

Van Dyke, D.L., Fluharty, A.L., Schafer, I.A. *et al.* (1981) Prenatal diagnosis of Maroteaux–Lamy syndrome. *American Journal of Medical Genetics*, 8, 235–42.

Vanier, M.T., Boue, J. and Dumez, Y. (1985) Niemann–Pick diseases type 8. First trimester prenatal diagnosis on chorionic villi. *Clinical Genetics*, 28, 348–50.

Vanier, M.T., Rodriguez Lafrasse, C., Rousson, R. *et al.* (1992) Prenatal diagnosis of Niemann–Pick type C disease: Current strategy from an experience of 37 pregnancies at risk. *American Journal of Human Genetics*, 51, 111–22.

Van Regemorter, H., Wilkin, P., Englert, Y. *et al.* (1984) Lethal multiple pterygium syndrome. *American Journal of Medical Genetics*, 17, 827–34.

Verma, I.C., Bhargava, S. and Agarwal, S. (1975) An autosomal recessive form of lethal chondrodystrophy with severe thoracic narrowing, rhizoactomelic type of micromelia, polydactyly, and genital anomalies. *Birth Defects*, **11**, 167–74.

Vermesh, M., Mayden, K.L., Confino, D. *et al.* (1986) Prenatal sonographic diagnosis of Hirschsprung's disease. *Journal of Ultrasound in Medicine*, **5**, 37–39.

Vesce, F., Guerrini, P., Perri, G. *et al.* (1987) Ultrasonographic diagnosis of ectasia of the umbilical vein. *Journal of Clinical Ultrasound*, **15**, 346–49.

Vimal, C.M., Fensom, A.H., Heaton, D. *et al.* (1984) Prenatal diagnosis of argininosuccinic aciduria by analysis of cultured chorionic villi. *Lancet*, **ii**, 521–22.

Vintners, H.V., Murphy, J., Wittman, B. and Norman, M.G. (1982) Intracranial teratoma: antenatal diagnosis at 31 weeks' gestation by ultrasound. *Acta Neuropathologica*, **58**, 233–36.

Vintzileos, A.M., Hovick, T.J., Escoto, D.T. *et al.* (1987) Congenital midline potencephaly: prenatal sonographic findings and review of the literature. *American Journal of Perinatology*, **4**, 125–28.

Viskochil, D., Buchberg, A.M., Xu, G. *et al.* (1990) Deletions and a translocation interrupted a cloned gene at the neurofobromatosis type I locus. *Cell*, **62**, 187–92.

Visser, G.H.A., Desmedt, M.C.H. and Meijboom, E.J. (1988) Altered fetal cardiac flow patterns in pure red cell anaemia (the Blackfan–Diamond syndrome). *Prenatal Diagnosis*, **8**, 525–29.

Vohra, N., Ghidini, A., Alvarez, M. and Lockwood, C. (1993) Walker–Warburg syndrome: Prenatal ultrasound findings. *Prenatal Diagnosis*, **13**, 575–79.

Von Figura, K., Van de Kamp, J.J. and Niermeijer, M.F. (1982) Prenatal diagnosis of Morquio's disease type A (*N*-acetyl-galactosamine 6-sulphate sulphatase deficiency). *Prenatal Diagnosis*, **8**, 525–29.

Von Koskull, H., Nordstrom, A.M., Salonen, R. and Peltonen, L. (1992) Prenatal diagnosis and carrier detection in fragile X. *American Journal of Medical Genetics*, **43**, 174–80.

Vora, S., Dimauro, S., Spear, D. *et al.* (1987) Characterisation of the enzymatic defect in late onset muscle phosphofructokinase deficiency: a new subtype of glycogen storage disease type VII. *Journal of Clinical Investigation*, **80**, 1479–85.

Voznyi, Y.V., Keulemans, J.L.M., Kleijer, W.J., Aula, P., Gray, G.R. and Van Diggelen, O.P. (1993) Applications of a new fluorimetric enzyme assay for the diagnosis of aspartylglucosaminuria. *Journal of Inherited Metabolic Disease*, **16**, 929–34.

Voznyi, Y.V., He, W., Huijmans, J.G.M., Geilen, G.C. *et al.* (1994) Prenatal diagnosis of Sanfilippo disease type C using a simple fluorometric enzyme assay. *Prenatal Diagnosis*, **14**, 17–22.

Wager, G.P., Couser, R.J., Edwards, O.P. *et al.* (1988) Antenal Ultrasound findings in a case of Uhl's anomaly. *American Journal of Perinatology*, **5**, 164–67.

Wallis, J., Shaw, J., Wilkes, D. *et al.* (1989) Prenatal diagnosis of Friedreich ataxia. *American Journal of Medical Genetics*, **34**, 458–61.

Wanders, P.J.A. and Ijlst, L. (1992) Long chain 3-hydroxyacyl CoA dehydrogenase in leucocytes and chorionic villus fibroblasts: potential for pre and postnatal diagnosis. *Journal of Inherited Metabolic Disease*, **15**, 356–58.

Wanders, R.J.A., Schelen, A., Feller, N. *et al.* (1990) First prenatal diagnosis of acyl-CoA oxidase deficiency. *Journal of Inherited Metabolic Disease*, **13**, 371–74.

Wang, I.M., Zhang, I., Wu, G. *et al.* (1986) First trimester prenatal diagnosis of severe alpha Thalassaemia. *Prenatal Diagnosis*, **6**, 89–95.

Ward, P.A., Hejmancik, J.F., Witkowski, J.A. *et al.* (1989) PND of Duchenne muscular dystrophy: prospective linkage analysis and retrospective dystrophin cDNA analysis. *American Journal of Human Genetics*, **44**, 270–81.

Warner, T.G., Robertson, A.D., Mock, A.K. *et al.* (1983) Prenatal diagnosis of G_{MI} gangliosidosis by detection of galactosyl-oligosaccharides in amniotic fluid with high performance liquid chromatography. *American Journal of Human Genetics*, **35**, 1034–45.

Weatherall, D.J., Old, J.M., Thein, S.L., *et al.* (1985) Prenatal diagnosis of the common haemoglobin disorders. *Journal of Medical Genetics*, **22**, 422–30.

Weaning, R.S., Bredius, R.G.M., Wolf, H. and van der Schoot, C.E. (1991) Prenatal diagnosis procedure for leucocyte adhesion deficiency. *Prenatal Diagnosis*, **11**, 193–97.

Weiner, C.P., Williamson, R.A. and Bonsib, S.M. (1986) Sonographic diagnosis of cloverleaf skull and thanatophoric dysplasia in the second trimester. *Journal of Clinical Ultrasound*, **14**, 463–65.

Weisman, Y., Jaccard, N., Legum, C. *et al.* (1990) Prenatal diagnosis of vitamin D-dependent rickets, type II: response to 1,25-dihydroxyvitamin D in amniotic fluid cells and fetal tissues. *Journal of Clinical Endocrinology and Metabolism*, **71**, 937–43.

Wellner, V.P., Sekura, R., Meister, A. and Larsson, A. (1974) Glutathione synthetase deficiency, an inborn error of metabolism involving the gamma-glutamyl cycle in patients with 5-oxoprolinuria (pyroglutamic aciduria). *Proceedings of the National Academy of Sciences of the USA*, **71**, 2505–509.

Wendel, U. and Claussen, U. (1979) Antenatal diagnosis of maple syrup urine disease. *Lancet*, **i**, 161–62.

Wendel, U., Claussen, U. and Diekmann, E. (1983) Prenatal diagnosis for methylene tetrahydrofolate reductase deficiency. *Journal of Pediatrics*, **102**, 938–40.

Wenstrom, K.D., Williamson, R.A., Hoover, W.W. and Grant, S.S. (1989) Achondrogenesis type II (Langer–Saldino) in association with jugular lymphatic obstruction sequence. *Prenatal Diagnosis*, **9**, 527–32.

Wenstrom, K.D., Williamson, R.A., Weiner, C.P. *et al.* (1991) Magnetic resonance imaging of fetuses with intracranial defects. *Obstetrics and Gynecology*, **77**, 529–32.

Westergaard, J.G., Chemnitz, J., Teisner, B. *et al.* (1983) Pregnancy associated plasma protein A: possible marker in the classification and prenatal diagnosis of Cornelia de Lange syndrome. *Prenatal Diagnosis*, **3**, 225–32.

Weston, M.J., Porter, H.J., Berry, P.J., Andrews, H.S. (1992) Ultrasonographic prenatal diagnosis of upper respiratory tract atresia. *Journal of Ultrasound in Medicine*, **11**, 673–75.

Wexler, S., Baruch, A., Ekshtein, N. *et al.* (1985) An acardiac acephalic anomaly detected on sonography. *Acta Obstetricia et Gynecologica Scandinavica*, **64**, 93–94.

Whitley, C.B., Burke, B.A., Granroth, G. and Gorlin, R.J. (1986) de la Chapelle dysplasia. *American Journal of Medical Genetics*, **25**, 29–39.

Wieacker, P., Griffin, J.E., Wienker, T. *et al.* (1987) Linkage analysis with RFLPs in families with androgen resistance syndromes: evidence for close linkage between the androgen receptor locus and the DXS1 segment. *Human Genetics*, **76**, 248–52.

Wiggins, J.W., Bowes, W., Clewell, W. *et al.* (1986) Echocardiographic diagnosis and intravenous digoxin management of fetal tachyarrhythmias and congestive heart failure. *American Journal of Diseases of Children*, **140**, 202–204.

Wijmenga, C., Frants, R.R., Brouwer, O.F. *et al.* (1990) Location of facioscapulohumeral muscular dystrophy gene on chromosome 4. *Lancet*, **336**, 651–53.

Wilson, R.H.J.K., Duncan, A., Hume, R. and Bain, A.D. (1985) Prenatal pleural effusion associated with congenital pulmonary lymphagiectasia. *Prenatal Diagnosis*, **5**, 73–76.

Winn, H.N., Gabrielli, S., Reece, F.A. *et al.* (1989) Ultrasonographic criteria for the prenatal diagnosis of placental chronicity in twin gestations. *American Journal of Obstetrics and Gynecology*, **161**, 1540–42.

Winter, R.M., Campbell, S., Wigglesworth, J.S. and Nevrkla, E.J. (1987) A previously undescribed syndrome of thoracic dysplasia and communicating hydrocephalus in two sibs, one diagnosed prenatally by ultrasound. *Journal of Medical Genetics*, **24**, 204–206.

Witter, F.R. and Molteni, R.A. (1986) Intrauterine intestinal volvulus with hemoperitoneum presenting as fetal distress at 34 weeks' gestation. *American Journal of Obstetrics and Gynecology*, **155**, 1080–81.

Woo, S.L.C., Gillam, S.S. and Woolf, L.I. (1974) The isolation and properties of phenylalaine hydrozylases from human liver. *Biochemical Journal*, **139**, 741–49.

Wood, S., Shukin, R.J., Yong, S.L. *et al.* (1987) Prenatal diagnosis in Becker muscular dystrophy. *Clinical Genetics*, **31**, 45–47.

Wright, A.F., Bhattacharya, S.S., Clayton, J.F. *et al.* (1987) Linkage relationships between X-linked retinitis pigmentosa and nine short arm markers: exclusion of the disease locus from Xp21 and localisation between DXS7 and DXS14. *American Journal of Human Genetics*, **41**, 653–44.

Yagel, S., Mandelberg, A., Hurwitz, A. and Jlaser, Y. (1986) Prenatal diagnosis of hypoplastic left ventricle. *American Journal of Perinatology*, **3**, 6–8.

Yang, B.-Z., Ding, J.-H., Brown, B.I. and Chen, Y.-T. (1990) Definitive prenatal diagnosis of type III glycogen storage disease. *American Journal of Human Genetics*, **47**, 735–39.

Yates, J.R.W., Affara, N.A., Jamieson, D.M. *et al.* (1986) Emery-Dreifus muscular dystrophy: localisation to Xq27.3-qter confirmed by linkage to factor VIII gene. *Journal of Medical Genetics*, **23**, 587–90.

Yates, J.R.W., Gillard, E.F., Cooke, A. *et al.* (1987) A deletion of Xp21 maps congenital adrenal hypoplasia distal to glycerol kinase deficiency. *Journal of Medical Genetics*, **24**, 241.

Yokota, I., Tanaka, K., Coates, P.M. and Ugarte, M. (1990) Mutations in medium chain acyl-CoA dehydrogenase deficiency. *Lancet*, **336**, 748.

Young, E.P. (1992) Prenatal diagnosis of Hurler disease by analysis of alpha-Iduronidase in chorionic villi *Journal of Inherited Metabolic Disease*, **15**, 224–30.

Yuen, M. and Fensom, A.H. (1985) Diagnosis of classical Morquio's disease: N-acetyl-galactosamine 6-sulphate sulphatase activity in cultured fibroblasis, leucocytes, amniotic fluid cells and chorionic villi. *Journal of Inherited Metabolic Disease*, **8**, 80.

Zanke, S. (1986) Prenatal ultrasound diagnosis of acardius. *Ultraschall in der Medizin*, **7**, 172–75.

Zeigler, M., Bargal, R., Suri, V., Meidan, B. and Bach, G. (1992) Mucolipidosis type IV: Accumulation of phospholipids and gangliosides in cultured amniotic cells. A tool for prenatal diagnosis. *Prenatal Diagnosis*, **12**, 1037–42.

Zeitune, M., Fejgin, M.D., Abramowicz, J. *et al.* (1988) Prenatal diagnosis of the pterygium syndrome. *Prenatal Diagnosis*, **8**, 145–49.

Zeng, Y.T. and Huang, S.Z. (1985) Alpha-globin gene organisation and prenatal diagnosis of alpha-thalassaemia in Chinese. *Lancet*, **i**, 304–307.

Zeng, Y.T., Zhang, M.-L., Ren, Z.-R. *et al.* (1987) Prenatal diagnosis of haemophilia B in the first trimester. *Journal of Medical Genetics*, **24**, 632.

Zerfowski, J. and Sandhoff, K. (1974) Juvenile GM$_2$ Gangliosidose mit veranderter Sub-stratspezifitat der Hexosaminidase A, *Acta Neuropathologica (Berlin)*, **27**, 225–32.

Zerres, K., Hansmann, M., Mallmann, R. and Gembruch, U. (1988) Autosomal recessive polycystic kidney disease. Problems of prenatal diagnosis. *Prenatal Diagnosis*, **8**, 215–29.

Zerres, K., Schwanitz, G., Niesen, M. *et al.* (1990) Prenatal diagnosis of acute non-lymphoblastic leukaemia in Down syndrome. *Lancet*, **i**, 117.

Zhao, H., Van Diggelen, D.P., Thoomes, R. *et al.* (1990) Prenatal diagnosis of Morquio disease type A using a simple fluorometric enzyme assay. *Prenatal Diagnosis*, **10**, 85–92.

Zimmer, E.Z., Bronshtein, M., Ophir, E. *et al.* (1993) Sonographic diagnosis of fetal congenital cataracts. *Prenatal Diagnosis*, **13**, 503–511.

Zimmerman, H.B. (1978) Prenatal demonstration of gastric and duodenal obstruction by ultrasound. *Journal of the Canadian Association of Radiologists*, **29**, 138–41.

Zlotogora, J., Granat, M. and Knowlton, R.G. (1994) Prenatal exclusion of Stickler syndrome. *Prenatal Diagnosis*, **14**, 145–47.

Zlotogora, J., Chakraborty, S., Knowlton, R.G. and Wenger, D.A. (1990) Krabbe disease locus mapped to chromosome 14 by genetic linkage. *American Journal of Human Genetics*, **47**, 37–44.

Zonana, J., Schinzel, A., Upadhyaya, M. *et al.* (1990) Prenatal diagnosis of X-linked hypohidrotic ectodermal dysplasia by linkage analysis. *American Journal of Medical Genetics*, **35**, 132–35.

Zoref-Shani, E., Bromberg, Y., Goldman, B. *et al.* (1989) Prenatal diagnosis of Lesch–Hyhan syndrome: experience with three fetuses at risk. *Prenatal Diagnosis*, **9**, 657–661.

Index